# Motor Neuron Disease

*Editors*

MAZEN M. DIMACHKIE
RICHARD J. BAROHN

# NEUROLOGIC CLINICS

www.neurologic.theclinics.com

*Consulting Editor*
RANDOLPH W. EVANS

November 2015 • Volume 33 • Number 4

**ELSEVIER**

1600 John F. Kennedy Boulevard • Suite 1800 • Philadelphia, Pennsylvania, 19103-2899

http://www.theclinics.com

**NEUROLOGIC CLINICS Volume 33, Number 4**
**November 2015 ISSN 0733-8619, ISBN-13: 978-0-323-41344-2**

Editor: Lauren Boyle
Developmental editor: Donald Mumford



*Neurologic Clinics* (ISSN 0733-8619) is published quarterly by Elsevier Inc., 360 Park Avenue South, New York, NY 10010–1710. Months of issue are February, May, August, and November. Periodicals postage paid at New York, NY, and additional mailing offices. Subscription prices are $300.00 per year for US individuals, $517.00 per year for US institutions, $145.00 per year for US students, $375.00 per year for Canadian individuals, $627.00 per year for Canadian institutions, $415.00 per year for international individuals, $627.00 per year for international institutions, and $210.00 for Canadian and foreign students/residents. To receive student/resident rate, orders must be accompanied by name of affiliated institution, date of term, and the *signature* of program/residency coordinator on institution letterhead. Orders will be billed at individual rate until proof of status is received. Foreign air speed delivery is included in all *Clinics* subscription prices. All prices are subject to change without notice. **POSTMASTER:** Send address changes to *Neurologic Clinics*, Elsevier Health Sciences Division, Subscription Customer Service, 3251 Riverport Lane, Maryland Heights, MO 63043. **Customer Service: Telephone: 1-800-654-2452 (U.S. and Canada); 314-447-8871 (outside U.S. and Canada). Fax: 314-447-8029. E-mail: journalscustomerservice-usa@elsevier.com (for print support); journalsonlinesupport-usa@elsevier.com (for online support).**

*Reprints.* For copies of 100 or more of articles in this publication, please contact the Commercial Reprints Department, Elsevier Inc., 360 Park Avenue South, New York, New York, 10010-1710; Tel.: +1-212-633-3874; Fax: +1-212-633-3820, and E-mail: reprints@elsevier.com.

*Neurologic Clinics* is also published in Spanish by Nueva Editorial Interamericana S.A., Mexico City, Mexico.

*Neurologic Clinics* is covered in *Current Contents/Clinical Medicine, MEDLINE/PubMed (Index Medicus), EMBASE/Excerpta Medica, and PsycINFO, and ISI/BIOMED.*

# Contributors

## CONSULTING EDITOR

**RANDOLPH W. EVANS, MD**
Clinical Professor, Department of Neurology, Baylor College of Medicine, Houston, Texas

## EDITORS

**MAZEN M. DIMACHKIE, MD**
Vice-Chair for Research; Director, Clinical Neurophysiology Division; Director, Neuromuscular Section; Professor of Neurology, Department of Neurology, University of Kansas Medical Center, Kansas City, Kansas

**RICHARD J. BAROHN, MD**
University Distinguished Professor, Gertrude & Dewey Ziegler Professor, Professor and Chair of Neurology, Department of Neurology, CEO, President of KU Neurological Foundation, Vice-Chancellor for Research, President, Research Institute, University of Kansas Medical Center, Kansas City, Kansas

## AUTHORS

**RICHARD J. BAROHN, MD**
University Distinguished Professor, Gertrude & Dewey Ziegler Professor, Professor and Chair of Neurology, Department of Neurology, CEO, President of KU Neurological Foundation, Vice-Chancellor for Research, President, Research Institute, University of Kansas Medical Center, Kansas City, Kansas

**RICHARD S. BEDLACK, MD, PhD**
Associate Professor, Department of Neurology, Duke University Medical Center, Durham, North Carolina

**KEVIN BOYLAN, MD**
Director, ALS Center, Department of Neurology, Mayo Clinic Jacksonville, Jacksonville, Florida

**GREGORY T. CARTER, MD, MS**
Medical Director, Department of Physical Medicine and Rehabilitation, St. Luke's Rehabilitation Institute, Spokane, Washington

**MAZEN M. DIMACHKIE, MD**
Vice-Chair for Research; Director, Clinical Neurophysiology Division; Director, Neuromuscular Section; Professor of Neurology, Department of Neurology, University of Kansas Medical Center, Kansas City, Kansas

**KENNETH H. FISCHBECK, MD**
Neurogenetics Branch, National Institute of Neurological Disorders and Stroke, National Institute of Health, Bethesda, Maryland

**MARY KAY FLOETER, MD, PhD**
Senior Clinician and Chief of the NINDS EMG Section, Human Spinal Physiology Unit, National Institute of Neurological Disorders and Stroke, Bethesda, Maryland

**CHRISTOPHER GRUNSEICH, MD**
Neurogenetics Branch, National Institute of Neurological Disorders and Stroke, National Institute of Health, Bethesda, Maryland

**D. KEVIN HORTON, DrPH, MSPH, CPH**
Chief, Environmental Health Surveillance Branch within the Division of Toxicology and Human Health Sciences, Agency for Toxic Substances and Disease Registry/Centers for Disease Control and Prevention, Atlanta, Georgia

**CARLAYNE E. JACKSON, MD, FAAN**
Professor of Neurology and Otolaryngology, Department of Neurology, University of Texas Health Science Center, San Antonio, Texas

**OMAR JAWDAT, MD**
Assistant Professor, Department of Neurology, University of Kansas Medical Center, Kansas City, Kansas

**NANETTE JOYCE, DO, MAS**
Assistant Professor, Department of Physical Medicine and Rehabilitation, University of California, Davis School of Medicine, Sacramento, California

**CHAFIC KARAM, MD**
Assistant Professor, Department of Neurology, University of North Carolina School of Medicine, Chapel Hill, North Carolina

**JONATHAN S. KATZ, MD**
Director of Neuromuscular Clinic, Forbes Norris MDA/ALS Center, Department of Neurology, California Pacific Medical Center (CPMC), San Francisco, California; Adjunct Professor of Neurology (KUMC), Department of Neurology, University of Kansas Medical Center, Kansas City, Kansas

**JOHN T. KISSEL, MD**
Professor and Chairman, Department of Neurology, The Ohio State University Wexner Medical Center, Columbus, Ohio

**STEPHEN J. KOLB, MD, PhD**
Assistant Professor, Departments of Neurology and Biological Chemistry and Pharmacology, The Ohio State University Wexner Medical Center, Columbus, Ohio

**TEERIN LIEWLUCK, MD**
Department of Neurology, University of Colorado School of Medicine, Aurora, Colorado; Department of Neurology, Mayo Clinic, Rochester, Minnesota

**APRIL L. McVEY, MD**
Professor, Department of Neurology, University of Kansas Medical Center, Kansas City, Kansas

**HIROSHI MITSUMOTO, MD, DSc**
Wesley J. Howe Professor of Neurology, The Eleanor and Lou Gehrig MDA/ALS Research Center, The Neurological Institute, Columbia University Medical Center, New York, New York

**BJÖRN OSKARSSON, MD**
Associate Professor of Clinical Neurology, Director of UC Davis Multidisciplinary ALS Clinic, An ALS Association Certified Center of Excellence, University of California Davis Medical Center, Sacramento, California

**SABRINA PAGANONI, MD, PhD**
Assistant Professor, Spaulding Rehabilitation Hospital, Harvard Medical School, Massachusetts General Hospital; Boston VA Health Care System, Boston, Massachusetts

**JOHN RAVITS, MD**
Department of Neurosciences, Head, ALS Translational Research, University of California, San Diego, La Jolla, California

**STACY RUDNICKI, MD, FAAN**
Professor of Neurology, Department of Neurology, University of Arkansas for Medical Sciences, Little Rock, Arkansas

**SHAHRAM SABERI, MD**
Department of Neurosciences, ALS Translational Research, University of California (San Diego), La Jolla, California

**DAVID S. SAPERSTEIN, MD**
Phoenix Neurological Associates, University of Arizona College of Medicine, Phoenix, Arizona

**DEREK J. SCHULTE, BS**
Department of Neurosciences, ALS Translational Research, University of California (San Diego), La Jolla, California

**JEFFREY M. STATLAND, MD**
Assistant Professor, Department of Neurology, University of Kansas Medical Center, Kansas City, Kansas

**JENNIFER E. STAUFFER, BA**
Department of Neurosciences, ALS Translational Research, University of California (San Diego), La Jolla, California

**MICHAEL J. STRONG, MD**
Department of Clinical Neurological Sciences, Schulich School of Medicine and Dentistry, Western University; University Hospital, London Health Sciences Centre, London, Ontario, Canada

**SUSAN C. WOOLLEY, PhD**
Forbes Norris MDA/ALS Research Center, California Pacific Medical Center, San Francisco, California

# Contents

**Progressive Muscular Atrophy** **761**

Teerin Liewluck and David S. Saperstein

Progressive muscular atrophy (PMA) is a rare, sporadic, adult-onset motor neuron disease, clinically characterized by isolated lower motor neuron features; however, clinically evident upper motor neuron signs may emerge in some patients. Subclinical upper motor neuron involvement is identified pathologically, radiologically, and neurophysiologically in a substantial number of patients with PMA. Patients with subclinical upper motor neuron involvement do not fulfill the revised El Escorial criteria to participate in amyotrophic lateral sclerosis clinical trials. Intravenous immunoglobulin therapy is only marginally beneficial in a small subgroup of patients with lower motor neuron syndrome without conduction block.

**Amyotrophic Lateral Sclerosis Regional Variants (Brachial Amyotrophic Diplegia, Leg Amyotrophic Diplegia, and Isolated Bulbar Amyotrophic Lateral Sclerosis)** **775**

Omar Jawdat, Jeffrey M. Statland, Richard J. Barohn, Jonathan S. Katz, and Mazen M. Dimachkie

Amyotrophic lateral sclerosis (ALS), a rapidly progressive, invariably fatal disease, involves mixed upper and lower motor neurons in different spinal cord regions. Patients with bulbar onset progress more rapidly than patients with limb onset or with a lower motor neuron presentation. Recent descriptions of regional variants suggest some patients have ALS isolated to a single spinal region for many years, including brachial amyotrophic diplegia, leg amyotrophic diplegia, and isolated bulbar palsy. Clearer definitions of regional variants will have implications for prognosis, understanding the pathophysiology of ALS, identifying genetic factors related to slower disease progression, and future planning of clinical trials.

**Frontotemporal Dysfunction and Dementia in Amyotrophic Lateral Sclerosis** **787**

Susan C. Woolley and Michael J. Strong

Although amyotrophic lateral sclerosis (ALS) is classically considered a disorder exclusively affecting motor neurons, there is substantial clinical, neuroimaging, and neuropathologic evidence that more than half of patients have an associated syndrome of frontotemporal dysfunction. These syndromes range from frontotemporal dementia to behavioral or cognitive syndromes. Neuroimaging and neuropathologic findings are consistent with frontotemporal lobar degeneration that underpins alterations in network connectivity. Future clinical trials need to be stratified based on the presence or absence of frontotemporal dysfunction on the disease course of ALS.

**Familial Amyotrophic Lateral Sclerosis** **807**

Kevin Boylan

Genes linked to amyotrophic lateral sclerosis (ALS) susceptibility are being identified at an increasing rate owing to advances in molecular genetic technology. Genetic mechanisms in ALS pathogenesis seem to exert major effects in about 10% of patients, but genetic factors at some level may be important components of disease risk in most patients with ALS. Identification of gene variants associated with ALS has informed concepts of

the pathogenesis of ALS, aided the identification of therapeutic targets, facilitated research to develop new ALS biomarkers, and supported the establishment of clinical diagnostic tests for ALS-linked genes.

**Spinal Muscular Atrophy** **831**

Stephen J. Kolb and John T. Kissel

Spinal muscular atrophy is an autosomal-recessive disorder characterized by degeneration of motor neurons in the spinal cord and caused by mutations in the survival motor neuron 1 gene, *SMN1*. The severity of SMA is variable. The *SMN2* gene produces a fraction of the SMN messenger RNA (mRNA) transcript produced by the *SMN1* gene. There is an inverse correlation between *SMN2* gene copy number and clinical severity. Clinical management focuses on multidisciplinary care. Preclinical models of SMA have led to an explosion of SMA clinical trials that hold great promise of effective therapy in the future.

**Spinal and Bulbar Muscular Atrophy** **847**

Christopher Grunseich and Kenneth H. Fischbeck

Spinal and bulbar muscular atrophy, or Kennedy disease, is a slowly progressive X-linked neuromuscular disease caused by a trinucleotide (CAG) repeat expansion in the androgen receptor gene. Affected males typically develop weakness in their mid-40s as well as evidence of androgen insensitivity with reduced fertility and gynecomastia. Diagnosis is often delayed because of decreased awareness of the disease, although genetic testing allows for direct diagnosis. Therapeutic strategies to block the toxicity of the mutant androgen receptor have been unsuccessful thus far, and evaluation of additional candidate therapies is underway.

**Neuropathology of Amyotrophic Lateral Sclerosis and Its Variants** **855**

Shahram Saberi, Jennifer E. Stauffer, Derek J. Schulte, and John Ravits

The neuropathologic molecular signature common to almost all sporadic amyotrophic lateral sclerosis (ALS) and most familial ALS is TDP-43 immunoreactive neuronal cytoplasmic inclusions. The neuropathologic and molecular neuropathologic features of ALS variants, primarily lateral sclerosis and progressive muscular atrophy, are less certain but also seem to share the primary features of ALS. Genetic causes, including mutations in SOD1, TDP-43, FUS, and C9orf72, all have distinctive molecular neuropathologic signatures. Neuropathology will continue to play an increasingly key role in solving the puzzle of ALS pathogenesis.

**Potential Environmental Factors in Amyotrophic Lateral Sclerosis** **877**

Björn Oskarsson, D. Kevin Horton, and Hiroshi Mitsumoto

The causes of amyotrophic lateral sclerosis (ALS) are largely unknown, and may always be multiple, including environmental factors. Monogenetic determinants of ALS are involved in roughly 20% of all cases (including 10% familial cases). Less well understood multigenetic causes may contribute to another 20% to 80%. Environmental factors likely play a role in the development of ALS in susceptible individuals, but proved causation remains elusive. This article discusses the possible factors of male gender

# NEUROLOGIC CLINICS

**FORTHCOMING ISSUES**

***February 2016***
**Neurobehavioral Manifestations of Neurological Diseases: Diagnosis and Treatment**
Alireza Minagar, Glen Finney, and Kenneth M. Heilman, *Editors*

***May 2016***
**Optimal Care for Patients with Epilepsy: Practical Aspects**
Steven C. Schachter, *Editor*

***August 2016***
**Case Studies in Neurology**
Randolph Evans, *Editor*

**RECENT ISSUES**

***August 2015***
**Emergency Neuro-Otology: Diagnosis and Management of Acute Dizziness and Vertigo**
David E. Newman-Toker, Kevin A. Kerber, William J. Meurer, Rodney Omron, Jonathan A. Edlow, *Editors*

***May 2015***
**Cerebrovascular Diseases: Controversies and Challenges**
William J. Powers, *Editor*

***February 2015***
**Movement Disorders**
Joseph Jankovic, *Editor*

# Preface
# Motor Neuron Disease

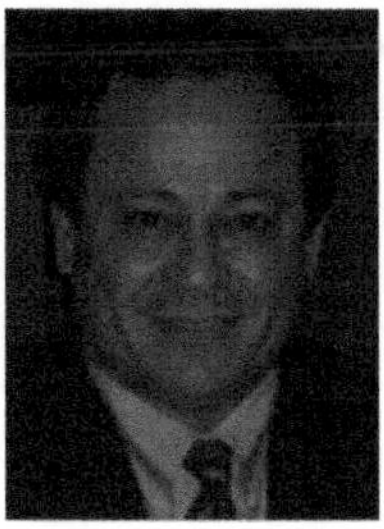 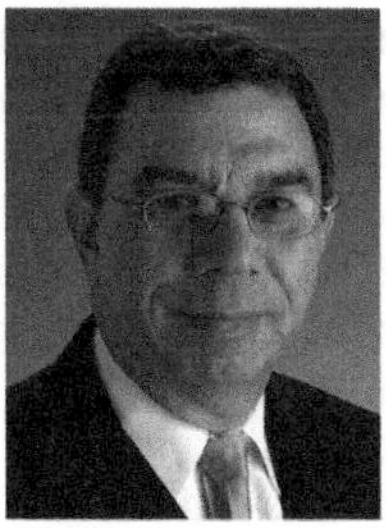

Mazen M. Dimachkie, MD   Richard J. Barohn, MD
*Editors*

We are pleased to have put together an issue of *Neurologic Clinics* on motor neuron disorders. We have assembled experts from throughout North America who have a great deal of experience and insight into these difficult diseases to provide the practicing neurologist a resource that can be used to help them approach patients. This is the third installment in neuromuscular disease we have coedited in the last 3 years for *Neurologic Clinics*.

To open this issue, we look back to the initial descriptions of amyotrophic lateral sclerosis (ALS) and related conditions from one the founders of neurology in France, Dr Charcot, and his trainees and contemporaries in Europe. It is perhaps not surprising that their observations over 150 years ago are still relevant today. We have introduced in 2013 and 2104 the pattern approach to evaluating neuropathies[1] and myopathies[2] to the audience of *Neurologic Clinics*. As a foundation, we are using the pattern-recognition approach, and we have referenced the various patterns that apply to the motor neuron disorders at every opportunity throughout the contributions in this issue. We believe using these clinical phenotypes as an anchor in approaching patients with these disorders greatly reduces the complexity in delivering health care, especially in trying to separate typical ALS from those with pure lower motor neuron findings (*progressive muscular atrophy*) and pure upper motor neuron findings (*primary lateral sclerosis*).

We also extend this approach to established genetic forms of motor neurononopathies with (familial ALS) or without upper motor neuron signs (*spinal muscular atrophy*) and with sensory manifestations (Kennedy disease). By focusing on a number of regional variants of acquired motor neuron disease that can remain confined to the arms (brachial amyotrophic diplegia), legs (leg amyotrophic diplegia), or bulbar region (isolated bulbar ALS), we suspect if we can first identify these phenotypes and then ultimately determine biologically why these patients have slowly progressive disorders, then we may be able to unlock the enigma of ALS. The same can be said of the well-recognized observation that many ALS patients also have frontotemporal dementia and vice versa. While the cause of ALS remains elusive, several advances have occurred since its original description by Charcot, including the role of TDP-43

Neurol Clin 33 (2015) xiii–xiv
http://dx.doi.org/10.1016/j.ncl.2015.09.001

0733-8619/15/$ – see front matter 

pathology and the description of C9ORF, the most common gene of familial ALS, which is also present in a small proportion of sporadic cases. While genetic factors form the basis of a small percentage of sporadic ALS, perhaps in time we will find that most ALS patients have a genetic basis. On the other hand, there is the possibility that a number of potential environmental influences may contribute to developing ALS, so we have an article on that as well as an article on the neuropathology of ALS.

Finally, while we still search for ways to phenotype, genotype, and understand ALS and *motor neuron diseases*, it is essential to care for our patients, so it is critically important to focus on symptomatic management, end-of-life care, complementary approaches, and the challenges of performing clinical trials to slow disease progression. Multidisciplinary clinics have emerged as the standard of care for optimizing quality of life and longevity and managing symptoms of patients with ALS. While there has been a growing interest by industry, foundations, and federal agencies in funding research in ALS, the only FDA-approved therapy for ALS in the last two decades remains riluzole. As researchers continue on the quest for new therapies, people with ALS often seek help from complementary and alternative medicine. It is important for patients, family, and physicians caring for victims of ALS to be aware of the ALSUntangled community and its website, which educates the ALS community about unconventional and often unproven interventions.

This issue offers a comprehensive review of all of these topics that we hope will be of interest to the ALS community. We tailored these discussions on motor neuron disease to be helpful to the practicing neurologist, health care provider, and also patients and families who are afflicted with these difficult conditions. We would like to thank all of the authors for their excellent contributions as well as the editorial team of *Neurologic Clinics* for their superb support, and importantly, all ALS patients and their caretakers, to whom we dedicate this issue.

Sincerely,

Mazen M. Dimachkie, MD
Department of Neurology
Neuromuscular Section
University of Kansas Medical Center
3901 Rainbow Boulevard
Mail Stop 2012
Kansas City, KS 66160, USA

Richard J. Barohn, MD
Department of Neurology
University of Kansas Medical Center
3901 Rainbow Boulevard
Mail Stop 2012
Kansas City, KS 66160, USA

E-mail addresses:
mdimachkie@kumc.edu (M.M. Dimachkie)
rbarohn@kumc.edu (R.J. Barohn)

## REFERENCES

1. Barohn RJ, Amato AA. Pattern-recognition approach to neuropathy and neuronopathy. Neurol Clin 2013;31:343–61.
2. Barohn RJ, Dimachkie MM, Jackson RJ. A pattern recognition approach to the patient with a suspected myopathy. Neurol Clin 2014;32(3):569–93.

# Amyotrophic Lateral Sclerosis: A Historical Perspective

Jonathan S. Katz, MD[a], Mazen M. Dimachkie, MD[b,*], Richard J. Barohn, MD[b]

**KEYWORDS**

• Amyotrophic lateral sclerosis • Jean-Martin Charcot • Phenotype • Genotype

**KEY POINTS**

- Jean-Martin Charcot is credited as the father of ALS, not because he was the first to report the disorder, but because he synthesized 50 years of prior work on progressive muscular weakness.
- Later work by Gowers and then by Charcot refined Charcot's basic description of the disease into a complete clinical spectrum with specific examination features.
- The history of ALS reminds us that there has been little change in the clinical understanding of the phenotypic disease description for nearly 150 years.
- The early work on ALS provides useful foundation for today's clinicians with respect to tying together genetic and biologic aspects of the disorder that have been discovered over the past few decades.
- The challenge today is to explore phenotype and genotype relationships and the pathophysiologic basis for slow and fast progression of disease.

For this issue of *Neurologic Clinics* we thought it was appropriate to look back in time to see where the foundational basis for the understanding of amyotrophic lateral sclerosis (ALS) originated. This foundation was created primarily in France by the great Jean-Martin Charcot and his fellow countrymen and disciples, along with key contributions from early clinicians in England and Germany.

Jean-Martin Charcot (1825–1893) is generally credited for first describing ALS (**Fig. 1**). During his Tuesday Lectures beginning in the late 1860s and culminating in a publication in 1874,[1–3] Charcot was able to link the disease to its pathology, and to culminate what was nearly a half century of slow scientific progress that ultimately led to an understanding of ALS as a distinct clinical entity.

To understand the genius of Charcot's contributions, one must consider the overall state of neurology in the middle to late nineteenth century. Clinicians were just

[a] Department of Neurology, Forbes Norris MDA/ALS Center, California Pacific Medical Center, 2324 Sacramento Street, Suite 111, San Francisco, CA 94115, USA; [b] Department of Neurology, The University of Kansas Medical Center, 3901 Rainbow Boulevard, Mail Stop 2012, Kansas City, KS 66160, USA

* Corresponding author.

*E-mail address:* mdmachkie@kumc.edu

Neurol Clin 33 (2015) 727–734

http://dx.doi.org/10.1016/j.ncl.2015.07.013 **neurologic.theclinics.com**

0733-8619/15/$ – see front matter 

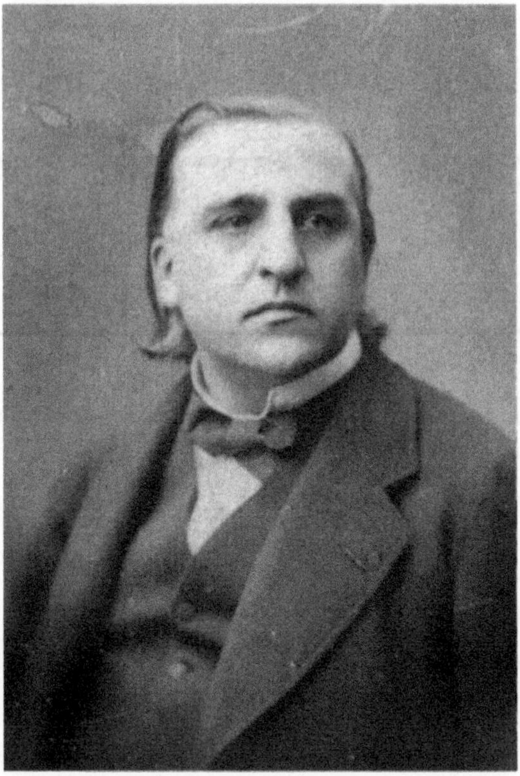

**Fig. 1.** Portrait of Charcot. http://vlp.mpiwg-berlin.mpg.de/library/data/lit38361?. (Max Planck Institute for the History of Science, Berlin.)

beginning to sort out the large number of conditions that resulted in progressive weakness and atrophy, but they were limited by several factors ranging from rudimentary examination skills to a meager understanding of how the nervous system was wired. To put this in context, Charcot lectured on ALS a few years before Wilhelm Heinrich Erb and Carl Otto Friedrich Westphal published separate papers on tendon reflexes in an 1875 issue of *Archiv fur Psychiatrie und Nervenkrankheiten*.[4] It was not until much later, in 1896, that Joseph Jules François Félix Babinski, a student of Charcot's, described the plantar reflex.[5] Scientifically, there was no understanding that two types of motor neurons had separate functions, nor was there a clear distinction between neurogenic and myopathic atrophy. Charcot worked years before Camillo Golgi's silver staining technique, which recognized the presence of dendrites and axons for the first time. As Charcot was lecturing, the nervous system was still understood to be a continuous single network, more like a mesh of a single thread, as opposed to interconnected cells. He also worked years before Santiago Ramón y Cajal published *Revista Trimestral de Histologiá Normal y Patológica*[6] where he theorized that nerve cells were not continuous, which was not proved until the later work of Sherrington in the early 1900s[7] and the invention of electron microscopy in the 1950s.

Charcot was probably not the first to describe a case of ALS. That designation is generally credited to Charles Bell in 1824,[8–10] who was interested in understanding the relationships between motor function and the anterior spinal nerves and describing cases of pure motor dysfunction. However, although the neurologists of the mid-nineteenth century developed a keen interest in cases of progressive muscle weakness, they were still uncertain about the distinction between muscle and nerve disorders. The term progressive muscular atrophy was first used by Aran in 1850,[11] and Duchenne had described a similar case the year earlier,[12] but both believed this was a muscle disorder. Aran actually described 11 patients with different patterns of progressive muscle weakness and atrophy of the limbs. He was the first to call the condition progressive muscular atrophy and described it as a condition that irregularly affects certain muscles, while sparing others. It eventually became clear that Aran was lumping numerous muscle and nerve diseases into a single entity. It is also noteworthy that one of Aran's cases, a 43-year-old sea captain who died of progressive wasting, had three sisters and a maternal uncle who died of the same condition.

The French anatomist Jean Cruveilhier first described a woman who suffered from the combination of progressive muscular atrophy and bulbar paralysis.[13] She died within a year, and on postmortem, Cruveilhier was surprised to find that there was no gross lesion of the central nervous system. Cruveilhier described another case of combined spinal and bulbar atrophy and suggested this was a myelopathic process. He described the atrophy of the anterior roots and pointed out that the lower lip and tongue were atrophic, and that there was wasting of the hypoglossal nerve with sparing of the lingual nerve. This led him to conclude this was a neurogenic process of motor nerves. It is likely that both Cruveilhier and Bell overlooked upper motor neuron findings because this concept had not yet been described.

The British physiologist and anatomist Jacob Augustus Lockhart Clarke was a pioneer in histologic techniques, and best known for his discovery of Clarke's columns. Along with Charles Bland Radcliffe, Clarke wrote "An important case of paralysis and muscular atrophy, with disease of the nervous centers" in 1862, nearly a decade before Charcot's Tuesday Lectures were published.[14,15] The subject of the work was a 43-year-old man with atrophy of the tongue and arms, increased tone, bulbar involvement, and diffuse fasciculations. Clarke found on autopsy that the gross spinal cord was not particularly remarkable, but clearly described marked histologic changes including loss of cells in the anterior cord, diffuse pallor of white matter columns, and loss of hypoglossal and lingual nuclei.

It was not until 1865, that Charcot published a description of a similar patient with lateral column sclerosis, intact cortical gray matter, and atrophy of some of the anterior roots.[16] With the door now open for further observation, the late 1860s included a flood of new cases adding to the work by Radcliffe, Charcot, and Lockhart Clarke. Charcot and Joffroy published two cases of progressive muscular atrophy where the lips and tongue, along with the limbs, were involved.[17] In each instance, they found, after death, atrophy of anterior spinal roots and of the hypoglossal and accessory nerves, with atrophy of the lateral columns, and extreme wasting of the ganglion cells of the anterior cornua. Still, it took a few more years for Charcot to formally theorize that the motor cells of the anterior gray matter were the locus for progressive muscular atrophy.[18]

The authors of these earlier papers were not yet fully certain how pathologic observations explained the clinical findings. Many of them, including Charcot's coauthor Joffroy, worked under the theory that motor nerves must possess two distinct functions, one trophic and the other motor. Without the understanding of upper and lower motor neurons, they had no way of linking the clinical findings to the disease.

At the same time that progressive atrophies of the limbs were being described, a parallel collection of observations were focusing on bulbar paralysis. These would eventually merge with descriptions of progressive muscular atrophy, but this was not immediate. In 1859, Dumenil recorded a case of progressive muscular atrophy, but it was associated with nonatrophic paralysis of the tongue.[19] In 1860, Duchenne described his experience with cases of bulbar paralysis and found autopsies demonstrated atrophy of anterior spinal roots and bulbar muscles.[20] To explain the lack of bulbar atrophy, he concluded that cranial motor nerves somehow differed from spinal motor nerves with respect to the "nutrition of muscles," and Duchenne worked under the assumption that bulbar paralysis was a completely different disease than progressive muscular atrophy. Wachsmuth, in an important monograph, gave to the disease the now generally accepted designation, "bulbar paralysis," and argued that the lesion must be in the medulla.[21]

Recent ALS historians have asked why it was Charcot who ultimately was credited with the disorder. A short answer is his shear dedication to the understanding. Charcot studied ALS for more than a decade, collecting cases from others, and drawing from other key observations so he could ultimately establish ALS as a unique disorder. Charcot went beyond case description and functioned more as a researcher than a clinician. According to Goetz, Charcot had personal experience with only five patients, and collected 15 others through communications. Learning about the disease was not simple.[18,22] ALS was even rarer at that time than it is today. Most descriptions suggest the most common age of onset was in the fourth or fifth decades, likely because of the shorter life expectancies. Patients were also not easily able to travel or follow up frequently and when autopsies were collected, the techniques were immature. Others have suggested that Charcot's main contribution was to finally name the condition and to separate it from other disorders with similar presentations.[15] Based on the poor understanding of the nervous system, this was not an easy task. Rowland[23] went further, offering the opinion that Charcot's contribution was greater than ALS. Charcot synthesized the abnormal bulbar syndrome, described clonus and focused on the abnormal tone, and reinforced that ALS was a disease of both the lateral columns and the spinal motor roots. He correlated clinical and pathologic observations and postulated a two-part motor nervous system with a lateral column causing spasticity and gray matter degeneration leading to atrophy and weakness. In short, Charcot provided a platform in clinicopathologic correlation that would help define diseases for future generations of neurologists.

Charcot described the prototype condition, with the brunt of the disease beginning in the cervical region. He saw ALS as having three stages, starting in the upper limbs with key features, such as "spasms of the arms, and principally the legs (without loss of sensation), together with progressive amyotrophy which was confined mostly to the upper limbs and trunk." In the next stage, the legs tend to become rigid beginning after 6 to 9 months. Walking became impossible, but there was no bladder involvement. In the third, and final stages bulbar symptoms worsen with death occurring after 2 or 3 years.

Charcot understood that this pattern was not ubiquitous, and that the disease can start in the bulbar regions or in legs, but he did not see these as the typical presentation. Charcot was synthesizing the varied presentations of a condition that takes different forms with respect to site of onset and the degrees to which upper and motor neurons may be involved. His primary goal was to distinguish ALS from other conditions with similar presentations, and these were mainly progressive atrophies and myopathies. Not surprisingly, Charcot split the disorder of classic ALS from other forms of progressive muscular atrophy and bulbar paralysis. Charcot made this division by using the term "protopathic" to describe cases with isolated anterior horn cell disease and "deuteropathic" for those cases with combined loss of anterior horns and lateral columns.[2] He saw the sclerosis in the lateral columns as the primary pathology, whereas the amyotrophy was the secondary phenomenon. His choice of the term "amyotrophic" lateral sclerosis actually reflects this point of view, where sclerosis somehow induced muscle atrophy.

Charcot's work set the stage for William Richard Gowers, the famed Queens Square neurologist, who over the next decade refined and expanded on Charcot's concepts. Gowers[24] understood ALS to be a single degenerative spectrum and noted that there was no clear division between the varied presentations. He saw that every combination of atrophy, spasticity, and combined "tonic wasting" existed, and could be seen across different cases and even within different limbs including the neck in individuals (**Fig. 2**; also discussed Ref.[25]). Gowers argued for a single condition by noting that typical clinical cases of progressive atrophy often had lateral column degeneration at autopsy. Like Charcot, Gowers placed the disease into different stages, and went on to detail how weakness spread, by pointing out that it begins in part of one limb and advances through that limb before tending to involve the same muscles on the contralateral side.

Gowers also first discussed treatments, thus offering the first hint of failed interventions that would continue to haunt patients with ALS for generations to come. In his 1886 work, Gowers describes his experience with strychnia and morphia, which may transiently improve "the power of swallowing." He also described symptomatic treatments with atropine or belladonna to control the flow of saliva (but suggested this did not work), and the need for dietary consistency changes and liquid feedings through a nasogastric tube, if necessary, in the setting of bulbar disease.

The description of ALS also opened the door to separate it from other conditions. Once ALS was described, Charcot was easily able to differentiate cases seen by Aran, who had forms of muscular atrophy that did not prove to be ALS. The conceptualization was also the basis for Charcot's student, Pierre Marie, and others, to define peroneal muscular atrophy as distinct from ALS[26] and for Erb[27] to describe primary lateral sclerosis in the mid-1870s.

With the disease finally described after three decades of observation, Marie[28] in his "Lessons on Diseases of the Spinal Cord" further refined the description of ALS. By this time, tendon reflexes had finally become integral in diagnosis and his description is clearly recognizable to today's clinician. He confirmed that amyotrophy is associated with "spastic phenomena," with diffuse increases in reflexes in "all parts of the body." He pointed out that "some sign of rigidity will be easily found in the upper or lower limbs in the great majority of cases." This included the pharyngeal reflex (gag), which may be increased or decreased; abnormal spread of "periosteal reflexes" in the arms; and ankle clonus. Marie saw the spread of ALS as slow and deliberate, as

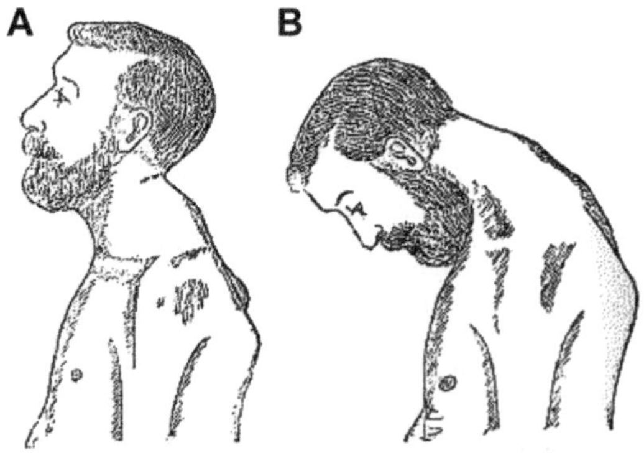


**Fig. 2.** Progressive muscular atrophy. Weakness of the muscles of the neck. (*A*) Habitual posture of the head inclined backward. (*B*) Position into which if falls if the patient attempts to keep it in the normal balance. (*From* Gowers WR. Manual of diseases of the nervous system. American edition. Philadelphia: P. Blakinston & Sons; 1888. p. 350–73.)

a disease that moved gradually "fasciculus after fasciculus, and so to speak, fiber after fiber." He focused on the distal predilection, with the small hand muscles involved first, so the hand becomes "claw like" (en patte de singe). He described the head drop, where the neck suffers from atrophy and paralysis with the head "bent forward over the sternum." Marie referred to ALS as a form of atrophy where "fibrillary contractions" (fasciculations) are "extremely pronounced" and may occur in muscles that have no sign of atrophy. He implored his colleagues "to investigate with great care, since it will indicate to you the muscles which will be affected in the course of the disease." He described tongue fasciculations that give way to atrophy with series of undulating or "rounded eminences" of the tongue, which resemble cerebral convolutions and noted that at the latest stages the vagus becomes affected with changes in respiration and a risk of pneumonia of deglutition.

Finally, Marie asked the question are "psychic functions altered in the course of ALS?" He pointed out that "most authors deny that this is the case" but explained that change is "frequent" and could even be thought as "constituting one of [ALS] ordinary symptoms." He noted that a tendency to laugh or weep is almost certainly found to exist and the "intellectual and moral condition of the patients are childish," in what was likely an early description of pseudobulbar affect. He implored his audience to "always mistrust the pronounced neurasthenia which occurs in an unexpected manner; when it is neither due to real misfortune, loss of money, nor excessive mental labor, it is almost always the unpleasant indication of a serious disease which affects the organism in its most important functions." He thought these symptoms often preceded the weakness.

It is remarkable to reflect on how, with the ability to focus on the disorder, 30 years had helped Marie move beyond the science of clinical investigation, into that of clinical observation and the art of medicine. With experience, he seems to have become a realist about the disease. Marie suggested that ALS "is like a certain goddess of antiquity" that "issued from the brain of its creator in a completely armed condition." He used fire as a metaphor in saying we must be "contented to observe as powerless witnesses the progress of a conflagration in the gray matter of the medulla and spinal cord which we can neither extinguish not limit" and went on with there is "nothing which indicates the reason for its existence," "we know nothing, absolutely nothing, of the treatment which should be employed against it" and finally, "How could it be otherwise when the two cardinal facts from which all efficient treatment starts, the cause and the nature of the affection are equally unknown to us."

Approximately 40 years later in his famous textbook *Neurology*,[29] Wilson had continued difficulty deciding if typical ALS and Aran-Duchenne progressive muscular atrophy and indeed primary lateral sclerosis are distinct entities or are on a spectrum. It is worthwhile to quote a paragraph from Wilson[29]:

*For these reasons various writers doubt the validity of the alleged distinctions, preferring to regard the two as variants of one affection, sometimes called "motor neurone disease," attacking upper or lower neurons, or both impartially. The term, however, has the default of being aetiologically vague and pathologically unspecific. Difficult as it is to reach the firm conclusion, the lesions of the Charcot type are so characteristic, and when advanced, so different from those of nuclear amyotrophy, that in my opinion the fact out-weight other considerations; they comprise much more than the mere addition of upper to lower motor neuronic disease. While I consider this divergence more striking than the similarities, the occurrence of gradations from one to the other, and also in the direction of "subacute anterior poliomyelitis" must be admitted; not all of either kind run true to type. For descriptive purposes it is best however to take the two varieties together inclusive of intermediate and aberrant clinical forms.*

The statements of Marie and Wilson remind us that, in regards to the phenotypic description, we have not moved far from where we stood then. Despite key advances in the understanding of the nature of the condition, clinicians are still standing against the same "armed goddess" that the masters alluded to in the late nineteenth century. The field has refined the ability to measure function and to collect data in the last 30 years. There is one Food and Drug Administration–approved drug for ALS, riluzole, which has been shown in trials to slow the disease progression slightly. The discovery of disease-associated genes in a small percentage of patients with ALS has been the other main breakthrough, while we have refined the nosology of progressive atrophy through clinical and genetic discoveries. Still, the statements of Marie remind us that in some ways clinicians have not moved to far from where they stood 125 years ago. Several groups are now in the process of taking the early clinical observations on ALS highlighted in this article to the next level in precision medicine programs, which it is hoped will allow for a more concise understanding of the disease and how it relates to genetic or biologic factors that have been discovered over the past few decades. For example, why do some patients die in 3 to 5 years, whereas others have a prolonged course for up to 10 or even 20 years? As clinicians move into a new millennium of ALS research, they are truly standing on the shoulders of the earliest observers and chroniclers of ALS.

## REFERENCES


1. Charcot J-M. De la sclérose latérale amyotrophique. Prog Med 1874;2:325–7, 341-342, 453-455.
2. Charcot JM. Lecture XI. Chronic spinal amyotrophies pp 163-179; Lecture XII. Deuteropathic spinal amyotrophies. Lateral amyotrophic sclerosis pp 180–191; Lecture XIII. On amyotrophic lateral sclerosis pp 192-204. In: Sigerson G, editor. Lectures on diseases of the nervous system. London: New Sydenham Society; 1881. p. 192–204. trans (Special Edition, copyright Classics of Neurology and Neurosurgery Library, Birmingham Alabama 1985).
3. Goetz CG. transcripts of Charcot J-M [with commentary]. Charcot the Clinician: The Tuesday Lessons. New York: Raven Press; 1987.
4. Louis ED. Erb and Westphal: simultaneous discovery of the deep tendon reflexes. Semin Neurol 2002;22:385–90.
5. Babinski J. Sur le réflexe cutané plantaire dans certains affections organique du système nerveux central. Comptes rendus de la Société de Biologie 1896;48: 207–8.
6. Finger S. Chapter 13: Santiago Ramon y Cajal. From nerve nets to neuron doctrine. In: Minds behind the brain: a history of the pioneers and their discoveries. New York: Oxford University Press; 2000. p. 197–216.
7. Sherrington CS. The integrative action of the nervous system. New Haven (CT): Yale University Press; 1906.
8. Bell C. The nervous system of the human body. London: Longman; 1830. p. 132–6 (Special Edition, copyright Classics of Neurology and Neurosurgery Library, Birmingham Alabama 1985).
9. Tyler HR, Shefner J. Amyotrophic lateral sclerosis. Handb Clin Neurol 1991;15: 169–215.
10. Goldblatt D. Motor neuron disease: historical introduction. In: Norris FH Jr, Kurland LT, editors. Motor neuron disease. New York: Grune & Stratton; 1968. p. 3–11.

11. Aran FA. Recherches sur une maladie non encore décrite du systemé musculaire (atrophie musculaire progressive). Arch Gen Med 1850;14:5–35, 172–214.
12. Duchenne de Boulogne GB. Recherches électro-physiologiques et thérapeutiques. Comp Rend Seances Acad Sci 1851;32:506.
13. Cruveilhier J. Sur le paralysie musculaire, progressive, atrophique. Bull Acad Med 1853;18:490–501, 546–83.
14. Radcliffe CB, Lockhart Clarke J. An important case of paralysis and muscular atrophy with disease of the nervous centres. Br Foreign Medico-Chirurgical Rev 1862;30:215–25.
15. Turner MT, Swash M, Ebers GC. Lockhart Clarke's contribution to the description of amyotrophic lateral sclerosis. Brain 2010;133:3470–9.
16. Charcot J-M. Sclérose des cordons latéraux de la moelle épinière chez une femme hystérique atteinte de contracture permanente des quatre membres. Bull de La Société Méd Des Hôpit de Paris 1865;10:24–35.
17. Charcot J-M, Joffroy A. Deus cas d'atrophie musculaire progressive avec lesions de la substance grise et des faisceaux antéro-latérale. Arch Physiol 1869;2: 354–67, 744–60.
18. Goetz CG. Amyotrophic lateral sclerosis: early contributions of Jean-Martin Charcot. Muscle Nerve 2000;23:336–43.
19. Dumenil DR. Atrophie des nerfs hypoglosses. Eaciaux et spinaux. Gax Hebd Med Chri 1859;390–2.
20. Duchenne G. Paralysie musculaire progressive de la langue, du voile du palais et des levres. Arch Gen Med 1860;16:283–96.
21. Wachsmuth A. Ueber progressive bulbär-paralyse (bulbus medullae): und die diplegia facialis. Dorpat: E.J. Karow; 1864.
22. Goetz CG, Bonduelle M, Gelfand T. Charcot. Constructing neurology. Oxford (England): Oxford University Press; 1995.
23. Rowland LP. How amyotrophic lateral sclerosis got its name. The clinical-pathologic genius of Jean-Martin Charcot. Arch Neurol 2001;58(3):512–5.
24. Gowers WR. Manual of diseases of the nervous system. American edition. Philadelphia: P. Blakinston & Sons; 1888. p. 350–73 (Special Edition Copyright: Birmingham, AL: Classics of Medicine Library; 1981).
25. ALS Regional Variants (Brachial Amyotrophic Diplegia, Leg Amyotrophic Diplegia, and Isolated Bulbar ALS), in press.
26. Marie P. Sur une forme particulière d'atrophie musculaire progressive, souvent familiale débutant par les pieds et les jambes et atteignant plus tard les mains. Revue médicale (Paris) 1886;6:97–138.
27. Erb W. Uber einen wenig bekannten spinalen symptomen complex. Berl Klin Wschr 1875;12:357–9.
28. Marie P. Amyotrophic lateral sclerosis, in Lessons in diseases of the spinal cord (English Translation of Lecons sur les maladies de la moelle). Montagu Lubbock. Paris; London: Masson; The New Sydenham Society; 1892. 1895 (Special Edition, copyright Classics of Neurology and Neurosurgery Library, Birmingham Alabama 1990).
29. Wilson K. Chapter LIV. Progressive spinal muscular atrophy. In: Ninian Bruce A, editor. Neurology, vol. 2. London: Edward Arnold Co; 1941. p. 1007. Special Edition, copyright Classics of Neurology and Neurosurgery Library, Birmingham Alabama 1989.

# Patterns of Weakness, Classification of Motor Neuron Disease, and Clinical Diagnosis of Sporadic Amyotrophic Lateral Sclerosis

Jeffrey M. Statland, MD[a,*], Richard J. Barohn, MD[a], April L. McVey, MD[a], Jonathan S. Katz, MD[a,b], Mazen M. Dimachkie, MD[a]

**KEYWORDS**

- Motor neuron disease • Upper motor neuron • Lower motor neuron
- Amyotrophic lateral sclerosis • Lou Gehrig disease

**KEY POINTS**

- Patterns of weakness can be useful when approaching a patient with suspected motor neuron disease (MND).
- MNDs exist on a spectrum: pure lower motor neuron ↔ mixed upper and lower motor neuron ↔ pure upper motor neuron.
- Amyotrophic lateral sclerosis (ALS) is a progressive mixed upper and lower MND that is most commonly sporadic and invariably fatal.
- A better understanding of the genetics and pathophysiology of heritable ALS may yield insights into possible therapies for sporadic ALS.

## PATTERNS OF WEAKNESS

Neuropathic disorders can be broadly divided into disorders affecting the peripheral nerve processes (neuropathy) or nerve cell body (neuronopathy), can be inherited or acquired, and have different clinical courses.[1] MNDs are neuronopathies. When

Disclosure: See last page of the article.

[a] Department of Neurology, University of Kansas Medical Center, 3901 Rainbow Boulevard, Mailstop 2012, Kansas City, KS 66160, USA; [b] Department of Neurology, California Pacific Medical Center, 475 Brannan Street, Suite 220, San Francisco, CA 94107, USA
* Corresponding author.
*E-mail address:* jstatland@kumc.edu

Neurol Clin 33 (2015) 735–748
http://dx.doi.org/10.1016/j.ncl.2015.07.006 neurologic.theclinics.com
0733-8619/15/$ – see front matter 

approaching a patient with a suspected neuropathy or neuronopathy, there are several key questions that can help further categorize the disorder:

- Which parts of the nervous system are involved: motor, sensory, or autonomic or a combination of more than 1 system?
- Where is the weakness (proximal, distal, or both) and is it symmetric or asymmetric?
- If there is sensory involvement, is there pain or proprioceptive loss?
- Over what time frame did symptoms evolve: acute (<4 weeks) or subacute (4–8 weeks) or is it chronic?
- Is there a family history of a similar disorder?
- If there is motor involvement, is it upper motor neuron, lower motor neuron, or both?

The neuropathic disorders can be confusing to a clinician first encountering them but several key patterns of involvement can help lead to the proper diagnosis (**Table 1**). For a full description of the neuropathic patterns (NP), readers are referred to Barohn and Amato.[1] Some of the myopathic patterns, including myopathy pattern (MP) 6 (neck extensor weakness) and MP7 (tongue, pharyngeal, or diaphragm), described previously, also overlap with MND.[2]

MNDs are typically motor syndromes (sensory sparing) that show insidious onset; are chronically progressive; can be distal, proximal, or mixed; and can have different combinations of upper and lower motor neuron findings. They can be inherited or sporadic. There several neuropathic patterns seen in the MNDs.

### *Asymmetric Distal Weakness Without Sensory Loss (NP5)*

If a patient comes in with asymmetric onset of distal weakness or muscle wasting and upper motor neuron findings on examination (brisk reflexes with spread to other regions, Babinski sign, Hoffmann reflex, or increased tone), ALS is a main consideration, in particular, if the onset was insidious and the weakness is painless. If there are only upper motor neuron findings on examination, then primary lateral sclerosis (PLS) needs to be considered in the differential diagnosis (see the article by Statland and colleagues[3]). If a patient only has lower motor neuron findings (muscle wasting or fasciculations), then the differential is broader and includes a motor neuron disorder, like progressive muscular atrophy (PMA) (see the article by Liewluck and colleagues[4]); acquired diseases of motor neurons, like multifocal motor neuropathy or multifocal acquired motor axonopathy; or para-infectious complications (polio-like illness). As the disease progresses, distal weakness may become symmetric and progress proximally and reflexes may be attenuated as can be seen with MP2 or NP7.[2]

### *Symmetric Weakness Without Sensory Loss (NP7)*

If weakness is proximal more than distal or both, then spinal muscular atrophy (SMA) and PMA are considerations. If weakness only includes upper motor neuron signs, then PLS is a consideration. If the weakness is distal only, then other heritable conditions, like distal SMA, hereditary motor neuropathy, and Charcot-Marie-Tooth disease become considerations. Sensory loss on examination in NP7 is evident, however, for Charcot-Marie-Tooth disease despite the absence of sensory symptoms, but when sensory symptoms are present, it is classified as NP2.

### *Focal Midline Proximal Symmetric (NP8)*

If the neck and trunk are prominently involved, ALS is the main consideration, also known as MP6. If the onset is mostly bulbar, as in MP7, then ALS and variants that include progressive bulbar palsy or PLS are considered. ALS can present with isolated respiratory involvement. Care needs to be taken, however, because there is overlap with this pattern of weakness and other MP6 and MP7 disorders of the neuromuscular junction (myasthenia gravis or the Lambert-Eaton myasthenic syndrome) or muscle (occulopharyngeal muscular dystrophy or isolated neck extensor myopathy).

- MNDs have insidious onset and are chronically progressive.
- They can be inherited or sporadic.
- Patterns of weakness include symmetric or asymmetric weakness without sensory loss or focal midline proximal symmetric.

## CLASSIFICATION OF MOTOR NEURON DISEASES

The classification of MNDs is broadly divided into heritable or sporadic and by the degree of upper or lower motor neuron involvement. MNDs exist on a spectrum from pure lower motor neuron syndromes to mixed upper and lower MNDs to pure upper MNDs (**Fig. 1**).

### *Pure Lower Motor Neuron Disease*

Heritable diseases include SMA (NP7) and spinobulbar muscular atrophy (SBMA) (NP8/MP7 or MP1 [proximal symmetric weakness without sensory loss or upper motor neuron signs]). SMA is characterized by progressive initially proximal weakness that can present at birth, in early childhood, or as an adult.[5] SMA is loosely divided based on whether patients develop the ability to walk or sit, and the vast majority are autosomal recessive due to deletion of the survival motor neuron gene. SBMA, on the other hand, typically presents in adulthood (third–fifth decades) and is characterized by prominent bulbar involvement but can have sensory loss with decreased reflexes and is X-linked due to CAG repeat expansion in the androgen receptor gene.[6] Sporadic progressive weakness confined to lower motor neurons is termed PMA and is more common in men, with slower disease progression than ALS (see the article on PMA by Liewluck and colleagues[4]) and presents initially at NP5 without upper motor neuron signs, followed in 40% by bulbar symptoms, but occasionally starts as MP1.[7] In addition, certain ALS regional variants present initially with isolated lower motor neuron involvement, including both leg (NP5 without upper motor neuron signs) and brachial (NP5 without upper motor neuron signs) amyotrophic diplegia (ALS regional variants) (see the article by Jawdat and colleagues[8]).

### *Mixed Upper and Lower Motor Neuron Diseases*

When a combination of both upper and lower MND is present and ancillary work-up fails to provide an alternative explanation, this almost invariably turns out to be ALS (NP5). Both familial and sporadic ALS present in a clinically similar fashion and cannot be distinguished by clinical history or signs alone with the exception of family history. In addition, isolated respiratory involvement (NP8/MP7) can have both upper and lower motor neuron components, and isolated bulbar palsy (NP8/MP7) also presents with mixed upper and lower motor neuron findings.[9]

### *Pure Upper Motor Neuron Diseases*

Both hereditary spastic paraplegias and PLS fall under NP5 with some distinctive clinical features. Patients who present with a pure upper motor neuron syndrome, with symmetric symptoms or signs largely confined to the legs, usually at an early age, with foot deformities (pes cavus or hammertoes), and with or without a known family history likely fall into the category of hereditary spastic paraplegias – these

**Table 1**
**Clinical patterns of neuropathic disorders**

| | Weakness | | | | | | | | |
|---|---|---|---|---|---|---|---|---|---|
| | Proximal | Distal | Asymmetric | Symmetric | Sensory Symptoms | Severe Proprioceptive Loss | Upper Motor Neuron Signs | Autonomic Symptoms/ Signs | Diagnosis |
| Pattern 1—symmetric proximal and distal weakness with sensory loss | + | + | — | + | + | — | — | — | GBS/CIDP |
| Pattern 2—distal sensory loss with/without weakness | — | + | — | + | + | — | — | — | CSPN, metabolic, drugs, hereditary |
| Pattern 3—distal weakness with sensory loss | — | + | + | — | + | — | — | — | Multiple – vasculitis, HNPP, MADSAM, infection<br>Single – Mononeuropathy, radiculopathy |
| Pattern 4—asymmetric proximal and distal weakness with sensory loss | + | + | + | — | + | — | — | — | Polyradiculopathy, plexopathy |
| Pattern 5—asymmetric distal weakness without sensory loss | — | + | + | — | — | — | +/– | — | + UMN: ALS, PLS<br>– UMN: MMN, PMA, MAMA, BAD, LAD |

| | | | | | | | | | |
|---|---|---|---|---|---|---|---|---|---|
| Pattern 6—symmetric sensory loss and upper motor neuron signs | — | + | — | + | + | + | + | — | $B_{12}$ deficiency; copper deficiency, Friedreich, adrenomyeloneuropathy |
| Pattern 7[a]—symmetric weakness without sensory loss | +/– | + | — | + | — | — | — | — | Proximal and distal SMA distal hereditary motor neuropathy |
| Pattern 8[a]—focal midline proximal symmetric weakness | + Neck/ extensor + bulbar | — | — | + + | — | — | + + | — | ALS |
| Pattern 9—asymmetric proprioceptive loss without weakness | — | — | + | — | + | + | — | — | Sensory neuronopathy (ganglionopathy) |
| Pattern 10—autonomic dysfunction | — | — | — | — | — | — | — | + | HSAN, diabetes, GBS, amyloid, porphyria, Fabry disease |

*Abbreviations:* BAD, brachial amyotrophic diplegia; CIDP, chronic inflammatory demyelinating polyneuropathy; CSPN, cryptogenic sensory polyneuropathy; GBS, Guillain-Barré syndrome; HNPP, hereditary neuropathy with liability to pressure palsy; HSAN, hereditary sensory and autonomic neuropathy; LAD, leg amyotrophic diplegia; LMN, lower motor neuron; MADSAM, multifocal acquired demyelinating sensory and motor; MAMA, multifocal acquired motor axonopathy; MMN, multifocal motor neuropathy; UMN, upper motor neuron.

[a] Overlap patterns with myopathy/NMJ disorders.

*From* Barohn RJ, Amato AA. Pattern-recognition approach to neuropathy and neuronopathy. Neurol Clin 2013;31(2):356–7; with permission.

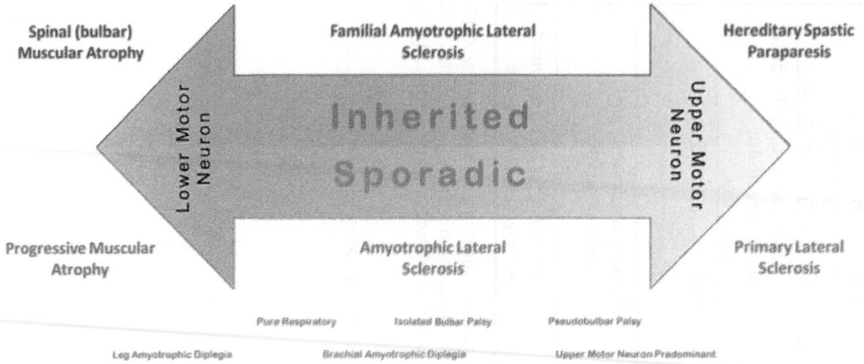


**Fig. 1.** The spectrum of MNDs.

disorders can be dominant or recessive and more than 60 genes have been described. Mutations in spastin are the most common dominant disorder, accounting for 30% to 50% families; and mutations in spatacsin are the most common recessive disorder with thinning of the corpus callosum, accounting for approximately 50% of cases.[10,11] PLS, on the other hand, is progressive, occurs at a later age, typically in the fifth to sixth decades, and often involves the arms or bulbar region, in addition to the legs asymmetrically.[12] In addition an upper motor neuron predominant presentation of ALS has been described.

## AMYOTROPHIC LATERAL SCLEROSIS

ALS is a progressive disorder of motor neurons in the brain and spinal cord that is invariably fatal. It can present with equal frequency as NP5 in the arms, NP of the legs or bulbar NP8/MP7 onset. Clinically patients have mixed upper and lower motor neuron findings on examination. A majority of patients have sporadic disease (approximately 85%) – the heritable causes of ALS are described elsewhere. ALS is fundamentally a clinical diagnosis, supported by neurophysiologic testing. There are no cures for ALS – but there are evidence-based guidelines for standards of care (see the article by Jackson and colleagues[13]). The epidemiology, clinical presentation, diagnosis, and progression of ALS are described.

### *Prevalence and Epidemiology*

The first major attempt to identify overall national US prevalence data for ALS used major national administrative databases (Medicare, Medicaid, Veterans Health Administration, and Veterans Benefits Administration), including more than 12,000 ALS cases identified by a standard algorithm (*International Classification of Diseases, Ninth Revision*, codes; Veterans Health Benefits codes; neurologist visits; and prescriptions for riluzole) between October 19, 2010, and December 31, 2011.[14] Using 2011 census data they estimated a US population prevalence for ALS of 3.9/100,000. The prevalence differed by age with highest prevalence between 70 and 79 years (17/100,000) and lowest between 18 and 39 years (0.5/100,000). There was a higher prevalence of ALS in men compared with women with a male-to-female ratio of 1.56. Overall ALS was twice as common in whites as blacks. Worldwide prevalence rates for ALS have varied – a meta-analysis of studies published since 1991 found 26 studies citing prevalence rates between 1.07 and 11.31 per 100,000.[15] Most studies report a male predominance with male-to-female ratios between 1.2 and 1.5.[16,17] There are fewer incidence data on ALS rates in the United States. But 1 large study in 3 states and 8 large metropolitan areas identified 5883 unique ALS cases (74.8% white, 9.3% African American, and 3.6% Asian). Most (77.5%) were non-Hispanic.[18] They estimated an average annual incidence rate of 1.52 per 100,000 person-years (an age-adjusted rate of 1.44 per 100,000 person-years). Worldwide incidence rates have varied between 0.42 and 5.3 per 100,000 person years.[15] The average age of onset is later in life, with means from 60.7 to 64.3 years and an average time from symptom onset to diagnosis between 10.8 and 16.9 months.[14,16,19–21] In the United States, African Americans may be affected slightly younger, with median age of onset of 58 years and more than half of African Americans diagnosed before 60 years.[18]

### *Clinical Findings*

Although there is considerable clinical variability in the presentation of ALS, several key patterns and clinical features are highly suggestive:

- Insidious onset of painless weakness and muscle wasting, which starts in one limb and then spreads typically to the contralateral limb
- Insidious onset of problems with speech or swallowing, followed by weakness or muscle wasting in the limbs
- Progressive muscle stiffness and spasticity with muscle cramps and fasciculations
- Unexplained restrictive respiratory disease, with a pattern suggestive of diaphragmatic weakness
- Head drop with weakness of trunk or paraspinal musculature with upper motor neuron signs on examination.

The classic ALS presentation is insidious onset of symptoms, which are progressive, and has a combination of both upper and lower motor neuron findings on clinical examination. The most common presentation is limb onset; bulbar onset accounts for between 30% and 32.5% of cases. Lower motor neuron findings include muscle wasting, weakness, and fasciculations. Upper motor neuron findings include spasticity, pathologically brisk reflexes, and weakness in antigravity muscles. Bulbar symptoms can include difficulty speaking (dysarthria), difficulty swallowing (dysphagia), and subsequent excess saliva (sialorrhea). Patients typically have a diaphragmatic pattern of respiratory weakness and may complain of feeling short of breath with activities or when lying on their back. In addition to the muscular complications of ALS, patients can experience pseudobulbar affect, which is characterized by excessive laughter or crying with minimal stimulation. Cognitive and behavioral changes have been described in up to 50% of patients with ALS, typically in the spectrum of changes seen with frontotemporal degeneration, with a smaller percentage meeting the frank diagnostic criteria for frontotemporal dementia.[22]

### *History of Amyotrophic Lateral Sclerosis Diagnostic Criteria*

Dr Edward Lambert published in 1957 the first attempt to help physicians diagnose ALS with electromyographic guidelines.[23] These criteria included (1) normal sensory nerve conduction studies, (2) motor nerve conduction velocities that are normal when recording from relatively unaffected muscles and not less than 70% of the age-based average normal value when recording from severely affected muscles, (3) fibrillation and fasciculation potentials in muscles of the upper and lower extremities or in the muscles of the extremities and the head, and (4) motor unit potentials that are reduced in number and increased in duration and amplitude. A 3-day workshop on "The Clinical Limits of ALS" was convened in El Escorial, Spain, in 1990 by the World Federation of Neurology Subcommittee on Motor Neuron Disease and developed the EEC.[24] In the original EEC criteria, when there are clear upper and lower motor neuron findings in 2 to 3 regions, EMG is not required for a patient to enter a study (**Box 1**). If EMG is required, fibrillation potentials must be present. For the EEC diagnostic categories, see **Box 2**.

In 1998, the Western ALS Study Group modified World Federation of Neurology diagnostic criteria for ALS to facilitate early diagnosis and used these criteria for enrollment of ALS patients in the recombinant human ciliary neurotrophic factor study trial.[25] The Western ALS criteria developed required lower motor neuron involvement in at least 2 limbs and upper motor neuron involvement in at least 1 region (bulbar, cervical, or lumbosacral). The EMG finding of fibrillation potentials was required for evidence of lower motor neuron involvement. Electrodiagnostic studies, neuroimaging, and laboratory studies were also used to exclude disorders that might mimic ALS. If no bulbar signs were present, a cervical MRI was needed for the patients to meet study criteria.

The revised EEC were specific although insensitive for early diagnosis. In 2006, a group of ALS researchers met in Awaji-shima, Japan, to revise ALS diagnostic criteria.[26] They made 2 significant changes to the El Escorial system (**Box 3**). First, signs of denervation on EMG were regarded as equivalent to clinical lower motor neuron signs and it was suggested to delete "laboratory supported probable ALS" and use only "probable ALS." Second, fasciculation potentials in muscles with chronic neurogenic EMG changes, in a clinical context fitting ALS, counted as a sign of active denervation, even in the absence of fibrillation potentials and positive sharp waves (see **Box 3**). The Awaji criteria (AC) improved the sensitivity of EMG studies considerably without increasing the rate of false-positive diagnoses, especially in bulbar-onset patients. One weakness of the AC was the requirement for 2 upper motor neuron signs for the clinically probable category. Although patients with upper motor neuron signs in 1 segment would be allowed into research studies by the revised El Escorial clinically probable–laboratory supported category, they would be downgraded to clinically possible by the AC requirement for 2 regions with UMN involvement.

**Box 1**
**The EEC diagnosis of ALS requires**

*Presence of*

(A:1) Signs of lower motor neuron degeneration by clinical, electrophysiologic or neuropathologic examination,

(A:2) Signs of upper motor neuron degeneration by clinical examination, and

(A:3) Progressive spread of signs within a region or to other regions

*Together with the absence of*

(B:1) Electrophysiologic evidence of other disease processes that might explain the signs of lower motor neuron and/or upper motor neuron degeneration, and

(B:2) Neuroimaging evidence of other disease processes that might explain the observed clinical and electrophysiologic signs

**Box 2**
**El Escorial Criteria diagnostic categories**

Definite ALS is defined on clinical grounds alone by the presence of upper motor neuron (UMN) as well as lower motor neuron (LMN) signs in the bulbar region and at least 2 of the other spinal regions or the presence of UMN and LMN signs in 3 spinal regions.

Probable ALS is defined on clinical grounds alone by UMN and LMN signs in at least 2 regions. Although the regions may be different, some UMN signs must be rostral to (above) the LMN signs. Multiple different combinations of UMN and LMN signs may be present in patients with probable ALS.

Possible ALS is defined on clinical grounds alone when the UMN and LMN signs are in only 1 region or UMN signs alone are present in 2 or more regions or LMN signs are rostral to UMN signs.

Suspected ALS manifest only LMN signs in 2 or more regions, although UMN pathology might be demonstrated at autopsy. Only clinical signs, however, are considered pertinent to the classification the time of diagnostic evaluation.

### *Diagnosis*

According to the revised El Escorial criteria (EEC), diagnosis of ALS[27] is suggested by the presence of

- Lower motor neuron dysfunction by physical, electrophysiologic, or neuropathologic examination
- Upper motor neuron dysfunction by clinical examination
- Progression of symptoms or signs over 6 months, as demonstrated by spread within a region or to other spinal regions

Diagnosis of ALS[27] is suggested by the absence of

- Electrophysiologic or pathologic evidence of other disease processes
- Neuroimaging evidence of other disease processes

**Box 3**
**Awaji criteria**

Clinically definite

UMN + LMN signs in bulbar region + ≥2 spinal regions; or

UMN + LMN signs in 3 spinal regions

Clinically probable

UMN + LMN signs in ≥2 spinal regions and "with some

UMN signs necessarily rostral to the LMN signs"

Clinically possible

UMN + LMN signs in 1 spinal region; or

UMN signs in ≥2 spinal regions; or

LMN signs are found rostral to UMN signs, only after the appropriate neuroimaging and laboratory tests are performed to exclude other possible differential diagnosis that may mimic ALS

The diagnosis is largely based on clinical history and physical examination findings and supported by electrodiagnostic testing. Evidence for widespread active denervation on electromyography includes fibrillations and positive sharp waves. Evidence for reinnervation on electromyography include large motor units, polyphasic motor unit morphology, reduced interference pattern with increased firing rates, or unstable motor unit potentials. The clinical diagnosis of ALS is often broken down by probabilities, and the revised EEC, which were developed for clinical trials, are widely used in clinics.[27] Patients are considered

- *Clinically definite* by the presence of upper and lower motor neuron signs in the bulbar region and 2 spinal cord levels or in 3 spinal cord levels
- *Clinically probable* if they have upper and lower motor neuron signs in 2 spinal cord levels, with some upper motor neuron signs rostral to the lower motor neuron signs
- *Clinically probable–laboratory supported* if they have upper and lower motor neuron signs in only 1 spinal cord level or when upper motor neuron signs are present alone in 1 region, and lower motor neuron signs are present on electromyography in 2 regions
- *Clinically possible* if they have have upper and lower motor neuron findings in only 1 region, or upper motor neuron signs are found alone in 2 regions, or lower motor neuron sings found rostral to upper motor neuron signs

For patients meeting clinically definite criteria who also have bulbar involvement, neuroimaging is not essential for the diagnosis. For other patients, additional evaluations that may be important include

- MRI of the brain and/or spine
- Complete metabolic profile, blood count and differential, and thyroid studies
- Autoimmune testing (eg, GM1 antibodies and serum protein electrophoresis)
- Screening for malignancy (eg, lymphoma and lung cancer)
- Cerebrospinal fluid testing
- Infectious work-up (eg, HIV, human T-lymphotropic virus 1, and Lyme disease)
- Toxins (eg, heavy metals)

The mimics of ALS include multifocal motor neuropathy, endocrinopathies, post-poliomyelitis syndromes, heavy metal toxicity, and paraneoplastic syndromes. Not all patients meet formal ALS criteria, and patients with motor neuron involvement and failure to find an alternative explanation should be followed in ALS multidisciplinary clinics.

### *Clinical Course*

ALS is a progressive disease that is invariably fatal. The median time from diagnosis to death ranges depending on the study but is generally reported to be approximately 2.5 to 3 years.[20,28,29] Due to delays in diagnosis, most patients show some respiratory involvement at the time of diagnosis, with more than half having a forced vital capacity less than 75% of predicted for age and gender at the time of first clinic visit.[20] Several factors have been associated with faster progression in ALS,[20,28–30] and these include

- Bulbar onset of symptoms
- Older age at symptom onset
- Shorter duration of symptoms
- Reduced forced vital capacity

Patients who present with symptoms isolated to either end of MND spectrum and regional ALS variants can have slower progression. Patients with PMA or lower motor neuron variants of ALS (brachial and leg amyotrophic diplegia) are more frequently male and have slower disease progression. On the other end of the spectrum, patients with upper motor neuron–dominant ALS also have slower progression than classic ALS.[31]

### *Therapeutic Strategies*

The only Food and Drug Administration (FDA)-approved therapy for ALS is riluzole, which is believed to act by decreasing glutamate toxicity on at-risk motor neurons and prolongs survival by approximately 3 months.[32] The main side effects of riluzole therapy are gastrointestinal upset, but it can cause elevation in liver transaminases. When starting riluzole therapy it is recommended to check liver profile at baseline, then 1 month after starting therapy, and then every 3 months for the first year. The only other FDA-approved therapy for ALS is the use of Nuedexta for pseudobulbar affect (bouts of sustained laughter or crying). Nuedexta is a combination medication containing dextromethorphan and quinidine. It is generally well tolerated but is contraindicated for use in patients taking monamine oxidase inhibitors, and caution should be used in patients on serotonin-specific reuptake inhibitors due to a slight increase in risk of serotonin syndrome with the dextromethorphan. The bottom line is that other than riluzole, there has not been a drug shown to slow ALS disease progression and that has led to FDA approval. Symptomatic management for ALS is discussed elsewhere (see the article by Jackson and colleagues[13]), but the authors recommend all patients with ALS be followed in a multidisciplinary clinic.[33,34] Regular surveillance and areas of symptom management include

- Respiratory therapy to monitor respiratory function – possible interventions include noninvasive positive pressure ventilation, cough assist, and oral suctioning
- Speech therapy to monitor swallow and speech – possible interventions include percutaneous gastrostomy tube for nutrition and assistive communication devices
- Assessment for excess salivation – possible interventions include anticholinergic medications, botulinum toxin, and irradiation
- Physical and occupational therapy to assess for the need for bracing, assistive devices, or power wheelchair
- Psychosocial counseling for patients and family members to deal with the emotional impact of ALS
- Case manager to review health benefits available to veterans and others

## SUMMARY AND FUTURE DIRECTIONS

MNDs exist on a spectrum of involvement with varying degrees of upper and lower motor neuron involvement. MNDs can be distinguished from other neuropathies or neuronopathies by the pattern of motor and/or sensory involvement. ALS is the most prevalent MND and can be inherited or sporadic. ALS is characterized by mixed upper and lower MND, with insidious onset of painless muscle wasting that spreads from one region of the body to another. Although variability exists based on the site of symptom onset, the regions of the body involved, and rate of progression, ALS is an invariably fatal disease. The only FDA-approved therapy prolongs survival by a few months. All patients with ALS should be followed in a multidisciplinary care clinic, which improves the quality of life in people with ALS. A better understanding of the genetics and pathophysiology in familial ALS, along with a better understanding of regional variants with faster or slower progression, may help develop more-effective future therapies.

## DISCLOSURE

Dr R.J. Barohn has served as a consultant and received consulting fees from Baxter, CSL Behring, Genzyme, Grifols, Novartis, and NuFactor. He has received research grants from Biomarin, Cytokinetics, Eli Lilly, FDA/OPD, GSK, MDA, MGFA, Neals, NIH, NINDS, Novartis, PTC, Sanofi/Genzyme, and Teva. Dr A.L. McVey has received research grants from Cytokinetics. J. Katz is a consultant and has received consulting fees from NuFactor. He has received research grants from ALSA, FDA, MDA, and Synapse. Dr J.M. Statland has no disclosures. Dr M.M. Dimachkie is on the speaker's bureau or is a consultant for Baxter, Biomarin, Catalyst, CSL-Behring, Depomed, Genzyme, Merck, NuFactor, and Pfizer. He has also received grants from Catalyst, CSL-Behring, FDA/OPD, GSK, MDA, NIH, and TMA. This publication was also supported by an Institutional Clinical and Translational Science Award, NIH/NCATS Grant Number UL1TR000001. J.M.Statland's work on this project was supported by a CTSA grant from NCATS awarded to the University of Kansas Medical Center for Frontiers: The Heartland Institute for Clinical and Translational Research #KL2TR000119. Its contents are solely the responsibility of the authors and do not necessarily represent the official views of the NIH.

## REFERENCES

1. Barohn RJ, Amato AA. Pattern-recognition approach to neuropathy and neuronopathy. Neurol Clin 2013;31(2):343–61.
2. Barohn RJ, Dimachkie MM, Jackson CE. A pattern recognition approach to patients with a suspected myopathy. Neurol Clin 2014;32(3):569–93.
3. Statland JM, Barohn RJ, Dimachkie MM, et al. Primary lateral sclerosis. Neurol Clin 2015, in press.
4. Liewluck T, Saperstein DS. Progressive muscular atrophy. Neurol Clin 2015, in press.
5. Wang CH, Finkel RS, Bertini ES, et al. Consensus statement for standard of care in spinal muscular atrophy. J Child Neurol 2007;22(8):1027–49.
6. Rhodes LE, Freeman BK, Auh S, et al. Clinical features of spinal and bulbar muscular atrophy. Brain 2009;132(Pt 12):3242–51.
7. Norris F, Shepherd R, Denys E, et al. Onset, natural history and outcome in idiopathic adult motor neuron disease. J Neurol Sci 1993;118(1):48–55.
8. Jawdat O, Statland JM, Barohn RJ, et al. Amyotrophic Lateral Sclerosis Regional Variant (Brachial Amyotrophic Diplegia, Leg Amyotrophic Diplegia, and Isolated Bulbar Amyotrophic Lateral Sclerosis). Neurol Clin 2015, in press.
9. Burrell JR, Vucic S, Kiernan MC. Isolated bulbar phenotype of amyotrophic lateral sclerosis. Amyotroph Lateral Scler 2011;12(4):283–9.
10. Hazan J, Fontaine B, Bruyn RP, et al. Linkage of a new locus for autosomal dominant familial spastic paraplegia to chromosome 2p. Hum Mol Genet 1994;3(9):1569–73.
11. Martinez Murillo F, Kobayashi H, Pegoraro E, et al. Genetic localization of a new locus for recessive familial spastic paraparesis to 15q13-15. Neurology 1999;53(1):50–6.
12. Zhai P, Pagan F, Statland J, et al. Primary lateral sclerosis: a heterogeneous disorder composed of different subtypes? Neurology 2003;60(8):1258–65.

13. Rudnicki S, McVey AL, Jackson CE, et al. Symptom management and end-of-life care. Neurol Clin 2015, in press.
14. Mehta P, Antao V, Kaye W, et al. Prevalence of amyotrophic lateral sclerosis - United States, 2010-2011. MMWR Surveill Summ 2014;63(Suppl 7):1–14.
15. Deenen J, Horlings C, Verschuuren J, et al. The epidemiology of neuromuscular disorders: a comprehensive overview of the literature. J Neuromuscul Dis 2015;2: 73–85.
16. Abhinav K, Stanton B, Johnston C, et al. Amyotrophic lateral sclerosis in South-East England: a population-based study. The South-East England register for amyotrophic lateral sclerosis (SEALS Registry). Neuroepidemiology 2007;29(1–2):44–8.
17. Chio A, Calvo A, Moglia C, et al. Phenotypic heterogeneity of amyotrophic lateral sclerosis: a population based study. J Neurol Neurosurg Psychiatry 2011;82(7): 740–6.
18. Rechtman L, Jordan H, Wagner L, et al. Racial and ethnic differences among amyotrophic lateral sclerosis cases in the United States. Amyotroph Lateral Scler Frontotemporal Degener 2015;16(1–2):65–71.
19. Chio A, Mora G, Calvo A, et al. Epidemiology of ALS in Italy: a 10-year prospective population-based study. Neurology 2009;72(8):725–31.
20. Traxinger K, Kelly C, Johnson BA, et al. Prognosis and epidemiology of amyotrophic lateral sclerosis: Analysis of a clinic population, 1997-2011. Neurol Clin Pract 2013;3(4):313–20.
21. Traynor BJ, Codd MB, Corr B, et al. Incidence and prevalence of ALS in Ireland, 1995-1997: a population-based study. Neurology 1999;52(3):504–9.
22. Giordana MT, Ferrero P, Grifoni S, et al. Dementia and cognitive impairment in amyotrophic lateral sclerosis: a review. Neurol Sci 2011;32(1):9–16.
23. Lambert EH, Mulder DW. Electromyographic studies in amyotrophic lateral sclerosis. Mayo Clinic 1957;32:441–6.
24. Brooks BR. El Escorial World Federation of Neurology criteria for the diagnosis of amyotrophic lateral sclerosis. Subcommittee on Motor Neuron Diseases/Amyotrophic Lateral Sclerosis of the World Federation of Neurology Research Group on Neuromuscular Diseases. J Neurol Sci 1994;124(Suppl):96–107.
25. Ross MA, Miller RG, Berchert L, et al. Toward earlier diagnosis of amyotrophic lateral sclerosis: revised criteria. rhCNTF ALS Study Group. Neurology 1998; 50(3):768–72.
26. de Carvalho M, Dengler R, Eisen A, et al. Electrodiagnostic criteria for diagnosis of ALS. Clin Neurophysiol 2008;119(3):497–503.
27. Brooks BR, Miller RG, Swash M, et al. El Escorial revisited: revised criteria for the diagnosis of amyotrophic lateral sclerosis. Amyotroph Lateral Scler Other Motor Neuron Disord 2000;1(5):293–9.
28. Chancellor AM, Slattery JM, Fraser H, et al. The prognosis of adult-onset motor neuron disease: a prospective study based on the Scottish Motor Neuron Disease Register. J Neurol 1993;240(6):339–46.
29. del Aguila MA, Longstreth WT Jr, McGuire V, et al. Prognosis in amyotrophic lateral sclerosis: a population-based study. Neurology 2003;60(5):813–9.
30. Kollewe K, Mauss U, Krampfl K, et al. ALSFRS-R score and its ratio: a useful predictor for ALS-progression. J Neurol Sci 2008;275(1–2):69–73.
31. Gordon PH, Cheng B, Katz IB, et al. Clinical features that distinguish PLS, upper motor neuron-dominant ALS, and typical ALS. Neurology 2009;72(22): 1948–52.
32. Miller RG, Mitchell JD, Moore DH. Riluzole for amyotrophic lateral sclerosis (ALS)/ motor neuron disease (MND). Cochrane Database Syst Rev 2012;(3):CD001447.

33. Bradley WG, Anderson F, Bromberg M, et al. Current management of ALS: comparison of the ALS CARE Database and the AAN Practice Parameter. The American Academy of Neurology. Neurology 2001;57(3):500–4.
34. Miller RG, Jackson CE, Kasarskis EJ, et al. Practice parameter update: the care of the patient with amyotrophic lateral sclerosis: multidisciplinary care, symptom management, and cognitive/behavioral impairment (an evidence-based review): report of the Quality Standards Subcommittee of the American Academy of Neurology. Neurology 2009;73(15):1227–33.

# Primary Lateral Sclerosis

Jeffrey M. Statland, MD[a,*], Richard J. Barohn, MD[a],
Mazen M. Dimachkie, MD[a], Mary Kay Floeter, MD, PhD[b], Hiroshi Mitsumoto, MD, DSc[c]

**KEYWORDS**

- Motor neuron disease • Upper motor neuron disease • Primary lateral sclerosis
- Spastic quadriparesis • Pseudobulbar affect • Neuroimaging

**KEY POINTS**

- Primary lateral sclerosis (PLS) is a progressive upper motor neuron disease in the absence of clinical signs of lower motor neuron involvement.
- PLS is a diagnosis of exclusion supported by a characteristic clinical history, examination findings, and diagnostic testing ruling out other causes.
- Key examination findings can include spasticity, upper motor neuron pattern weakness, and pseudobulbar findings.
- The pathophysiologic hallmark is dysfunction of corticospinal tracts leading to upper motor neuron signs and symptoms.
- Patients with absence of lower motor neuron signs on electromyogram after 4 years are unlikely to progress to amyotrophic lateral sclerosis.

## INTRODUCTION

Primary lateral sclerosis (PLS) is a disorder of progressive upper motor neuron dysfunction, in the absence of clinical signs of lower motor neuron involvement or family history suggestive of hereditary spastic paraplegia. PLS is a diagnosis of exclusion. PLS exists on a spectrum of sporadic motor neuron disorders, including progressive muscular atrophy (lower motor neuron only), and amyotrophic lateral sclerosis (mixed upper and lower motor neuron involvement). PLS is a rare disorder, representing approximately 1% to 4% of all patients with motor neuron disease.[1–3] Although controversy exists as to whether PLS is a distinct pathologic disease from

Disclosure: See last page of article.

[a] Department of Neurology, University of Kansas Medical Center, 3901 Rainbow Boulevard, Mailstop 2012, Kansas City, KS 66160, USA; [b] Human Spinal Physiology Unit, National Institute of Neurological Disorders and Stroke, Building 10, Room 7-5680, 10 Center Drive, Bethesda, MD 20892, USA; [c] Department of Neurology, Columbia University Medical Center, 710 West 168th Street, New York City, NY 10032, USA
* Corresponding author.
*E-mail address:* jstatland@kumc.edu

Neurol Clin 33 (2015) 749–760
http://dx.doi.org/10.1016/j.ncl.2015.07.007 neurologic.theclinics.com

amyotrophic lateral sclerosis (ALS), it is clinically distinct, and portends a more benign clinical prognosis, making this a useful clinical category.

- PLS is a progressive upper motor neuron disorder
- From 1% to 3% of patients presenting with motor neuron disease
- Diagnosis of exclusion
- More benign prognosis than ALS

## CLINICAL FINDINGS

Although considerable heterogeneity exists between patients, symptoms usually begin in the fifth to sixth decade, unlike hereditary forms of spastic paresis, which usually present earlier and are associated with foot deformities, which are not present in PLS.[4] Most patients present at more than 20 years of age. As is seen in ALS, there may be a slight male predominance. The most common clinical presentation matches Erb's[5] original description of patients with spastic spinal paralysis from the early twentieth century, which included spasticity, hyperreflexia, and mild weakness. Patients may report stiffness, clumsiness, and poor coordination. Most patients report balance difficulties, and, as the disease progresses, increasing falls. Bulbar symptoms can include dysarthria, dysphagia, and emotional lability (fits of laughing or crying, termed pseudobulbar affect). Typically the examination shows only upper motor neuron signs, spasticity, spread of reflexes, and absence of lower motor neuron findings (fasciculations and muscle wasting). Stiffness as a presenting symptom is seen more commonly in PLS than in ALS (47% vs 4%), and limb wasting is rare in PLS (~2%).[6] An upper motor neuron pattern of weakness may be seen (extensors in upper extremity, flexors in lower extremity), but what the patient describes as weakness is often a combination of increased tone, decreased coordination, and mild weakness.

Although visual symptoms are not reported, some abnormalities of eye movements have been described, including saccadic breakdown of smooth pursuits, or supranuclear paralysis.[1,3] Urinary frequency or urgency can be seen in around one-third to one-half of patients.[2,3,7] In general, cognition is reported as being unaffected in PLS; however, some frontal lobe dysfunction can be seen in 10% to 20% of patients. Case reports have described cognitive changes in cases termed PLS plus, or overlap with parkinsonian syndromes.[8,9]

PLS is typically slowly progressive. Patterns of progression most commonly show spread from side to side, and from region to region, with many patients ultimately developing spastic quadriparesis with bulbar involvement. In one series an ascending progression was noted in patients with limb onset, with progression from one side to the other occurring first, followed by ascending progression (average 3.5 years from onset to arm involvement, 5 years from onset to bulbar involvement).[10,11] Other series have described bulbar onset then skipping the arms to appear in the legs.[3] However, overall the rate of progression is much slower than is typically encountered in ALS. The average symptom duration from various case series ranged from 7.2 to 14.5 years.[4] In many patients, progression seems to halt after several years, with varied levels of disability.

Clinical hallmarks of PLS include:

- Insidious onset of stiffness, clumsiness, or mild weakness; or dysarthria, dysphagia, and emotional lability
- Symptoms begin most commonly in the legs, but can begin in the bulbar region or multiple areas of the body
- Signs include spasticity, hyperreflexia, and upper motor neuron pattern weakness

- The absence of diffuse fasciculations or muscle wasting, or sensory symptoms or signs
- PLS is progressive, spreading from side to side and from region to region
- Urinary urgency or frequency may be reported

## CASE HISTORY

At age 46 years, a healthy right-handed woman developed a mild left foot drop that caused occasional tripping. An orthopedic examination, electromyogram (EMG), and rheumatologic evaluation at that time were unrevealing. Stiffness and mild weakness of her left leg progressed, and by age 49 years she noted stiffness in her right leg. Increasing difficulty with balance occasionally resulted in a fall. Neurologic examination at that time revealed mild hip and ankle flexor weakness, with bilateral leg spasticity, but no sensory loss or ataxia. An extensive work-up was done, as described later, and she was given a working diagnosis of progressive multiple sclerosis.

When first seen in our PLS clinic at age 51 years (year 5 of her disease), her examination was notable for spastic gait and spasticity of the left arm. Her right upper extremity was normal, as were speech and swallowing. She had symptoms of bladder urgency and an increased startle response. Over the next 5 years, spasticity gradually progressed to involve both upper extremities, as seen in the decline in annual measures of finger tapping, timed gait, and ALS functional rating scale (**Table 1**). Handwriting first became slower in year 7 of her disease, pseudobulbar affect and occasional choking when eating in year 8, and dysarthria in year 9. As her gait and balance worsened, she experienced more frequent falls with injuries: a scalp laceration requiring stitches, a concussion, a broken nose. She progressed from using a cane outside the home in year 6, to dependence on a wheeled walker in year 8, to occasional use of a power scooter outside the home in year 9. However, throughout her course, she has had no respiratory difficulties, no weight loss, and no muscle atrophy. She has reported occasional fasciculations, although none were observed during clinical or EMG examinations.

Her evaluations included multiple brain and spine MRI scans; aortic arch magnetic resonance angiography; abdominal computed tomography scan; cerebrospinal fluid (CSF) examination; and visual, auditory, and somatosensory evoked potentials, all unrevealing. Blood was negative for paraneoplastic autoantibodies, various metabolic and enzymatic measures associated with rare causes of spasticity, and genes known to cause hereditary spastic paraplegia. EMGs done in years 3 and 5 showed no denervation, only incomplete recruitment of motor units in leg muscles.

She began oral baclofen at increasing doses, eventually reaching 60 mg/d. A baclofen pump was placed, with improvement in spasticity and leg cramps.

**Table 1**
**Case history measures of function at annual visits**

| Disease Year | Age (y) | ALSFRS-R | Finger Taps/s Right | Finger Taps/s Left | Timed 6-m (20′) Gait (s) | FVC % Predicted |
|---|---|---|---|---|---|---|
| 5 | 51 | 44 | 5.1 | 3.2 | 10 | — |
| 6 | 52 | 44 | 3.8 | 3.5 | 12 | 88 |
| 7 | 53 | 42 | 3.1 | 1.9 | 19 | 87 |
| 8 | 54 | 36 | 2.3 | 1.7 | 18 | 85 |
| 9 | 55 | 36 | 2.1 | 1.5 | 17 | — |

*Abbreviation:* ALSFRS-R, Revised ALS Functional Rating Scale.

This case features several points that are common in PLS:

- Very slow progression of spasticity and motor slowing, often beginning in the legs
- Balance problems leading to falls
- Mild pyramidal weakness
- Often with sparing of respiratory function
- Possible benefit from intrathecal baclofen and treatment of pseudobulbar affect

## DIAGNOSIS

The diagnosis of PLS includes the presence of upper motor neuron dysfunction, in the absence of other neurologic findings, or alternative explanations on diagnostic testing. Ultimately PLS is a diagnosis of exclusion. Although structural, infectious, and demyelinating diseases can cause an upper motor neuron syndrome. After a thorough clinical history and examination the 2 most common differential considerations for PLS are an upper motor neuron presentation of ALS, and the hereditary spastic paraplegias. Additional differential considerations include structural lesions, infection, and demyelinating disease (**Box 1**). Several diagnostic criteria have been proposed.[3,4] In the Pringle criteria, symptoms had to be present for greater than or equal to 3 years; in the Singer criteria greater than or equal to 4 years; and in our ongoing cohort study of multicenter oxidative stress (COSMOS) study in PLS, patients had to have symptoms for greater than or equal to 5 years.[2,3,12] However, common features include the clinical presence of:

- Upper motor dysfunction on examination: spasticity, pathologic reflexes, and upper motor neuron pattern of weakness
- Presentation most commonly in the legs, but can be in the bulbar region, or mixed limb and bulbar
- Slow progression of symptoms ($\geq$4 years) with an age of onset greater than or equal to 20 years

Absence of:

- Marked fasciculations or muscle atrophy
- Sensory signs on examination
- Family history of similar disorder

In addition, laboratory or diagnostic studies must be negative for an alternative explanation for the symptoms. Additional normal studies supportive of PLS include:

- $B_{12}$, copper, HTLV1/HTLV2, human immunodeficiency virus (HIV) testing, paraneoplastic work-up
- MRI of brain and spine
- CSF evaluation
- EMG (normal, or minimal denervation that does not fulfill El Escorial criteria)

Basic laboratory studies, including serum chemistries, serum $B_{12}$, and complete blood count, should be normal. Additional studies recommended in patients based on clinical suspicion could include testing for Lyme disease, human T-cell lymphocytotropic virus-1, paraneoplastic panel, HIV testing, polyglucosan body disease, and CSF evaluation. Serum long-chain fatty acids can be evaluated to exclude adrenomyeloneuropathy. Serum creatine kinase level is not particularly useful in the

**Box 1**
**Differential diagnosis for PLS ALS Functional Rating Scale**

*Structural*

Tumor

Cervical spondylomyelopathy

Spinal arteriovenous fistula

Arnold-Chiari malformation

*Demyelinating*

Multiple sclerosis/primary progressive multiple sclerosis

Vitamin E deficiency

*Hereditary*

Hereditary spastic paraplegia

Leukodystrophy (metachromatic, adrenoleukodystrophy)

Polyglucosan body disease

*Infectious/inflammatory*

Tropical spastic paraparesis (HTLV1/HTLV2)

Human immunodeficiency virus

Syphilis

Sarcoidosis

*Metabolic/toxic*

Subacute combined degeneration ($B_{12}$ deficiency)

Vitamin E deficiency

Lathyrism

*Neurodegenerative*

ALS

*Abbreviation*: HTLV, human T-lymphotropic virus.

work-up of PLS, although case series suggest that it may be increased in fewer patients than in ALS.[4]

### *Electromyogram*

Although patients with PLS lack lower motor neuron signs on clinical examination, several studies report minor or transient changes with needle EMG in some patients with PLS. These changes include sparse fibrillations, generally limited to 1 or 2 muscles; fasciculations; and enlarged motor unit potentials.[1,2,7,13] After 4 years the probability of developing new lower motor neuron findings on EMG is low (~20%).[14]

### *Imaging*

The criteria proposed for a clinical diagnosis of PLS include brain imaging without structural abnormalities, although atrophy of the precentral gyrus is allowed.[3,4] Occasionally, clinical MRI scans show T2 hyperintensity within the corticospinal tracts, although this is a variable and nonspecific finding thought to result from wallerian degeneration, and T2 shortening within the gray matter of the precentral gyrus, which is likely caused by iron uptake by activated microglia.[15,16]

A common theme that has emerged from quantitative MRI studies is that imaging changes in PLS are less diffuse than in patients with ALS, being more restricted to motor regions. Within motor structures, the severity of changes is often greater in patients with PLS than in patients with ALS, possibly reflecting the longer duration of disease. Quantitative MRI has shown that brain atrophy affects gray and white matter in patients with PLS.[17] The precentral cortex and underlying white matter are particularly affected.[18] The precentral gray matter becomes thinner and thinning continues to progress for many years.[18,19] Metabolic markers show dysfunction of the motor cortex. With fluorodeoxyglucose-PET, a stripe of hypometabolism may be seen in the precentral gyrus.[20] *N*-Acetyl aspartate, a neuronal marker measured in magnetic resonance spectroscopy studies, was reduced in the precentral cortex.[10,21,22] Flumazenil-PET, which binds to receptors for gamma-aminobutyric acid on cortical neurons, was decreased in patients with PLS, particularly in motor regions, whereas patients with ALS also had decreased binding in frontal regions.[23]

White matter integrity in PLS has been compared with groups of healthy controls, patients with ALS, and patients with hereditary spastic paraparesis in several studies using diffusion tensor imaging (DTI). All agree that fractional anisotropy is reduced and mean diffusivity is increased within the corticospinal tracts and midbody of the corpus callosum in PLS.[24–29] Patients with PLS had a more restricted distribution of affected white matter tracts compared with the widespread pattern seen in patients with ALS, and the magnitudes of diffusion changes were greater. Some studies also note greater diffusion changes in subcortical white matter and proximal portions of the corticospinal tract in patients with PLS.[24,25,28] Longitudinal studies showed that the same tracts were affected 6 months and 2 years later, but progressive thinning of the corticospinal tract occurred.[18,28] Most DTI studies have not found significant group-level differences outside motor tracts in DTI; however, in patients who have mild cognitive impairment, small and scattered diffusion changes may be seen in extramotor association tracts.[30,31] MRI sequences specific for myelin also show a broader distribution of white matter changes than are seen with DTI.[32]

Imaging findings in PLS include the following:

- Diagnostically, MRI in PLS should be without structural abnormalities, with the exception of atrophy of the precentral gyrus
- MRI T2 imaging hyperintensity can be seen in the corticospinal tracts, which corresponds with decreased fractional anisotropy and increased mean diffusivity on DTI
- Metabolic imaging shows decreased function in the precentral gyrus (magnetic resonance spectroscopy, PET)

### *Summary*

The diagnosis of PLS requires a characteristic clinical history and neurologic examination suggesting insidious onset of slowly progressive upper motor neuron dysfunction in the absence of family history, diagnostic testing, or signs suggesting another disorder.

## PATHOPHYSIOLOGY

- The fundamental defect in PLS is dysfunction of descending corticospinal tracts.

Motor unit estimation studies showed either normal or mild reduction in motor unit numbers in hand muscles.[22,33] During voluntary movement, recruitment is incomplete. The motor neurons tend to have slower and less variable firing rates than in patients with ALS or controls, which may reflect expression of channels that promote stable membrane states.[34,35]

Transcranial magnetic stimulation (TMS) has been used to assess the excitability of the motor cortex in patients with PLS. TMS most commonly finds that motor evoked potentials from muscles of affected limbs are unobtainable or have slightly delayed central motor conduction times.[10,12,36,37] When surface evoked potentials can be elicited by TMS, thresholds for excitation are increased, although intracortical inhibition is reduced.[10,36] The relative inexcitability of the cortex particularly affects the fastest conducting corticospinal axons that synapse directly on lower motor neurons. TMS evoked cortical peaks were delayed and prolonged in peristimulus time histograms of motor unit firing, produced by desynchronized impulses of dying corticomotoneuronal axons.[37]

Loss of functional motor cortical neurons has also been revealed by other physiologic measures. In a longitudinal study of one patient with PLS, beta-band intramuscular coherence during precision grip disappeared concurrently with cortical inexcitability measured with TMS.[38] Intramuscular coherence between hand and forearm muscles is thought to arise from common corticospinal inputs. Movement-related cortical potentials, measured from back-averaged electroencephalograms, were reduced in 10 patients with PLS.[39] The reduction affected components of the potentials generated by the motor cortex and components generated by premotor and supplementary cortical motor areas. The loss of fast-conducting corticospinal axons results in slow and effortful voluntary movements in PLS that are likely to use slower conducting or indirect descending cortical projections or to be relayed through more primitive motor pathways. For example, startle produced by descending brainstem pathways is enhanced in PLS.[10]

The long duration of disease in PLS may allow adaptive changes in brain function. Two studies have examined functional connectivity in patients with PLS using resting state functional MRI. This method measures correlated signals associated with blood deoxygenation as a surrogate for neuronal activity in brain regions. Both studies found functional connectivity was increased in PLS compared with controls. Sensorimotor regions of the 2 sides had increased connectivity that was correlated with disability; functional connectivity was also increased in frontal networks and was associated with executive function.[40] The other study, which searched for new patterns of function connectivity, found increased functional connectivity between the cerebellum and several cortical regions that were not structurally connected.[41] It is not clear whether the increased functional connectivity reflects loss of selective activation or develops as a form of compensation for the loss of motor cortical circuits.

## *Autopsy*

Autopsy findings in PLS are rare, and only a few have been performed after the discovery of Bunina bodies and ubiquitinated neuronal inclusions as being key pathologic features in ALS. In autopsy reports since 1997 common features include degeneration of the corticospinal tracts, absence of Betz cells, or decreased pyramidal cells in the precentral gyrus. However, most cases were described as complicated PLS, including dementia, and some reports had Bunina bodies, or ubiquitinated inclusions, which, because of the overlap in symptoms between ALS and PLS, make it possible that these were cases of upper motor neuron presentation of ALS, or other neurodegenerative disorders.[4]

### Genetics

PLS is a sporadic disease. The main differential consideration is hereditary spastic paraplegia (HSP). HSP can show autosomal dominant, recessive, or X-linked inheritance, and to date more than 50 different genes have been described. The most common autosomal dominant form is caused by mutations in SPG4 (spastin), accounting for 30% to 40% of families, and the most common recessive mutation in SPG11 (spatacsin) accounts for up to 50% of recessive cases.[42] In general, in pure HSP the legs are most commonly affected, with variable bladder spasticity, and some vibratory loss in the feet. HSP generally presents younger than PLS, in the 20-year to 30-year range, but considerable variability exists. There is also potentially overlap between juvenile ALS, early onset HSP, and what is termed juvenile PLS (all caused by mutations in the alsin gene, ALS2).[43]

A couple of large case series have looked for genetic mutations in patients with PLS. One study looking for *C9orf72* repeat expansions found mutations in 0.9% of 110 patients with PLS.[44] A more recent study by the PLS CSOMOS study group found *C9orf72* mutation in 2.9% of 34 patients with PLS.[12] Only 1 patient had a mutation associated with HSP in *SPG7*. Additional pathologic mutations were identified in *DCTN1* and *PARK2*. Ultimately, as it becomes possible to more specifically define the phenotype in PLS, the ability to identify pathogenic mutations may increase. However, most patients meeting clinical criteria for PLS are sporadic.

### Summary

Although there is no pathognomonic pathologic change in PLS, several changes are consistent with the diagnosis:

- TMS reveals unobtainable or slightly delayed central motor conduction times, with increased thresholds for activation
- Loss of fast-conducting corticospinal axons may shift to slower conducting or indirect descending corticospinal projections
- Although autopsy data are limited, loss of descending corticospinal pathways is common
- Only a minority of patients with PLS meeting clinically definite criteria have pathologic mutations

## PROGNOSIS

A question of great concern to patients with PLS is whether their condition will convert to ALS. A small fraction of patients with ALS initially present with pure upper motor neuron findings, but most develop lower motor neuron signs and EMG findings within 4 years.[6,14,45] Patients who do not have lower motor neuron findings after 4 years typically remain with clinically pure upper motor neuron dysfunction with a normal lifespan.[2,6,11] However, there are a few reported cases of patients with PLS developing late slowly progressive lower motor neurons and EMG findings, even several decades later.[46]

## THERAPEUTIC STRATEGIES

There is no cure for PLS. Most treatment strategies are intended to alleviate symptoms and improve functioning. Nonmedication approaches to PLS include physical and occupational therapy for range of motion exercises, gait and balance training, and evaluation for assistive devices. Riluzole, the only US Food and Drug Administration approved drug for ALS, which provides a modest increase in survival (about 3 months), has not shown any clear benefit in patients with PLS. For spasticity, first-line oral agents include baclofen, tizanidine, or valium. For patients who achieve some benefit with antispasticity drugs but are limited by sedating side effects of oral agents, a trial of intrathecal baclofen may be useful, with subsequent baclofen pump placement. Management of excess oral secretions or drooling is similar to that used for ALS. Most patients are first tried on oral anticholinergic medications: amitriptyline, scopolamine, glycopyrrolate, or atropine drops. For drooling unresponsive to oral therapies, botulism toxin injections into submandibular glands may be beneficial.[47] For pseudobulbar affect (bouts of uncontrollable laughter and crying) the combination of dextromethorphan and quinidine (Nuedexta) may prove beneficial. Tricyclic antidepressants may prove beneficial for patients in whom Nuedexta does not work. For further discussion of symptom management, the reader is referred elsewhere in this issue.[48]

Recommendation:

- Periodic evaluation with physical and occupational therapy
- Oral antispasticity drugs
- Consider baclofen pump
- Oral anticholinergic agents for drooling, or botulism toxin injections
- Combination dextromethorphan and quinidine, or tricyclic antidepressants for pseudobulbar affect

## SUMMARY AND FUTURE DIRECTIONS

PLS is a sporadic and progressive disorder of upper motor neuron dysfunction. Despite being functionally debilitating, lack of lower motor neuron findings after 4 years portends a more benign prognosis than ALS. There are several characteristic patterns of progression in PLS, suggesting the possibility for an underlying, as-yet undefined genetic contribution to the disease. However, the largest case series to date identified mutations in only a minority of patients. Treatment of PLS remains supportive, including physical therapy and drugs for spasticity, drooling, and pseudobulbar affect. A better understanding of the pathophysiology of PLS may help guide development of future disease-directed therapies. A large multicenter study is ongoing to gain a better understanding of the natural history, genetics, and pathophysiology of PLS.[12]

## DISCLOSURE

This publication was supported by an Institutional Clinical and Translational Science Award, NIH/NCATS Grant Number UL1TR000001. J.M. Statland's work on this project was supported by a CTSA grant from NCATS awarded to the University of Kansas Medical Center for Frontiers: The Heartland Institute for Clinical and Translational Research #KL2TR000119. M.K Floeter's work on this project was supported by the intramural program of NIH, NINDS, grant # Z01 NS002976. Its contents are solely the responsibility of the authors and do not necessarily represent the official views of the NIH.

## REFERENCES

1. Le Forestier N, Maisonobe T, Piquard A, et al. Does primary lateral sclerosis exist? A study of 20 patients and a review of the literature. Brain 2001;124(Pt 10): 1989–99.
2. Singer MA, Kojan S, Barohn RJ, et al. Primary lateral sclerosis: clinical and laboratory features in 25 patients. J Clin Neuromuscul Dis 2005;7(1):1–9.

3. Pringle CE, Hudson AJ, Munoz DG, et al. Primary lateral sclerosis. Clinical features, neuropathology and diagnostic criteria. Brain 1992;115(Pt 2):495–520.
4. Singer MA, Statland JM, Wolfe GI, et al. Primary lateral sclerosis. Muscle Nerve 2007;35(3):291–302.
5. Erb W. Concerning spastic and syphilitic spinal paralysis. Br Med J 1902;2(2180): 1114–9.
6. Tartaglia MC, Rowe A, Findlater K, et al. Differentiation between primary lateral sclerosis and amyotrophic lateral sclerosis: examination of symptoms and signs at disease onset and during follow-up. Arch Neurol 2007;64(2):232–6.
7. Kuipers-Upmeijer J, de Jager AE, Hew JM, et al. Primary lateral sclerosis: clinical, neurophysiological, and magnetic resonance findings. J Neurol Neurosurg Psychiatry 2001;71(5):615–20.
8. Caselli RJ, Smith BE, Osborne D. Primary lateral sclerosis: a neuropsychological study. Neurology 1995;45(11):2005–9.
9. de Koning I, van Doorn PA, van Dongen HR. Slowly progressive isolated dysarthria: longitudinal course, speech features, and neuropsychological deficits. J Neurol 1997;244(10):664–6.
10. Zhai P, Pagan F, Statland J, et al. Primary lateral sclerosis: A heterogeneous disorder composed of different subtypes? Neurology 2003;60(8):1258–65.
11. Floeter MK, Mills R. Progression in primary lateral sclerosis: a prospective analysis. Amyotroph Lateral Scler 2009;10(5–6):339–46.
12. Mitsumoto H, Nagy P, Gennings C, et al. Phenotypic and molecular analyses of primary lateral sclerosis. Neurol Genet 2015;1:e3.
13. Brown WF, Ebers GC, Hudson AJ, et al. Motor-evoked responses in primary lateral sclerosis. Muscle Nerve 1992;15(5):626–9.
14. Gordon PH, Cheng B, Katz IB, et al. The natural history of primary lateral sclerosis. Neurology 2006;66(5):647–53.
15. Peretti-Viton P, Azulay JP, Trefouret S, et al. MRI of the intracranial corticospinal tracts in amyotrophic and primary lateral sclerosis. Neuroradiology 1999; 41(10):744–9.
16. Kwan JY, Jeong SY, Van Gelderen P, et al. Iron accumulation in deep cortical layers accounts for MRI signal abnormalities in ALS: correlating 7 Tesla MRI and pathology. PLoS One 2012;7(4):e35241.
17. Tartaglia MC, Laluz V, Rowe A, et al. Brain atrophy in primary lateral sclerosis. Neurology 2009;72(14):1236–41.
18. Kwan JY, Meoded A, Danielian LE, et al. Structural imaging differences and longitudinal changes in primary lateral sclerosis and amyotrophic lateral sclerosis. Neuroimage Clin 2012;2:151–60.
19. Butman JA, Floeter MK. Decreased thickness of primary motor cortex in primary lateral sclerosis. AJNR Am J Neuroradiol 2007;28(1):87–91.
20. Claassen DO, Josephs KA, Peller PJ. The stripe of primary lateral sclerosis: focal primary motor cortex hypometabolism seen on fluorodeoxyglucose F18 positron emission tomography. Arch Neurol 2010;67(1):122–5.
21. Chan S, Shungu DC, Douglas-Akinwande A, et al. Motor neuron diseases: comparison of single-voxel proton MR spectroscopy of the motor cortex with MR imaging of the brain. Radiology 1999;212(3):763–9.
22. Mitsumoto H, Ulug AM, Pullman SL, et al. Quantitative objective markers for upper and lower motor neuron dysfunction in ALS. Neurology 2007;68(17):1402–10.
23. Turner MR, Hammers A, Al-Chalabi A, et al. Cortical involvement in four cases of primary lateral sclerosis using [(11)C]-flumazenil PET. J Neurol 2007;254(8): 1033–6.

24. Ciccarelli O, Behrens TE, Johansen-Berg H, et al. Investigation of white matter pathology in ALS and PLS using tract-based spatial statistics. Hum Brain Mapp 2009;30(2):615–24.
25. Iwata NK, Kwan JY, Danielian LE, et al. White matter alterations differ in primary lateral sclerosis and amyotrophic lateral sclerosis. Brain 2011;134(Pt 9):2642–55.
26. Muller HP, Unrath A, Huppertz HJ, et al. Neuroanatomical patterns of cerebral white matter involvement in different motor neuron diseases as studied by diffusion tensor imaging analysis. Amyotroph Lateral Scler 2012;13(3):254–64.
27. Tzarouchi LC, Kyritsis AP, Giannopoulos S, et al. Voxel-based diffusion tensor imaging detects pyramidal tract degeneration in primary lateral sclerosis. Br J Radiol 2011;84(997):78–80.
28. Unrath A, Muller HP, Riecker A, et al. Whole brain-based analysis of regional white matter tract alterations in rare motor neuron diseases by diffusion tensor imaging. Hum Brain Mapp 2010;31:1727–40.
29. van der Graaff MM, Sage CA, Caan MW, et al. Upper and extra-motoneuron involvement in early motoneuron disease: a diffusion tensor imaging study. Brain 2011;134(Pt 4):1211–28.
30. Canu E, Agosta F, Galantucci S, et al. Extramotor damage is associated with cognition in primary lateral sclerosis patients. PLoS One 2013;8(12):e82017.
31. Meoded A, Kwan JY, Peters TL, et al. Imaging findings associated with cognitive performance in primary lateral sclerosis and amyotrophic lateral sclerosis. Dement Geriatr Cogn Dis Extra 2013;3(1):233–50.
32. Kolind S, Sharma R, Knight S, et al. Myelin imaging in amyotrophic and primary lateral sclerosis. Amyotroph Lateral Scler Frontotemporal Degener 2013;14(7–8):562–73.
33. Craciun L, Floeter MK. Motor unit number estimation in primary lateral sclerosis. Muscle and Nerve 2009;40(4):710.
34. de Carvalho M, Turkman A, Swash M. Motor unit firing in amyotrophic lateral sclerosis and other upper and lower motor neurone disorders. Clin Neurophysiol 2012;123(11):2312–8.
35. Floeter MK, Zhai P, Saigal R, et al. Motor neuron firing dysfunction in spastic patients with primary lateral sclerosis. J Neurophysiol 2005;94(2):919–27.
36. Geevasinga N, Menon P, Sue CM, et al. Cortical excitability changes distinguish the motor neuron disease phenotypes from hereditary spastic paraplegia. Eur J Neurol 2015;22(5):826–31.
37. Weber M, Stewart H, Hirota N, et al. Corticomotoneuronal connections in primary lateral sclerosis (PLS). Amyotroph Lateral Scler Other Motor Neuron Disord 2002; 3(4):190–8.
38. Fisher KM, Zaaimi B, Williams TL, et al. Beta-band intermuscular coherence: a novel biomarker of upper motor neuron dysfunction in motor neuron disease. Brain 2012;135(Pt 9):2849–64.
39. Bai O, Vorbach S, Hallett M, et al. Movement-related cortical potentials in primary lateral sclerosis. Ann Neurol 2006;59(4):682–90.
40. Agosta F, Canu E, Inuggi A, et al. Resting state functional connectivity alterations in primary lateral sclerosis. Neurobiol Aging 2014;35(4):916–25.
41. Meoded A, Morrissette AE, Katipally R, et al. Cerebro-cerebellar connectivity is increased in primary lateral sclerosis. Neuroimage Clin 2015;7:288–96.
42. Fink JK. Hereditary spastic paraplegia: clinico-pathologic features and emerging molecular mechanisms. Acta Neuropathol 2013;126(3):307–28.
43. Rowland LP. Primary lateral sclerosis, hereditary spastic paraplegia, and mutations in the alsin gene: historical background for the first International Conference. Amyotroph Lateral Scler Other Motor Neuron Disord 2005;6(2):67–76.

44. van Rheenen W, van Blitterswijk M, Huisman MH, et al. Hexanucleotide repeat expansions in C9ORF72 in the spectrum of motor neuron diseases. Neurology 2012;79(9):878–82.
45. Gordon PH, Cheng B, Katz IB, et al. Clinical features that distinguish PLS, upper motor neuron-dominant ALS, and typical ALS. Neurology 2009;72(22):1948–52.
46. Bruyn RP, Koelman JH, Troost D, et al. Motor neuron disease (amyotrophic lateral sclerosis) arising from longstanding primary lateral sclerosis. J Neurol Neurosurg Psychiatry 1995;58(6):742–4.
47. Jackson CE, Gronseth G, Rosenfeld J, et al. Randomized double-blind study of botulinum toxin type B for sialorrhea in ALS patients. Muscle Nerve 2009;39(2):137–43.
48. Symptom Management and End of Life Care, in press.

# Progressive Muscular Atrophy

Teerin Liewluck, MD[a,b,*], David S. Saperstein, MD[c]

**KEYWORDS**

- Lower motor neuron syndrome • Lower motor neuron-onset ALS • PMA
- Progressive muscular atrophy

**KEY POINTS**

- Progressive muscular atrophy (PMA) is a rare, sporadic, adult-onset motor neuron disease (MND), clinically characterized by isolated lower motor neuron (LMN) features; however, clinically evident upper motor neuron (UMN) signs may emerge in 20% to 30% of patients with the initial diagnosis of PMA within typically 5 years from onset and up to 10 years.
- Subclinical UMN involvement is identified pathologically, radiologically, and neurophysiologically in a substantial number of patients with PMA.
- Imaging and electrophysiologic biomarkers of UMN involvement should be easily accessible in clinical practice. Patients with PMA with subclinical UMN involvement do not fulfill the revised El Escorial criteria to participate in amyotrophic lateral sclerosis (ALS) clinical trials and may follow a different trajectory. Intravenous immunoglobulin (IVIg) therapy is only marginally beneficial in a small subgroup of patients with LMN syndrome without conduction block (CB).
- There continues to be debate regarding whether PMA is a unique variant of MNDs or belongs on an ALS spectrum.

## INTRODUCTION

PMA is a rare, sporadic, adult-onset, clinically isolated LMN syndrome due to the degeneration of LMNs, including anterior horn cells and brainstem motor nuclei. It is clinically characterized by progressive flaccid weakness, muscle atrophy, fasciculations, and reduced or absent tendon reflexes. The term PMA was first coined by the French neurologist Aran in 1850 to describe patients with progressive muscle atrophy

Disclosure: T. Liewluck has nothing to disclose. D.S. Saperstein is a consultant for Baxter and on the Speaker's bureau for Griffols.

[a] Department of Neurology, University of Colorado School of Medicine, Anschutz Medical Campus, 12631 East 17th Avenue, Mail Stop B-185, Aurora, CO 80045, USA; [b] Department of Neurology, Mayo Clinic, 200 First Street SW, Rochester, MN 55905, USA; [c] Phoenix Neurological Associates, University of Arizona College of Medicine, 5090 North 40th Street, Suite 250, Phoenix, AZ 85018, USA
* Corresponding author. Department of Neurology, Mayo Clinic, 200 First Street SW, Rochester, MN 55905.
*E-mail address:* liewluck.teerin@mayo.edu

Neurol Clin 33 (2015) 761–773
http://dx.doi.org/10.1016/j.ncl.2015.07.005 neurologic.theclinics.com
0733-8619/15/$ – see front matter 

of presumed myopathic cause.[1] Later, Duchenne also claimed the first description of PMA. Therefore, PMA is sometimes referred to as Aran-Duchenne or Duchenne-Aran disease. In 1853, Cruveilhier provided the first evidence of PMA being a neurogenic disorder based on the atrophy of the ventral spinal roots and the motor nerves found on autopsy of Aran's patients. Nearly 2 decades later, Charcot described the first patients with ALS and highlighted the pathologic differences between PMA and ALS. Charcot concluded that degeneration affected only the LMNs in PMA but affected both LMNs and corticospinal tracts (UMNs) in ALS.[1] At that time, PMA was considered a distinct entity of pure LMN syndrome. PMA can be distinguished from ALS by the absence of clinical evidence of UMN dysfunction (spasticity, hyperreflexia, preserved tendon reflexes in atrophic limbs, pathologic reflexes, and pseudobulbar affect). It has been recognized that a substantial number of patients with the initial diagnosis of PMA progress to a diagnosis of ALS through the development of UMN signs or may have UMN pathology at autopsy despite the absence of clinical UMN features during their lifetime.[2]

Recent studies have shown that patients with PMA often have subclinical UMN involvement identified radiographically or neurophysiologically despite the absence of UMN findings on examination.[3–8] Mutations in genes responsible for familial ALS (FALS) may also cause clinically isolated LMN syndrome phenotypes, mimicking PMA.[9–12] Patients with PMA have been considered to have longer life expectancy than patients with ALS, but recent studies show that the difference in life span may not be as long as previously reported.[13–15] These observations support the notion of PMA belonging to an ALS spectrum rather than being a unique variant of MNDs. However, there remains a significant proportion of patients with PMA who have no clinical or subclinical evidence of UMN dysfunction, supporting the existence of PMA as a separate entity. At present, the term PMA is reserved for sporadic patients with MND with pure LMN findings on examination, who may or may not later develop clinically defined UMN features. Patients who subsequently developed UMN signs are reclassified as having ALS.

There are a limited number of studies dedicated to the epidemiology and natural course of PMA. Most of these studies have grouped patients with PMA with or without later clinical UMN features together. Earlier studies predated the description of multifocal motor neuropathy (MMN) and hereditary MNDs, which may mimic PMA. Several studies suggest the usefulness of ancillary tests to detect subclinical corticospinal tract degeneration, but epidemiologic studies of PMA have not used such testing. These factors affect the interpretation of available studies.

## EPIDEMIOLOGY

PMA accounts for 2.5% to 11% of MND.[13,15–18] Its incidence is estimated at 0.02 per 100,000.[13] PMA is more common in men than in women (male/female ratio, 3:1–7.5:1).[13,15] Age of onset is generally older than for patients with ALS, with the mean being $63.4 \pm 11.7$ years.[15] Previous studies report an earlier age of onset, but many of these earlier studies may have included patients with other LMN syndromes mimicking PMA.[13]

## CLINICAL PRESENTATION

Patients with PMA develop a constellation of LMN features, namely, progressive flaccid weakness, muscle atrophy, fasciculations, and hyporeflexia or areflexia. Weakness and atrophy typically starts in distal limb muscles in an asymmetric manner following neuropathy pattern 5 (NP5)[19] and then spreads over months and years. There is a mean delay of approximately 23 months between the onset and the diagnosis.[15] Symmetric proximal limb weakness (myopathy pattern 1 [MP1]) occurs in only 20% of patients.[15] Bulbar muscles are generally spared at onset but may be involved in up to 40% of patients within a median of 19 months from onset of limb weakness. Patients with bulbar involvement (NP8/MP7) are more likely to progress to ALS or run a relentless course, as seen in ALS.[14] It is uncommon for axial or respiratory muscles (NP8/MP6) to be involved at the onset of PMA.[14,18]

About 22% to 35% of patients with the initial diagnosis of PMA develop UMN features at a later time.[15] UMN findings mostly emerge within the first 2 years of diagnosis; however, it could range from a half month to 5 years (median, 8.5 months)[15] or even a decade after the onset of LMN weakness.[20] This subset of patients, in fact, has LMN-onset ALS. Patients with LMN-onset ALS have an earlier age of onset compared with patients with PMA who have no UMN sings throughout their clinical course (mean ± standard deviation, 58.8 ± 11.2 vs 64.8 ± 11.7 years).[15] Patients with LMN-onset ALS are more likely to need noninvasive ventilation compared with patients with PMA without subsequent UMN signs (60% vs 30%). A feeding tube is used in a similar proportion (10%–15%) of patients with PMA or LMN-onset ALS.[15]

Cognitive impartment affects about one-third of nondemented patients with ALS and was reported in 8 of 9 nondemented patients with PLS.[21,22] A neuropsychological study of 12 patients with PMA identified no patients with cognitive dysfunction.[23] Therefore, the cognitive impairment in MND is initially thought to be linked to UMN involvement. A subsequent study identified executive dysfunction in 4 of 23 nondemented patients with PMA; moreover, the degree of UMN involvement in cognitively impaired patients with ALS does not correlate with cognitive dysfunction.[24] Functional MRI showed impaired recruitment of left inferior frontal gyrus in patients with PMA with letter fluency impairment.[25] This impaired prefrontal activation is similar to what is observed in patients with ALS with executive dysfunction.[25]

The rate of progression in patients with PMA varies from slow (over years and decades) to very rapid (months to a year). The median survival duration after onset in patients with PMA is about 12 months longer than in patients with ALS (48.3 vs 36 months).[15] An earlier study estimated the mean survival duration in patients with PMA at 200 months. Survival duration could have been overestimated due to a fewer subjects and the inclusion of other LMN syndromes.[13] The 3-year and 5-year survival rate is 67% to 73.3% and 40.7% to 45%, respectively.[14,15] There is no significant difference in the survival time between patients with PMA with and without subsequent UMN signs (median, 47.2 vs 63.2 months from onset).[15] However, this could be in part due to the inclusion of patients with radiographic or neurophysiologic evidence of subclinical UMN degenerations in the category of patients with PMA without interval development of UMN signs. Several factors have been shown to be associated with shorter survival, including axial onset, involvement of more segmental regions, ALSFRS-R at diagnosis less than 38, baseline forced vital capacity (FVC) less than 80% of the predicted value, and a sharp decline in FVC within the first 6 months.[14,15] Patients with PMA who have weakness restricted to distal or proximal muscles for at least 4 years typically have a more favorable prognosis.[20] Restricted arm (brachial amyotrophic diplegia) and leg (leg amyotrophic diplegia) variants[26] carry a more favorable prognosis.

## PATHOPHYSIOLOGY

Like other sporadic adult-onset MNDs, the pathogenesis of PMA is unknown. Isolated anterior horn cell degeneration has long been thought to be the pathologic hallmark of PMA; however, postmortem studies identified not only LMNs harboring ubiquitinated inclusion bodies, similar to ALS, but also corticospinal degeneration in 50% to 85% of patients with PMA. These patients with autopsy findings of UMN degeneration have mostly had a rapidly progressive course despite the absence of clinically detectable UMN features antemortem[2,27–29]; however, corticospinal tract degeneration has also been reported in patients with PMA with a slow progressive course over 4 to 10 years.[28,30–32] The aggregation of macrophages is more sensitive than the presence of myelin pallor in detecting the corticospinal tract pathology.[2,27] This series of autopsy findings highlights the difficulty in detecting UMN signs in patients with severe LMN weakness. Most inclusion body–containing LMNs are also positive for TAR DNA-binding protein 43 (TDP-43) immunoreactivity, similar to findings in patients with ALS.[27,28] A recent study has classified PMA into 3 different pathologic conditions: (1) ALS-like pathology (combined UMN and LMN degeneration with TDP-43-positive cytoplasmic inclusions) in 61.5% of patients, (2) isolated LMN degeneration with TDP-43-positive inclusions in 23% of patients, and (3) combined UMN and LMN degeneration with FUS-positive inclusions in 15.5% of patients.[27]

It has long been known that patients with mutations in genes responsible for FALS may present with a familial or sporadic, purely or predominantly LMN syndrome, mimicking PMA. The initial descriptions of such cases were mostly attributed to SOD1 mutations.[10–12] Mutations in other FALS genes have also been identified in patients with sporadic PMA, including C9orf72 hexanucleotide repeat expansions, *ANG*, CHMP2B, *FUS*, and *TARDBP*.[33–35] The C9orf72 repeat expansions account for 1.6% of patients with sporadic PMA.[33] About 3% of patients with sporadic PMA carry mutations in *ANG*, CHMP2B, *FUS*, SOD1, or *TARDBP*.[34] Analysis of *VCP* and *TRPV4* mutations in patients with PMA revealed no pathogenic mutations.[36,37] It is unknown to what extent overlap exists between hereditary adult-onset LMN diseases[38,39] and PMA with symmetric proximal weakness. The absence of family history does not necessarily exclude hereditary disorders.[40]

## DIAGNOSIS

There is no biological marker for the diagnosis of PMA. Diagnosis requires clinical and electrophysiologic features of LMN dysfunction in 2 or more different myotomal distributions (bulbar, cervical, thoracic, and lumbosacral), evidence of disease progression over time, and the exclusion of other LMN syndromes. Needle electromyography (EMG) could help to show fasciculations in deep muscles that are not visible on examination and provide evidence of LMN dysfunction (large polyphasic motor unit potentials with reduced recruitment) in clinically affected and nonaffected areas. Other ancillary tests may be applied to exclude PMA mimickers. PMA should be differentiated from LMN diseases that affect only 1 myotome, either the cervical (flail arm syndrome or brachial amyotrophic diplegia) or the lumbosacral (flail leg syndrome or leg amyotrophic diplegia) area, for at least 1 to 2 years without spreading to other body areas.[26,41,42] Patients with flail arm or flail leg syndrome generally have a better prognosis than patients with PMA.[41,42] PMA is included in the category of suspected ALS according to the 1994 El Escorial criteria; however, this category no longer exists with the 1998 revision of El Escorial criteria.[43,44] Therefore, patients with PMA have now been excluded from ALS clinical trials and other research studies.

## SUBCLINICAL UPPER MOTOR NEURON INVOLVEMENT IN PROGRESSIVE MUSCULAR ATROPHY

PMA is a clinical diagnosis. It encompasses patients with MND with pure LMN signs, some of which may later develop into UMN signs (ALS with LMN onset). Needle EMG is the only mandatory ancillary test included in the revised El Escorial criteria. It could enhance the detection of LMN dysfunction in clinically unaffected or minimally affected body areas, but it cannot detect subclinical UMN dysfunction. Over the years, several radiologic and neurophysiologic techniques, outline later, have been developed to identify subclinical UMN involvement in patients with MND with clinically isolated LMN dysfunction. However, none of these techniques are included in the revised El Escorial criteria.

### *Imaging Biomarkers of Upper Motor Neuron Involvement*

The data on radiographic biomarkers of UMN lesions are inconclusive. Two different techniques have been applied to identify UMN involvement in patients with MND: diffusion tensor MRI and magnetic resonance spectroscopy (MRS).

Diffusion tensor MRI studies of the structural integrity of neuronal fibers showed modest reduction of fractional anisotropy, suggesting axonal degeneration and myelin breakdown in the corticospinal tract in all 12 patients with PMA,[7] and may predate the clinical evidence of UMN lesions in some patients.[3] However, another study showed no significant abnormal fractional anisotropy in 8 patients with PMA.[45] White matter involvement in patients with PMA may be involved beyond the corticospinal tract. Voxel-based analysis identified fractional anisotropy reduction in nonmotor white matter including the prefrontal area.[7]

MRS showed reduced *N*-acetyl aspartate (NAA) concentration and ratio of NAA to creatine, markers of neuronal health, in the primary motor cortex, suggesting UMN involvement, in about 60% of patients with PMA.[4,15] The corticospinal tract degeneration was pathologically confirmed when autopsy was available.[4] However, normal results on MRS does not exclude UMN pathology.[4] Another MRS study showed only modest, nonsignificant changes in patients with PMA, which could be due to the slightly different imaging technique.[5]

### *Neurophysiologic Biomarkers of Upper Motor Neuron Involvement*

Transcranial magnetic stimulation (TMS) assesses the electrophysiologic integrity of central motor pathways. Prolonged central motor conduction time occurred in 30% to 60% of patients with PMA.[4,6,15,18] A new neurophysiologic technique, β-band intermuscular coherence, has shown to be a reliable marker of UMN degeneration in patients with PLS, a clinically isolated UMN disorder. This technique aims to assess the propagation of oscillatory activity between the motor cortex and the contralateral limb muscles. In a study of patients with PLS with abnormal results on TMS, β-band intermuscular coherence was absent. TMS and β-band intermuscular coherence were normal in patients with PMA in this study.[8]

## DIFFERENTIAL DIAGNOSIS

Unlike ALS, in which the combination of UMN and LMN signs presents a rather distinctive clinical presentation, PMA can be difficult to distinguish from other LMN syndromes, including disorders affecting motor neurons, motor nerves, neuromuscular junctions, and muscle fibers.

### *Motor Neuron Diseases*

Hereditary LMN diseases encompass spinal muscular atrophy (SMA) (MP1 or NP7; Table 1 in Ref.[19]) and spinobulbar muscular atrophy (SBMA) (Kennedy disease; MP1 or NP8/MP7). Obviously, positive family history, when present, provides an invaluable clue. SMA and SBMA produce symmetric, predominately proximal weakness (MP1), which is different from asymmetric distal weakness (NP5), typically seen in PMA. SMA generally presents in young patients, but there is overlap with the age groups in whom PMA is seen. Distal variants of SMA (NP7) have been reported. Although weakness in these patients with distal SMA is predominant distally, it is symmetric. In SBMA, there are additional distinguishing features such as prominent bulbar involvement (NP8/MP7), perioral fasciculations, gynecomastia, testicular atrophy, and subtle sensory abnormalities. In one series, SBMA made up 13% of patients initially misidentified as having ALS.[46] The creatine kinase (CK) levels can be elevated in any chronic MND.[47] HyperCKemia has been observed in about 25% of patients with ALS and 85% of patients with SBMA. CK levels more than 1000 U/L are more common in patients with SBMA than in patients with ALS.[47] The range of CK levels in patients with PMA is unknown. Hexosaminidase A deficiency is a multisystem lysosomal storage disease. Late-onset patients may present with predominant LMN dysfunction, mimicking PMA.[48] Careful neurologic examination may identify, in addition to progressive proximal weakness (MP1), ataxia and in some psychiatric symptoms.

Acquired LMN degeneration can rarely be a result of a paraneoplastic process, a long-term complication of radiotherapy or viral illness.[49–51] The absence of conventional paraneoplastic antibodies does not exclude a paraneoplastic process.[49] In postradiation LMN syndrome, the onset of weakness may occur months to years, or even decades, after exposure, and can affect any body areas depending on what part of the neuraxis was irradiated.[51] LMN disease due to viral infection (poliovirus, West Nile virus, and enterovirus D68) or poliomyelitis should be considered in patients with febrile illness preceding LMN weakness.[52–54] Polio survivors may develop progressive weakness years after the initial polio attack in initially affected or nonaffected body areas, so-called postpolio syndrome.[52]

A rather unique motor neuron disorder that is part of the differential diagnosis of PMA is monomelic amyotrophy. In this clinical entity, there is usually weakness and denervation restricted to 1 limb, usually the arm. The contralateral limb may appear unaffected clinically, yet show denervation on needle EMG. Some cases of monomelic amyotrophy are simply early cases of PMA and, with more time, the typical phenotype may become apparent. There are also regional variants of PMA.[55] What has been referred to as monomelic amyotrophy in the literature for the most part is Hirayama disease. Hirayama disease, also referred to as juvenile muscular atrophy of the distal upper extremity, affects mainly young men. The average age of onset is approximately 20 years (13–28 years).[56] Weakness tends to progress over 1 to 4 years and then often plateaus. Hirayama has strong geographic proclivities, occurring most often in parts of India, Japan, and other East Asian countries. Weakness usually involves just 1 upper limb, distally in the C7-T1 myotomes (NP5). Atrophy is typical, and there is more hypothenar than thenar involvement; this is observed both clinically and on nerve conduction studies.[57] Fasciculations and tremor are common. An interesting phenomenon that may be seen is cold paresis wherein cold exposure increases weakness. There may be progression to the contralateral arm, which occurs 20% to 40% of the time and tends to occur within 3 to 4 years (range 2–120 months) after onset in the initial limb.[56] When this occurs, weakness tends to be much less than in the initial limb. More often, needle EMG shows subclinical involvement in the contralateral arm. Hirayama disease has a unique imaging finding consisting of an increase in the posterior epidural space and a compressive flattening of the lower cervical cord due to forward displacement of the cervical dural sac induced by neck flexion.[58,59] Madras disease is another LMN disorder affecting young adults in India.[60] In contrast to Hirayama disease, patients with Madras disease may have cranial nerve involvement, manifest weakness in multiple limbs, and exhibit UMN findings.

Spinocerebellar ataxias and Creutzfeldt-Jakob disease may rarely mimic PMA due to LMN involvement[61–63]; however, there are other clinical features pointing away from a purely LMN process in both disorders.

### *Motor Neuropathies*

Probably the most difficult differential diagnosis challenge comes from distinguishing PMA from motor neuropathies. Motor neuropathies could be due to immune-mediated disorder, MMN, or hereditary motor neuropathies (HMNs).

MMN, in most cases, exhibits features that permit clear diagnosis based on the clinical, electrodiagnostic, or laboratory features. MMN typically affects men between ages 30 and 50 years.[64,65] Weakness commonly involves the upper extremities (NP5) but follows a motor nerve distribution as opposed to a myotomal pattern. Fasciculations may be present, making differentiation from MND difficult. CB has been considered the electrophysiologic hallmark of MMN; however, CB is not necessary for diagnosis.[66,67] It is often not emphasized, but most patients with MMN, even if they lack CB, have other features of demyelination, such as slow nerve conduction velocity or prolonged distal latencies.[66] IgM antibodies directed against ganglioside-monosialic acid (GM1), when present at a high titer, are specific for MMN. However, GM1 antibodies are identified in only 30% to 50% of patients with MMN.[65] The treatment of MMN is typically IVIg. Cyclophosphamide is also of demonstrated effectiveness but is infrequently used because of morbidity. Corticosteroids and plasmapheresis do not help and make the condition worse in some patients.[64]

The most difficult diagnostic conundrum is posed by cases of MMN that lack clear-cut electrodiagnostic features. In the literature as well as in clinical practice, there is concern about when to consider a trial of immunotherapy (usually IVIg) in patients presenting with an LMN syndrome.[68–73] A careful review of these reported cases illustrates that IVIg is not warranted in most patients with an LMN syndrome, so liberal use of IVIg brings about expense and risk of complications. The biggest issue with these studies is that patients with high-titer GM1 antibodies, CB, or prolonged F-wave latencies were not excluded. Such patients can be considered to have MMN or demyelinating motor neuropathies and, therefore, warrant treatment with IVIg. Aside from GM1 antibodies and CB, factors that favored a response to IVIg were distal upper limb–onset weakness, normal CK levels, and needle EMG showing denervation only in clinically affected muscles.[72] Important considerations to keep in mind when approaching the electrodiagnosis of MMN have been outlined by Bromberg and Franssen.[74] Imaging studies, MRI or ultrasonography, may help identify patients with MMN,[65,75] but more studies are needed.

HMNs (NP7) are a rare form of hereditary neuropathies affecting only motor nerves. These can manifest with asymmetric features, but the age of onset is often early enough to steer the clinician toward this diagnosis away from PMA.[76] In addition to HMN, other hereditary neuropathies, such as Charcot-Marie-Tooth disease (CMT; NP7) can mimic PMA. Although most patients with CMT have sensory signs and symptoms, some patients can have purely motor phenotypes but have subtle sensory deficits on examination or nerve conduction studies. Amyloid neuropathy and porphyria-related neuropathy rarely may present with PMA-like phenotype.[77,78]

More prosaic conditions can be mistaken for PMA, such as radiculopathies. Most commonly, this is cervical spondylotic disease. In this condition, there are usually sensory symptoms and signs but presentation can be purely motor. Cervical spine MRI should facilitate the diagnosis along with needle EMG to show that denervation is restricted to myotomes that could be affected by the abnormal imaging findings.

### *Neuromuscular Junction Disorders*

Myasthenia gravis generally affects oculobulbar (MP5 ocular and NP8/MP7 bulbar) and proximal limb muscles (MP1); however, a subset of patients with isolated limb weakness can sometimes be mistaken as having PMA, especially if weakness is distal (NP7) or asymmetric (NP5).[79,80] In such cases, routine electrodiagnostic testing may not readily point to a diagnosis of neuromuscular transmission defects, but the absence of denervation on needle EMG would at least direct the clinician away from a diagnosis of PMA. If findings of myopathy are also lacking, then more specialized electrodiagnostic testing, such as repetitive stimulation and single-fiber EMG, can be obtained as can serologic testing for myasthenia gravis antibodies.

### *Myopathies*

Myopathies are more likely to be confused with PMA than with neuromuscular transmission disorders. In older individuals, inclusion body myositis (IBM) should be considered. IBM typically produces asymmetric proximal and distal weakness and muscle atrophy (MP4), mimicking PMA, but fasciculation is absent. Nevertheless, the unique pattern of weakness affecting finger flexors and knee extensors usually guides the clinician to this diagnosis. Similarly, needle EMG findings in IBM usually point to a myopathic process. However, in some patients, there may be neurogenic features, making definitive diagnosis difficult.[81] In selected circumstances, muscle biopsy can help determine whether one is dealing with a myopathic or neurogenic process. The symmetric proximal weakness seen in most cases of polymyositis and dermatomyositis (MP1) should not lend to confusion with PMA, but some patients with myositis may have regional presentations, such as those affecting bulbar and upper body/limb muscles.[82]

There are several genetic distal myopathies and muscular dystrophies (MP2) that could potentially be confused for PMA.[83] However, CK levels in some of these distal muscular dystrophies are markedly elevated. Electrodiagnostic testing should clearly differentiate these myopathic changes from neurogenic features of PMA. In rare circumstances, muscle biopsy can be useful.[84]

## MANAGEMENT

The principles of managing the patient with PMA do not differ from those for the patient with ALS.[85] As previously mentioned, patients with PMA are excluded from clinical trials. This area is being carefully reconsidered by the ALS research community.[15]

## SUMMARY

PMA poses several difficulties as a diagnostic construct. In clinical practice, 20% to 30% of patients initially identified as having PMA may develop ALS with UMN features, typically within 5 years from onset and up to 10 years, and many more have subclinical UMN involvement. However, there are patients who have a benign clinical course distinctly different from that of ALS. Patients with deficits that remain restricted to upper or lower limbs, brachial amyotrophic diplegia or leg amyotrophic diplegia, generally are grouped into this category. However, clinicians also encounter patients with progressive, asymmetric multilimb weakness who have diseases showing long duration and survival. For such patients, the term PMA remains valuable to emphasize to these patients (and providers) that these individuals do not share the grave prognosis of a typical ALS patient. Another consideration is that the absence of UMN signs can make it difficult to be certain that a patient has PMA as opposed to other LMN syndromes. Potentially treatable disorders, such as MMN, remain important considerations and may be considered in a small subgroup of cases with distal upper limb–onset weakness, normal CK levels, and needle EMG showing denervation only in clinically affected muscles, but liberal use of treatment trials with IVIg is not appropriate. Last but not least, more clinically accessible means for identifying UMN involvement in patients with PMA are needed.

## ACKNOWLEDGMENTS

The authors thank Sarrah Knause for providing help with article preparation.

## REFERENCES

1. Visser J, de Jong JM, de Visser M. The history of progressive muscular atrophy: syndrome or disease? Neurology 2008;70:723–7.
2. Ince PG, Evans J, Knopp M, et al. Corticospinal tract degeneration in the progressive muscular atrophy variant of ALS. Neurology 2003;60:1252–8.
3. Sach M, Winkler G, Glauche V, et al. Diffusion tensor MRI of early upper motor neuron involvement in amyotrophic lateral sclerosis. Brain 2004;127:340–50.
4. Kaufmann P, Pullman SL, Shungu DC, et al. Objective tests for upper motor neuron involvement in amyotrophic lateral sclerosis (ALS). Neurology 2004;62:1753–7.
5. Mitsumoto H, Ulug AM, Pullman SL, et al. Quantitative objective markers for upper and lower motor neuron dysfunction in ALS. Neurology 2007;68:1402–10.
6. Floyd AG, Yu QP, Piboolnurak P, et al. Transcranial magnetic stimulation in ALS: utility of central motor conduction tests. Neurology 2009;72:498–504.
7. van der Graaff MM, Sage CA, Caan MW, et al. Upper and extra-motoneuron involvement in early motoneuron disease: a diffusion tensor imaging study. Brain 2011;134:1211–28.
8. Fisher KM, Zaaimi B, Williams TL, et al. Beta-band intermuscular coherence: a novel biomarker of upper motor neuron dysfunction in motor neuron disease. Brain 2012;135:2849–64.
9. Cervenakova L, Protas II, Hirano A, et al. Progressive muscular atrophy variant of familial amyotrophic lateral sclerosis (PMA/ALS). J Neurol Sci 2000;177:124–30.
10. Cudkowicz ME, McKenna-Yasek D, Chen C, et al. Limited corticospinal tract involvement in amyotrophic lateral sclerosis subjects with the A4V mutation in the copper/zinc superoxide dismutase gene. Ann Neurol 1998;43:703–10.
11. Restagno G, Lombardo F, Sbaiz L, et al. The rare G93D mutation causes a slowly progressing lower motor neuron disease. Amyotroph Lateral Scler 2008;9:35–9.
12. Suzuki M, Irie T, Watanabe T, et al. Familial amyotrophic lateral sclerosis with Gly93Ser mutation in Cu/Zn superoxide dismutase: a clinical and neuropathological study. J Neurol Sci 2008;268:140–4.
13. Norris F. Adult progressive muscular atrophy and hereditary spinal muscular atrophies. Handbook Clin Neurol 1991;59:13–34.
14. Visser J, van den Berg-Vos RM, Franssen H, et al. Disease course and prognostic factors of progressive muscular atrophy. Arch Neurol 2007;64:522–8.
15. Kim WK, Liu X, Sandner J, et al. Study of 962 patients indicates progressive muscular atrophy is a form of ALS. Neurology 2009;73:1686–92.
16. Rowland LP. Progressive muscular atrophy and other lower motor neuron syndromes of adults. Muscle Nerve 2010;41:161–5.
17. Mackay R. Course and prognosis in amyotrophic lateral sclerosis. Arch Neurol 1963;8:17–27.

18. de Carvalho M, Scotto M, Swash M. Clinical patterns in progressive muscular atrophy (PMA): a prospective study. Amyotroph Lateral Scler 2007;8:296–9.
19. Statland JM, Barohn RJ, McVey AL, et al. Patterns of weakness, classification of motor neuron disease & clinical diagnosis of sporadic ALS. Neurol Clin 2015, in press.
20. Van den Berg-Vos RM, Visser J, Kalmijn S, et al. A long-term prospective study of the natural course of sporadic adult-onset lower motor neuron syndromes. Arch Neurol 2009;66:751–7.
21. Ringholz GM, Appel SH, Bradshaw M, et al. Prevalence and patterns of cognitive impairment in sporadic ALS. Neurology 2005;65:586–90.
22. Caselli RJ, Smith BE, Osborne D. Primary lateral sclerosis: a neuropsychological study. Neurology 1995;45:2005–9.
23. Wicks P, Abrahams S, Leigh PN, et al. Absence of cognitive, behavioral, or emotional dysfunction in progressive muscular atrophy. Neurology 2006;67:1718–9.
24. Raaphorst J, de Visser M, van Tol MJ, et al. Cognitive dysfunction in lower motor neuron disease: executive and memory deficits in progressive muscular atrophy. J Neurol Neurosurg Psychiatry 2011;82:170–5.
25. Raaphorst J, van Tol MJ, Groot PF, et al. Prefrontal involvement related to cognitive impairment in progressive muscular atrophy. Neurology 2014;83:818–25.
26. Brachial amyotrophic diplpegia, leg amyotrophic diplegia, and isolated bulbar ALS, inpress.
27. Riku Y, Atsuta N, Yoshida M, et al. Differential motor neuron involvement in progressive muscular atrophy: a comparative study with amyotrophic lateral sclerosis. BMJ Open 2014;4:e005213.
28. Geser F, Stein B, Partain M, et al. Motor neuron disease clinically limited to the lower motor neuron is a diffuse TDP-43 proteinopathy. Acta Neuropathol 2011;121:509–17.
29. Brownell B, Oppenheimer DR, Hughes JT. The central nervous system in motor neurone disease. J Neurol Neurosurg Psychiatry 1970;33:338–57.
30. Tsuchiya K, Sano M, Shiotsu H, et al. Sporadic amyotrophic lateral sclerosis of long duration mimicking spinal progressive muscular atrophy exists: additional autopsy case with a clinical course of 19 years. Neuropathology 2004;24:228–35.
31. Iwanaga K, Hayashi S, Oyake M, et al. Neuropathology of sporadic amyotrophic lateral sclerosis of long duration. J Neurol Sci 1997;146:139–43.
32. Tsuchiya K, Shintani S, Kikuchi M, et al. Sporadic amyotrophic lateral sclerosis of long duration mimicking spinal progressive muscular atrophy: a clinicopathological study. J Neurol Sci 1999;162:174–8.
33. van Rheenen W, van Blitterswijk M, Huisman MH, et al. Hexanucleotide repeat expansions in C9ORF72 in the spectrum of motor neuron diseases. Neurology 2012;79:878–82.
34. van Blitterswijk M, Vlam L, van Es MA, et al. Genetic overlap between apparently sporadic motor neuron diseases. PLoS One 2012;7:e48983.
35. Cox LE, Ferraiuolo L, Goodall EF, et al. Mutations in CHMP2B in lower motor neuron predominant amyotrophic lateral sclerosis (ALS). PLoS One 2010;5:e9872.
36. Koppers M, van Blitterswijk MM, Vlam L, et al. VCP mutations in familial and sporadic amyotrophic lateral sclerosis. Neurobiol Aging 2012;33:837.e7–13.
37. Vlam L, Schelhaas HJ, van Blitterswijk M, et al. Mutations in the TRPV4 gene are not associated with sporadic progressive muscular atrophy. Arch Neurol 2012;69:790–1.

38. Kolb SJ, Kissel JT. Spinal muscular atrophy. Neurol Clin 2015, in press.
39. Kennedy disease, inpress.
40. Boylan K. Familial Amyotrophic Lateral Sclerosis. Neurol Clin 2015, in press.
41. Wijesekera LC, Mathers S, Talman P, et al. Natural history and clinical features of the flail arm and flail leg ALS variants. Neurology 2009;72:1087–94.
42. Dimachkie MM, Muzyka IM, Katz JS, et al. Leg amyotrophic diplegia: prevalence and pattern of weakness at US neuromuscular centers. J Clin Neuromuscul Dis 2013;15:7–12.
43. Brooks BR. El Escorial World Federation of Neurology criteria for the diagnosis of amyotrophic lateral sclerosis. Subcommittee on Motor Neuron Diseases/Amyotrophic Lateral Sclerosis of the World Federation of Neurology Research Group on Neuromuscular Diseases and the El Escorial "Clinical limits of amyotrophic lateral sclerosis" workshop contributors. J Neurol Sci 1994;124(Suppl):96–107.
44. Brooks BR, Miller RG, Swash M, et al, World Federation of Neurology Research Group on Motor Neuron Diseases. El Escorial revisited: revised criteria for the diagnosis of amyotrophic lateral sclerosis. Amyotroph Lateral Scler Other Motor Neuron Disord 2000;1:293–9.
45. Cosottini M, Giannelli M, Siciliano G, et al. Diffusion-tensor MR imaging of corticospinal tract in amyotrophic lateral sclerosis and progressive muscular atrophy. Radiology 2005;237:258–64.
46. Traynor BJ, Codd MB, Corr B, et al. Amyotrophic lateral sclerosis mimic syndromes: a population-based study. Arch Neurol 2000;57:109–13.
47. Chahin N, Sorenson EJ. Serum creatine kinase levels in spinobulbar muscular atrophy and amyotrophic lateral sclerosis. Muscle Nerve 2009;40:126–9.
48. Parnes S, Karpati G, Carpenter S, et al. Hexosaminidase-A deficiency presenting as atypical juvenile-onset spinal muscular atrophy. Arch Neurol 1985;42:1176–80.
49. Flanagan EP, Sandroni P, Pittock SJ, et al. Paraneoplastic lower motor neuronopathy associated with Hodgkin lymphoma. Muscle Nerve 2012;46:823–7.
50. Struck AF, Salamat S, Waclawik AJ. Motor neuron disease with selective degeneration of anterior horn cells associated with non-Hodgkin lymphoma. J Clin Neuromuscul Dis 2014;16:83–9.
51. van der Sluis RW, Wolfe GI, Nations SP, et al. Post-radiation lower motor neuron syndrome. J Clin Neuromuscul Dis 2000;2:10–7.
52. Boyer FC, Tiffreau V, Rapin A, et al. Post-polio syndrome: Pathophysiological hypotheses, diagnosis criteria, drug therapy. Ann Phys Rehabil Med 2010;53: 34–41.
53. Debiasi RL. West Nile virus neuroinvasive disease. Curr Infect Dis Rep 2011;13: 350–9.
54. Messacar K, Schreiner TL, Maloney JA, et al. A cluster of acute flaccid paralysis and cranial nerve dysfunction temporally associated with an outbreak of enterovirus D68 in children in Colorado, USA. Lancet 2015;385(9978):1662–71.
55. Jawdat O, Statland JM, Barohn RJ, et al. Regional variants: leg amyotrophic diplegia (LAD); brachial amyotropic diplegia (BAD); isolated bulbar ALS (IBALS). Neurol Clin 2015, in press.
56. Zhou B, Chen L, Fan D, et al. Clinical features of Hirayama disease in mainland China. Amyotroph Lateral Scler 2010;11:133–9.
57. Jin X, Jiang JY, Lu FZ, et al. Electrophysiological differences between Hirayama disease, amyotrophic lateral sclerosis and cervical spondylotic amyotrophy. BMC Musculoskelet Disord 2014;15:349.
58. Pradhan S, Gupta RK. Magnetic resonance imaging in juvenile asymmetric segmental spinal muscular atrophy. J Neurol Sci 1997;146:133–8.

59. Hirayama K. Juvenile muscular atrophy of distal upper extremity (Hirayama disease). Intern Med 2000;39:283–90.
60. Nalini A, Thennarasu K, Yamini BK, et al. Madras motor neuron disease (MMND): clinical description and survival pattern of 116 patients from Southern India seen over 36 years (1971-2007). J Neurol Sci 2008;269:65–73.
61. Worrall BB, Rowland LP, Chin SS, et al. Amyotrophy in prion diseases. Arch Neurol 2000;57:33–8.
62. Manabe Y, Shiro Y, Takahashi K, et al. A case of spinocerebellar ataxia accompanied by severe involvement of the motor neuron system. Neurol Res 2000;22:567–70.
63. Tan CF, Yamada M, Toyoshima Y, et al. Selective occurrence of TDP-43-immunoreactive inclusions in the lower motor neurons in Machado-Joseph disease. Acta Neuropathol 2009;118:553–60.
64. Saperstein DS. Chronic acquired demyelinating polyneuropathies. Semin Neurol 2008;28:168–84.
65. Joint Task Force of the EFNS and the PNS. European Federation of Neurological Societies/Peripheral Nerve Society guideline on management of multifocal motor neuropathy. Report of a joint task force of the European Federation of Neurological Societies and the Peripheral Nerve Society–first revision. J Peripher Nerv Syst 2010;15:295–301.
66. Katz JS, Wolfe GI, Bryan WW, et al. Electrophysiologic findings in multifocal motor neuropathy. Neurology 1997;48:700–7.
67. Pakiam AS, Parry GJ. Multifocal motor neuropathy without overt conduction block. Muscle Nerve 1998;21:243–5.
68. Tan E, Lynn DJ, Amato AA, et al. Immunosuppressive treatment of motor neuron syndromes. Attempts to distinguish a treatable disorder. Arch Neurol 1994;51:194–200.
69. Katz JS, Barohn RJ, Kojan S, et al. Axonal multifocal motor neuropathy without conduction block or other features of demyelination. Neurology 2002;58:615–20.
70. Strigl-Pill N, Konig A, Schroder M, et al. Prediction of response to IVIg treatment in patients with lower motor neurone disorders. Eur J Neurol 2006;13:135–40.
71. Burrell JR, Yiannikas C, Rowe D, et al. Predicting a positive response to intravenous immunoglobulin in isolated lower motor neuron syndromes. PLoS One 2011;6:e27041.
72. Simon NG, Ayer G, Lomen-Hoerth C. Is IVIg therapy warranted in progressive lower motor neuron syndromes without conduction block? Neurology 2013;81:2116–20.
73. Ellis CM, Leary S, Payan J, et al. Use of human intravenous immunoglobulin in lower motor neuron syndromes. J Neurol Neurosurg Psychiatry 1999;67:15–9.
74. Bromberg MB, Franssen H. Practical rules for electrodiagnosis in suspected multifocal motor neuropathy. J Clin Neuromuscul Dis 2015;16:141–52.
75. Grimm A, Decard BF, Athanasopoulou I, et al. Nerve ultrasound for differentiation between amyotrophic lateral sclerosis and multifocal motor neuropathy. J Neurol 2015;262:870–80.
76. Hanemann CO, Ludolph AC. Hereditary motor neuropathies and motor neuron diseases: which is which. Amyotroph Lateral Scler Other Motor Neuron Disord 2002;3:186–9.
77. Cappellari M, Cavallaro T, Ferrarini M, et al. Variable presentations of TTR-related familial amyloid polyneuropathy in seventeen patients. J Peripher Nerv Syst 2011;16:119–29.

78. Albertyn CH, Sonderup M, Bryer A, et al. Acute intermittent porphyria presenting as progressive muscular atrophy in a young black man. S Afr Med J 2014;104: 283–5.
79. Nations SP, Wolfe GI, Amato AA, et al. Distal myasthenia gravis. Neurology 1999; 52:632–4.
80. Rubin DI, Litchy WJ. Severe, focal tibialis anterior and triceps brachii weakness in myasthenia gravis: a case report. J Clin Neuromuscul Dis 2011;12:219–22.
81. Dabby R, Lange DJ, Trojaborg W, et al. Inclusion body myositis mimicking motor neuron disease. Arch Neurol 2001;58:1253–6.
82. Pestronk A. Acquired immune and inflammatory myopathies: pathologic classification. Curr Opin Rheumatol 2011;23:595–604.
83. Dimachkie MM, Barohn RJ. Distal myopathies. Neurol Clin 2014;32:817–42.
84. Alanazy MH, White C, Korngut L. Diagnostic yield and cost-effectiveness of investigations in patients presenting with isolated lower motor neuron signs. Amyotroph Lateral Scler Frontotemporal Degener 2014;15:414–9.
85. Rudnicki S, McVey AL, Jackson CE, et al. Symptoms management and end of life care. Neurol Clin 2015, in press.

# Amyotrophic Lateral Sclerosis Regional Variants (Brachial Amyotrophic Diplegia, Leg Amyotrophic Diplegia, and Isolated Bulbar Amyotrophic Lateral Sclerosis)

Omar Jawdat, MD[a], Jeffrey M. Statland, MD[a,*],
Richard J. Barohn, MD[a], Jonathan S. Katz, MD[a,b],
Mazen M. Dimachkie, MD[a]

**KEYWORDS**

- Motor neuron disease • Amyotrophic lateral sclerosis • Flail arm • Flail leg
- Leg amyotrophic diplegia • Brachial amyotrophic diplegia • Isolated bulbar ALS

**KEY POINTS**

- Regional variants of ALS include brachial amyotrophic diplegia, leg amyotrophic diplegia, and isolated bulbar ALS, and can overlap with classic ALS presentations.
- Regional ALS variants have symptoms isolated to a single spinal cord region for periods of time greater than 1 year.
- Brachial and leg amyotrophic diplegia are regional variants of progressive muscular atrophy.
- Regional ALS variants may have slower disease progression so are important clinical distinctions.

## INTRODUCTION

ALS is a rapidly progressive disease characterized by degeneration of motor nerves in the brain and spinal cord; it is invariably fatal, with overall median survival between 3 and 4 years.[1,2] Three classic clinical presentations have been described; they have clear

---

Disclosure statement: See last page of article.

[a] Department of Neurology, University of Kansas Medical Center, 3901 Rainbow Boulevard, Mailstop 2012, Kansas City, KS 66160, USA; [b] Department of Neurology, California Pacific Medical Center, 475 Brannan Street, Suite 220, San Francisco, CA 94107, USA
* Corresponding author.
*E-mail address:* jstatland@kumc.edu

Neurol Clin 33 (2015) 775–785
http://dx.doi.org/10.1016/j.ncl.2015.07.003 neurologic.theclinics.com
0733-8619/15/$ – see front matter 

prognostic correlates in survival: bulbar onset disease is more rapidly progressive than limb onset disease; and both progress more rapidly than pure lower motor neuron disease (progressive muscular atrophy).[1–3] The average prevalence for ALS in the United States is 3.9/100,000.[4] Approximately two-thirds present with limb onset and one-third with bulbar onset.[2] A much smaller frequency of patients with motor neuron disease present with progressive muscular atrophy (~5%).[2,5] In addition to the classic presentations of ALS, many other variants have been described at lower frequency, including flail arm or flail leg, respiratory or bulbar only, and pure upper motor neuron presentations. Clinical experience has shown that some patients have disease isolated to a single spinal region for many years. Although only limited case series to date have tried to better delineate these slow progressors, what is clear is that a group of patients do not progress as rapidly as classic ALS, and these patients seem to have extended survival (**Table 1**).[5–9] Brachial amyotrophic diplegia (BAD) and leg amyotrophic diplegia (LAD) are variants of progressive muscular atrophy with disease confined to 1 spinal region. Isolated bulbar ALS (IBALS) has symptoms confined to speech and swallowing and can involve both upper and lower motor neurons but, as in BAD and LAD, symptoms remain confined to the bulbar region for extended periods. Here we describe the clinical presentations, diagnostic considerations, and prognosis for these regional ALS variants, and conclude with pathologic considerations, and future directions.

- Classic clinical presentations for sporadic ALS include limb onset (about two-thirds), bulbar onset (about one-third), and pure lower motor neuron (~5%)
- These patterns have implications for prognosis, with bulbar onset faster than limb onset, and both faster than progressive muscular atrophy
- Some patients have disease isolated to single spinal regions for years
- These potentially slower progressing regional variants include
  - Brachial amyotrophic diplegia (BAD)
  - Leg amyotrophic diplegia (LAD)
  - Isolated bulbar ALS (IBALS)

### Case Vignette 1 (Brachial Amyotrophic Diplegia)

*A 55-year-old man presented with a 6-month history of progressive painless proximal arm weakness. There were no associated sensory complaints. Weakness started in the right arm and progressed to involve the left arm after 3 months. Within a year his weakness spread over the proximal arms and shoulder girdles in a symmetric fashion. There was no bladder involvement.*

*On examination, there was significant atrophy and weakness of the shoulder girdles casing the arms to hang on the sides (man-in-the-barrel picture). Muscle strength testing demonstrated symmetric 2/5 (Medical Research Council [MRC]) strength on shoulder abduction, shoulder flexion, and extension and elbow flexion, 4/5 wrist and finger flexion, and 3/5 wrist and finger extension and finger abduction. Facial strength, neck flexion and extension, and strength in the lower extremities were normal. Fasciculations were noted over the upper extremities. Sensation was normal. Muscle stretch reflexes were absent in the upper extremities and normal at the lower extremities. This case illustrates NP 5 without upper motor neuron signs restricted to the arms. But BAD, as in this case, starts with proximal rather than distal asymmetric weakness. For full pattern description, please refer to Ref.*[10]

*Nerve conduction studies showed low amplitude median and ulnar compound muscle action potentials (CMAP). There was no electrodiagnostic evidence of conduction block or demyelination. Median, ulnar, and radial sensory nerve action potentials (SNAP) were normal. Needle electromyography (EMG) showed active and chronic denervation changes with reduced recruitment throughout the upper extremities and cervical paraspinal muscles, with leg sparing. Creatine kinase (CK) level was mildly increases at 250 IU/L. Magnetic resonance imaging (MRI) scans of the brain and cervical spine were unremarkable. GM1 Ab titers were normal.*

*Over the following 3 years, weakness in the arms progressed to 0/5 MRC in the deltoid, biceps, elbow and wrist extension, and hand intrinsic muscles with 3/5 strength at the wrist and finger flexion. His physical examination remained restricted for 6 years when he developed 4/5 neck flexion weakness and diffuse 4/5 lower extremity weakness. Respiratory and bulbar function remained normal.*

*This case of NP 5 without upper motor neuron signs eventually evolved from arm restricted to leg involvement.*

## BRACHIAL AMYOTROPHIC DIPLEGIA

### *Clinical Features*

Patients with BAD have motor neuron disease confined to the cervical spinal cord region. This regional variant has also been described as flail arm or man-in-the-barrel syndrome. The differential diagnosis for BAD includes bilateral cortical watershed infarcts, spinal cord infarction, and infectious causes. Most can be distinguished based on clinical history and basic diagnostic testing. The main differential for BAD in the absence of other clinical or diagnostic abnormalities is regional presentation of classic ALS. BAD accounts for between 2% and 11.4% of patients presenting with motor neuron disease and the mean age of onset is similar to ALS at 53.3 to 57.3 years.[8,9,11,12] Patients are more likely to be male than the general ALS population, for which the male to female ratio ranges from 1.5 to 5 to 1. Symptoms can begin asymmetrically but usually progress to include both arms (70%) (**Figs. 1** and **2**). Unlike ALS with arm onset, which usually presents with distal weakness, most patients with BAD have proximal weakness at presentation (70%).[8,11,12] In most series, patients with BAD have only lower motor neuron involvement at presentation, with decreased or absent reflexes (47%–90%), and some series define this group as a variant of progressive muscular atrophy. Progression of symptoms after 12 months has been variable from case series to case series. In 1 of the largest series (UK and Melbourne study), the time until second spinal region involvement was 34.3 months[9] (**Fig. 3**). In another case series (US study) limiting inclusion to patients with BAD after 18 months without signs of progression, only 20% developed subclinical denervating changes in the lower extremity over 3 to 11 years of follow-up.

**Table 1**
**Clinical Features of Regional ALS Variants**

| | BAD | LAD | IBALS |
|---|---|---|---|
| Isolated symptoms for ≥ | 12–18 mo | 12–24 mo | 6–24 mo |
| LMN/UMN | LMN | LMN | LMN/UMN |
| Symmetry | Can start asymmetric; most progress to symmetric | Asymmetric | — |
| Pattern | Proximal | Pelviperineal; or distal | Bulbar restricted |
| Months until second region involved | 34.3 | 37.9 | NR |
| 5-year survival | 52%–52.6% | 63.9%–76.9% | 75%[a] |

*Abbreviations:* LMN, lower motor neurons; NR, not reported; UMN, upper motor neurons.
[a] Only 1 study; 75% at 54 months.
*Adapted from* Byrne S, Bede P, Elamin M, et al. Proposed criteria for familial amyotrophic lateral sclerosis. Amyotroph Lateral Scler 2011;12(3):157–9.

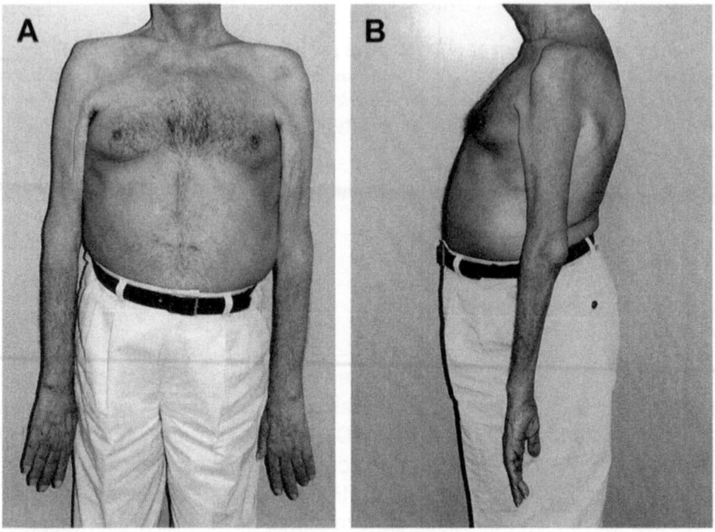


**Fig. 1.** A 59-year-old man with brachial amyotrophic diplegia 7 years after the onset of his initial symptoms. (*A*) BAD phenotype causing the arms to hang flaccidly at his sides. (*B*) Note the severe neurogenic atrophy throughout the arm and shoulder girdle with normal bulk in the sternocleidomastoid. (*From* Katz JS, Wolfe GI, Andersson PB, et al. Brachial amyotrophic diplegia: a slowly progressive motor neuron disorder. Neurology 1999;53(5):1071; with permission.)

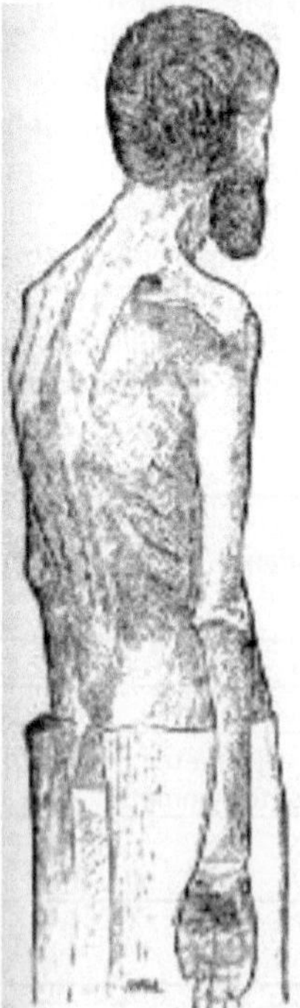

**Fig. 2.** Flail arm syndrome from Gower's original description in 1888. (*From* Gowers WR. A manual of diseases of the nervous system: spinal cord and nerves. American Edition Philadelphia: P. Blakiston, Son & Co; 1888; special edition copyright The Classics of Medicine Library; Birmingham: Leslie B Abrams, Jr, 1981. p. 354.)

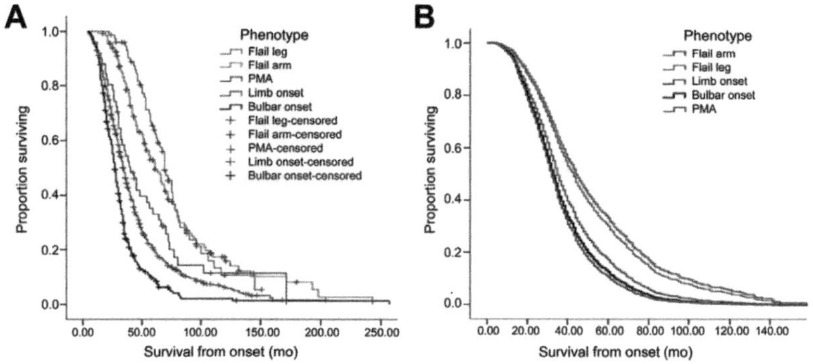


**Fig. 3.** (*A*) Kaplan-Meier survival curves for each phenotype category in the London population. (*B*) Survival curves for each phenotype after adjusting for age at onset, gender, riluzole use, El Escorial category at presentation, and diagnostic delay at the covariate means using the Cox regression model. PMA, progressive muscular atrophy. (*From* Wijesekera LC, Mathers S, Talman P, et al. Natural history and clinical features of the flail arm and flail leg ALS variants. Neurology 2009;72(12):1090; with permission.)

- Patients with BAD present with proximal arm weakness
- Reflexes are reduced or absent
- May be more common in male patients

### *Diagnosis*

The definitions for BAD differ by case series but common features include

- Insidious onset of weakness in the proximal arm muscles
- Decreased or absent reflexes
- Symptoms confined to 1 spinal region for 12 to 18 months

In the absence of

- Sensory symptoms or signs

Diagnostic testing should include

- Normal MRI of the cervical spinal cord
- Negative GM1 antibody testing
- Consideration for genetic testing for spinal muscular atrophy and/or spinobulbar muscular atrophy

Electrodiagnostic testing reveals normal sensory studies. Motor conduction studies may show axonal changes but conduction velocities should be normal with no conduction block. Multifocal motor neuropathy, which needs to be ruled out with serologic testing, is more commonly asymmetric and distal than BAD. EMG should support a denervating process in the cervical region (including fibrillation potentials, positive sharp waves, fasciculations, and large polyphasic motor units), without involvement of other spinal cord regions. Patients most frequently do not meet El Escorial criteria for ALS at presentation. However, case series have varied on the length of time symptoms need to be isolated, and some patients may meet probable or possible ALS criteria (70% in the UK and Melbourne study).

Genetic testing is not required. That said, a brachial amyotrophic presentation of spinal muscular atrophy or spinobulbar muscular atrophy must be considered. These disorders can sometimes be delineated by electrodiagnostic testing (sensory changes in spinal bulbar muscular atrophy) or family history. Several case series have described patients with SOD1 mutations described in sporadic ALS in patients with BAD.[13,14] It is unclear whether this simply represents the natural frequency of SOD1 mutations in motor neuron disease or is particular for BAD.

### *Prognosis*

Overall, the prognosis for BAD is better than classic ALS. Although a large Italian study of ALS suggested that the survival of patients with flail arm presentation was no different than patients with classic ALS, they included patients with upper motor neuron findings at presentation.[5] Other case series have shown a clear benefit in survival; in the UK and Melbourne study of patients with BAD limited to 1 region for at least 12 months, mean survival was 76.8 to 79.9 months, with 52% to 52.6% alive at 5 years and 13% to 15.8% alive at 10 years; in the US study, there were no deaths in 3 to 11 years of follow-up (n = 10 patients)[8]; and in 2 additional smaller studies, there were no deaths in 2 to 10 years of follow-up.[11,12]

- There is increased 5-year and 10-year survival in patients with BAD compared with classic ALS

**Case Vignette 2 (Leg Amyotrophic Diplegia)**

*A 65-year-old man presented with a 1-year history of falls. His toes caught when walking. He first noticed weakness in the left foot, which progressed to involve the right foot. There were no pain or sensory complaints. Over the following year, he developed difficulty getting out of a chair and climbing stairs.*

*On examination, muscle strength testing showed hip flexion of 4+/5 on the right and 4/5 on the left, hip abduction 4+/5 on the right and 4/5 on the left, ankle dorsiflexion 4/5 on the right and 4+/5 on the left with sparing of knee flexion and extension and of ankle plantar flexion. Upper extremity strength was also normal, as were facial strength and neck flexion and extension. Sensory examination was normal to pinprick and vibration testing. Muscle stretch reflexes were absent in the lower extremities and normal in the upper extremities.*

*Laboratory testing demonstrated a normal chemistry profile, sedimentation rate, antinuclear antibodies, but the CK level was mildly increased at 340 IU/L. GM1 Ab titers were normal.*

*Nerve conduction studies showed normal median and ulnar motor studies. Peroneal CMAPs showed asymmetrically reduced amplitude. Tibial CMAPs and sural SNAPs were normal. Needle EMG showed active and chronic denervation changes with reduced recruitment in the lower extremities with sparing of the arms. There were active denervation changes in the lumbar paraspinal muscles.*

*His weakness remained restricted to the lower extremities throughout 5 years of follow-up.*

*This case illustrates NP 5 without upper motor neuron signs, restricted to the legs with distal asymmetric weakness. For full pattern description, please refer to Ref.*[10]

## LEG AMYOTROPHIC DIPLEGIA

### *Clinical Features*

Patients with LAD have weakness confined to the lumbosacral spinal cord region. A lower motor neuron syndrome in the legs was first described by Pierre Marie and his student Patrikios in 1918, known as a pseudopolyneuritic variant of ALS, the Marie-Patrikios form, or the peroneal form of ALS.[15] LAD has also been described as flail leg. LAD accounts for between 2.5% and 6.3% of cases of motor neuron disease, and has a similar mean age of symptom onset to classic ALS, between 55 and

57 years of age.[7,9] Similar to BAD, there seems to be a greater male predominance in LAD than classic ALS, with a male to female ratio of between 1 and 7 to 1. Onset is asymmetric in about half of patients but typically progresses to include both lower extremities, and muscle stretch reflexes are absent or diminished. Two large case series evaluated patients with LAD: the UK and Melbourne study, in which symptoms were confined to the lumbar region for 12 months; and a US and major academic center study, in which symptoms were confined to the lumbar region for 24 months.[7,9] In the UK and Melbourne study, about two-thirds of patients met El Escorial criteria for probable or possible ALS. In contrast in the US study, none of the patients met the criteria for probable ALS. About half of patients showed an initial pattern of weakness described as pelviperoneal, with sparing of the quadriceps and ankle plantarflexors.[7] The remaining patients showed either diffuse weakness or a distal pattern of weakness. Progression of disease was seen more commonly than in BAD. In the UK and Melbourne study, the mean time for progression to a second spinal cord region was 37.9 months.[9] In the US and major academic centers study, 25% of patients progressed to include a second spinal cord region at 2 years of follow-up.

- Patients with LAD present with a pelviperoneal pattern of weakness or diffuse or distal weakness
- Reflexes are reduced or absent
- May be more common in male patients
- About 25% progress to include a second spinal cord region at 2 years of follow-up

### *Diagnosis*

The definitions for LAD differ by case series but common features include

- Insidious onset of weakness isolated to the legs
- Decreased or absent reflexes at presentation
- Symptoms confined to 1 spinal region for 12 to 24 months

In the absence of

- Sensory symptoms or signs

Diagnostic testing should include

- MRI of the spine
- Negative GM1 antibody testing

Nerve conduction studies demonstrate only age-appropriate sensory changes, and motor conduction studies reveal reduced CMAP amplitude, without evidence of demyelination or conduction block. EMG shows denervating changes, including fibrillation potentials, positive sharp waves, and long-duration polyphasic motor units.

Like classic ALS, serum CK levels may be increase; patient values in previous studies range from 100 to 500 IU/L.

### *Prognosis*

Similar to patients with BAD, patients with LAD have a better overall prognosis than classic ALS. Mean survival was reported to be between 75.9 and 87 months.[7,9] The UK and Melbourne study reported a 5-year survival rate of 63.9% to 76.9% and 10-year survival of 5.3% to 23.1%.[9] The US and major academic centers study showed an 8-year survival of 92%, the increased survival likely a result of limiting the inclusion of participants to patients with isolated lumbosacral symptoms for 24 months.[7]

- Survival in LAD is longer than in classic ALS

**Clinical Vignette 3 (Isolated Bulbar Amyotrophic Lateral Sclerosis)**

*A 48-year-old man presented with a 6-month history of dysphagia. He had been having speech difficulties for the past 4 months. He had been using a handkerchief for the past couple of months because of drooling. There was no associated shortness of breath, arm weakness, or leg weakness. He had no sensory complaints. There was no double vision or droopy eyelids. Within the first year, he needed to use a communication device and a percutaneous endoscopic gastrostomy (PEG) tube was placed to support his nutritional needs.*

*On examination, there was atrophy and fasciculations of the tongue. Palatal elevation was minimal. He had marked spastic dysarthria. His muscle strength testing showed orbicularis oculi was 5/5, orbicularis oris was 3/5, and tongue was 2/5 as he was unable to protrude his tongue through his cheek. Neck flexion and extension were 5/5 and the rest of his motor examination was full. Sensation was normal large and small fiber modalities. Jaw jerk was 3+ but otherwise muscle stretch reflexes were 2/4 all over.*

*Nerve conduction studies of the right arm and leg were normal. Needle electrode examination showed active and chronic denervation changes at the genioglossus muscle. EMG examination of the cervical, thoracic, and lumbar regions was normal.*

*His CK level was mildly increased at 240 IU/L. MRI of the brain was unremarkable.*

*His examination remained restricted for 7 years before he developed shortness of breath.*

*This case illustrates NP 8 with upper and lower motor neuron focal midline symmetric bulbar dysfunction. For full pattern discussion, please refer to Ref.*[10]

## ISOLATED BULBAR AMYOTROPHIC LATERAL SCLEROSIS

Patients with bulbar onset ALS often have a less favorable prognosis with short survival time of about 24 months.[3,5] However, clinical experience has shown there is a minority of patients who seem to have symptoms restricted to the bulbar region, often for many years. A large California study, although not identifying this group of patients for their study, mentions their anecdotal experience with at least 2 patients in this clinic.[3] Although limited literature exists at this time, there seem to be a group of patients with bulbar presentation who have isolated symptoms for extended periods of time (IBALS). Two series have been published or presented at national meetings: an Australian study of 12 patients and a study at the University of Kansas of 7 patients (KU study).[6,16,17] Patients with IBALS represent about 4% of patients presenting with motor neuron disease.[6,16,17] Age at onset is slightly older than classic ALS, with 1 study reporting a mean age of 61 years.[6] Unlike BAD and LAD, the Australian study reported a female predominance, with a female to male ratio of 3 to 1.[6] Patients with IBALS may have upper motor neuron and/or lower motor neuron signs in the bulbar region. Patients may demonstrate a flaccid or mixed dysarthria, or spastic dysarthria, and may have diffuse hyper-reflexia. About half show emotional lability, whereas only one-third demonstrate tongue wasting. The KU study only included patients if the initial EMG did not show denervating changes in any region outside the bulbar region.[16] Respiratory function is usually preserved initially. PEG tube placement may be required early in the course of the disease because of difficulty swallowing and risk of aspiration.

- Patients with IBALS have weakness confined to the bulbar region
- Patients may have difficulty with speech or swallowing but respiration is usually preserved
- Patients may show flaccid or spastic dysarthria
- Possibly more common in female patients

### *Diagnosis*

The diagnosis of IBALS is suggested by the presence of

- Insidious onset of symptoms isolated to the bulbar region for at least 6 months
- Spastic or flaccid dysarthria, or mixed dysarthria
- Preserved respiration at presentation

In the absence of

- Sensory symptoms or signs

Diagnostic testing should include

- MRI of the brain
- Consider autoantibody screening (acetylcholine receptor antibodies, Lambert–Eaton myasthenic syndrome antibody possibly)

Examination may show pathologically brisk reflexes, including positive jaw jerk or Hoffman sign. EMG should show denervating changes isolated to the bulbar region (fibrillation potentials, positive sharp waves, large polyphasic motor units). Despite the denervating changes in the bulbar region, CMAP amplitudes in the limb should be preserved. The Australian study found several differences between patients with IBALS and those with bulbar ALS including larger CMAP amplitudes at the abductor pollicis brevis and smaller motor evoked potentials on transcranial magnetic stimulation.[6]

### *Prognosis*

Although there are more limited data on survival than for BAD or LAD, IBALS also seems to have a more benign prognosis compared with classic ALS, and with bulbar ALS in particular. Survival of patients with IBALS was prolonged in the Australian study compared with those with bulbar ALS, with 75% alive at 54 months, compared with 45% for bulbar ALS. The inclusion criteria were less restrictive in the KU study; all patients who presented with isolated bulbar symptoms and no evidence of involvement of other regions on EMG were included. But they still saw benefits in survival; 75% were still living after 2 and 8 years of follow-up and 40% still had symptoms isolated to the bulbar region.[16]

- Patients with IBALS may have increased survival compared with those with bulbar ALS

## SUMMARY AND FUTURE DIRECTIONS

BAD, LAD, and IBALS are unique regional variants of motor neuron disease. Understanding the natural history of these phenotypes may help to provide guidance regarding prognosis for patients with an otherwise bleak prognosis. These regional variants do not meet clinical trial diagnostic criteria for definite ALS; and identifying them may be important for clinical trials that include patients with El Escorial probable or possible criteria. Including patients with regional variants in ALS clinical trials may obscure the effectiveness of a therapy as a result of their slower progression, or increase the variability in response. Future trials including these patients should consider stratifying their inclusion between groups. There are currently no predictive features that suggest the diagnosis of BAD, LAD, or IBALS early in the process so all 3 are really diagnosis based on time: the longer symptoms remain confined to 1 spinal cord region, the better the prognosis. Understanding the genetic and environmental factors that predispose patients to these regional variants may yield important information about the pathogenesis of ALS and may reveal potential protective modifying genes.

- A better understanding of the natural history of regional variants is essential for ALS management and for understanding genetic and environmental modifiers of ALS

## DISCLOSURE STATEMENT

O. Jawdat and J.M. Statland have no disclosures to report. R.J. Barohn has served as a consultant and received consulting fees from Baxter, CSL Behring, Genzyme, Grifols, Novartis, and NuFactor. He has received research grants from Biomarin, Cytokinetics, Eli Lilly, FDA/OPD, GSK, MDA, MGFA, Neals, NIH, NINDS, Novartis, PTC, Sanofi/Genzyme. T.J. Katz is a consultant and has received consulting fees from NuFactor. He has received research grants from ALSA, FDA, MDA, and Synapse. M.M. Dimachkie is on the speaker's bureau or is a consultant for Baxter, Biomarin, Catalyst, CSL-Behring, Depomed, Genzyme, Merck, NuFactor, and Pfizer. He has also received grants from Catalyst, CSL-Behring, FDA/OPD, GSK, MDA, NIH, and TMA. This publication was also supported by an Institutional Clinical and Translational Science Award, NIH/NCATS Grant Numbers UL1TR000001. J.M. Statland's work on this project was supported by a CTSA grant from NCATS awarded to the University of Kansas Medical Center for Frontiers: The Heartland Institute for Clinical and Translational Research # KL2TR000119. Its contents are solely the responsibility of the authors and do not necessarily represent the official views of the NIH.

## REFERENCES

1. Chancellor AM, Slattery JM, Fraser H, et al. The prognosis of adult-onset motor neuron disease: a prospective study based on the Scottish Motor Neuron Disease Register. J Neurol 1993;240(6):339–46.
2. del Aguila MA, Longstreth WT Jr, McGuire V, et al. Prognosis in amyotrophic lateral sclerosis: a population-based study. Neurology 2003;60(5):813–9.
3. Norris F, Shepherd R, Denys E, et al. Onset, natural history and outcome in idiopathic adult motor neuron disease. J Neurol Sci 1993;118(1):48–55.
4. Mehta P, Antao V, Kaye W, et al. Prevalence of amyotrophic lateral sclerosis - United States, 2010-2011. MMWR Surveill Summ 2014;63(Suppl 7):1–14.
5. Chio A, Calvo A, Moglia C, et al. Phenotypic heterogeneity of amyotrophic lateral sclerosis: a population based study. J Neurol Neurosurg Psychiatry 2011;82(7): 740–6.
6. Burrell JR, Vucic S, Kiernan MC. Isolated bulbar phenotype of amyotrophic lateral sclerosis. Amyotroph Lateral Scler 2011;12(4):283–9.
7. Dimachkie MM, Muzyka IM, Katz JS, et al. Leg amyotrophic diplegia: prevalence and pattern of weakness at US neuromuscular centers. J Clin Neuromuscul Dis 2013;15(1):7–12.
8. Katz JS, Wolfe GI, Andersson PB, et al. Brachial amyotrophic diplegia: a slowly progressive motor neuron disorder. Neurology 1999;53(5):1071–6.

9. Wijesekera LC, Mathers S, Talman P, et al. Natural history and clinical features of the flail arm and flail leg ALS variants. Neurology 2009;72(12):1087–94.
10. Statland JM, Barohn RJ, McVey AL, et al. Patterns of weakness, classification of motor neuron disease and clinical diagnosis of sporadic amyotrophic lateral sclerosis. Neurol Clin N Am 2015, in press.
11. Orsini M, Catharino AM, Catharino FM, et al. Man-in-the-barrel syndrome, a symmetrical proximal brachial amyotrophic diplegia related to motor neuron diseases: a survey of nine cases. Rev Assoc Med Bras 2009;55(6):712–5.
12. Yoon BN, Choi SH, Rha JH, et al. Comparison between flail arm syndrome and upper limb onset amyotrophic lateral sclerosis: clinical features and electromyographic findings. Exp Neurobiol 2014;23(3):253–7.
13. Di Vito L, de Biase D, Pession A, et al. Brachial amyotrophic diplegia associated with the a140a superoxide dismutase 1 mutation. Neurogenetics 2013;14(3–4):255–6.
14. Robberecht W, Aguirre T, Van den Bosch L, et al. D90A heterozygosity in the SOD1 gene is associated with familial and apparently sporadic amyotrophic lateral sclerosis. Neurology 1996;47(5):1336–9.
15. Patrikios J. Contributions to the study of the clinical presentations and pathologic anatomy of amyotrophic lateral sclerosis [in French]. Paris: Paris University; 1918.
16. Dumitru D, Wang Y, Syed K, et al. Isolated bulbar ALS (IBALS): clinical and electrophysiological features. J Clin Neuromuscular Dis 2007;8(3):183.
17. Wang Y, Dumitru HL, McVey D, et al. Isolated bulbar amyotrophic lateral sclerosis (IBALS): Clinical and electrophysiological features. Amyotroph Lateral Scler 2007;5(Suppl 1):117.

# Frontotemporal Dysfunction and Dementia in Amyotrophic Lateral Sclerosis

Susan C. Woolley, PhD[a], Michael J. Strong, MD[b,*]

**KEYWORDS**

- Frontotemporal dementia • Frontotemporal lobar degeneration
- Cognitive impairment • Neural network • Theory of mind • TDP-43 • Tau

**KEY POINTS**

- Syndromes of frontotemporal dysfunction in amyotrophic lateral sclerosis (ALS) affect up to 50% to 60% of patients irrespective of the presence or absence of an underlying genetic basis for the disease.
- The syndromes of ALS include frontotemporal dementia (FTD), behavioral impairment, and/or cognitive impairment, which are best diagnosed through formal neuropsychological testing.
- The presence of frontotemporal dysfunction reduces the disease course in ALS by approximately 1 year, specifically in patients with FTD or executive dysfunction.
- Language impairment is a sensitive indicator of frontotemporal dysfunction in ALS.

## INTRODUCTION

The classic description of amyotrophic lateral sclerosis (ALS) has little to do with the presence of neuropsychological dysfunction, and instead focuses largely on the motor manifestations of the disorder. However, the contemporary view of ALS is that a significant proportion of patients have evidence of frontotemporal dysfunction that can include a frontotemporal dementia (FTD), syndromes of ALS with behavioral impairment (ALSbi) or ALS with cognitive impairment (ALSci), deficits in social cognition, or language impairment.[1–3] Although clinically manifest dementia was historically thought to be rare in ALS, when carefully examined, 45% to 55% of patients with ALS show extramotor deficits. Although in most cases frontotemporal dysfunction

[a] Forbes Norris MDA/ALS Research Center, California Pacific Medical Center, 2324 Sacramento Street, Suite 111, San Francisco, CA 94115, USA; [b] Department of Clinical Neurological Sciences, Schulich School of Medicine & Dentistry, Western University, London, Ontario, Canada
* Corresponding author. University Hospital, London Health Sciences Centre, 339 Windermere Road, Room C7-120, London, Ontario N6A 5A5, Canada.
*E-mail address:* Michael.Strong@Schulich.uwo.ca

Neurol Clin 33 (2015) 787–805
http://dx.doi.org/10.1016/j.ncl.2015.07.011 neurologic.theclinics.com

precedes the development of ALS, the converse is also true.[4] International consensus criteria have been developed to aid in differentiating among these individual syndromes, and, when applied prospectively, suggest that approximately a third will develop ALSci, 4% ALSbi, 9% ALS-FTD, and 4% probable Alzheimer disease.[2,5] Less than half would be considered neuropsychologically intact. These figures have remained remarkably consistent across several contemporary studies, although, as reviewed here, with refinements in neuropsychological tools, further clarity is arising regarding the exact nature of these syndromes.[6–8]

The presence of frontotemporal dysfunction is of more than academic interest. When present, frontotemporal dysfunction is associated with a significant reduction in ALS survival.[6,9,10] Although the basis of this is not clear, there is increasing evidence that the nature of the frontotemporal syndrome is key. For instance, the presence of executive dysfunction is a greater risk factor for poor prognosis than FTD.[6] This greater risk is independent of age at onset, delay to diagnosis, baseline disease severity, education, and respiratory status. Patients with nonexecutive cognitive impairment do not have significantly worse prognosis. In a study of prognosis,[6] patients with ALS-FTD survived 23 months from the time of symptom onset compared with 34 months for patients with ALS without dementia. Those with executive dysfunction survived an average of 24 months, compared with 38 months for nonexecutive cognitively impaired or cognitively normal ALS. The presence of abnormal behavior is similarly a negative prognostic variable.[10]

Longitudinal studies regarding the evolution of cognitive impairment are difficult to conduct while maintaining adequate statistical power, contributing in part to the lack of consensus as to whether cognitive deficits progress over time. Although impairments in verbal fluency are key markers of altered cognition in ALS, there is no evidence that such deficits progress over time.[11] In contrast, a recent longitudinal study observed clear evidence of progression.[12]

Region of onset does not improve prognostication related to cognition or behavior. Similar to neuroimaging studies, neuropsychological testing is more feasible with patients with limb onset over time and therefore longitudinal studies tend to capture more data for limb onset. Studies are mixed about whether bulbar onset increases risk for cognitive impairment,[13,14] but studies with larger cohorts do not support increased prevalence of cognitive impairment in patients with bulbar onset.[15–18]

This article reviews the characteristics of frontotemporal dysfunction in ALS from both a clinical and molecular vantage.

## ILLUSTRATIVE CASE

A 53-year-old male accountant first presented with reduced organizational skills, increasing inattention, word-finding difficulties, and an inability to perform his daily banking. Within a month, he developed a marked increase in his appetite, increasingly obsessive behavior, and stubbornness. Two months later, he develop choking, slurring of his speech, and a reduced speech volume. Neuropsychological studies revealed intact auditory and verbal comprehension, naming, and repetition, whereas impairments were noted in verbal fluency and spelling, and visuospatial task performance. His clinical examination and electrophysiologic studies were consistent with a diagnosis of ALS. MRI showed prominent atrophy of the mesial frontal lobes and the anterior superior temporal gyrus (**Fig. 1**A). He died 1 year following symptom onset from respiratory failure.

At autopsy, prominent atrophy of the mesial frontal lobe was observed (see **Fig. 1**B). Spinal motor neurons showed TAR DNA binding protein of 43 kDa (TDP-43),

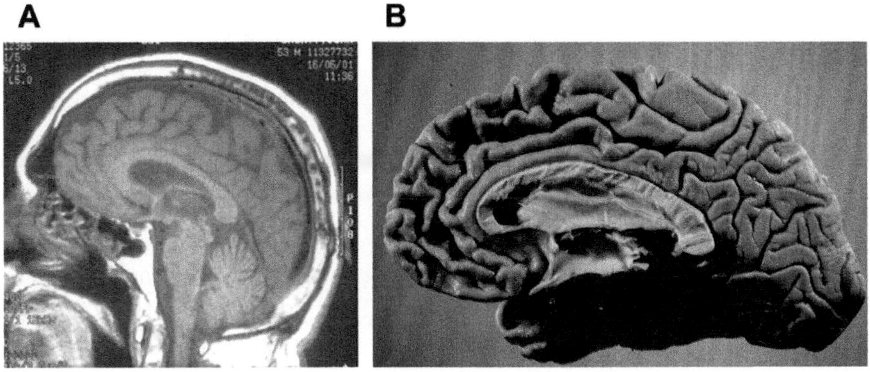


**Fig. 1.** Prominent atrophy of the mesial frontal lobes was observed on both T1-weighted MRI (*A*) and at gross examination of the brain at autopsy (*B*).

neurofilamentous and peripherin immunoreactive neuronal cytoplasmic inclusions (NCIs) that were ubiquitinated. Corticospinal tract degeneration was evident. Throughout the mesial frontal lobe, and to a lesser degree the entorhinal cortex, superficial linear spongiosis with astrocytic and microglial activation within layers II/III and deeper cortical layers was observed. Although diffusely increased cytoplasmic TDP-43 immunoreactivity was observed within neurons, no inclusions were observed.

One year following symptom onset in this index case, his 56-year-old sister developed marked behavior alteration consisting of reduced verbal output and emotional expression, repetitious activities, poor task completion, and a marked deterioration in personal hygiene. She became increasingly unkempt, and developed an insatiable appetite and inappropriate sexuality. Her muscle bulk was globally reduced in the absence of fasciculations or focal weakness. Spasticity was noted in all limbs, accompanied by spastic speech and prominent primitive reflexes. Neuropsychological examination showed impairment in executive functioning, attention and concentration, language, visuospatial construction, memory, and facial recognition. Electrophysiologic studies were normal. At year 3 following symptom onset, she had markedly deteriorated with whispering, repetitive behavior, perseveration of word phrases, oral apraxia, and a marked tendency to wander. Although she remained spastic throughout, her electrophysiology continued to be repeatedly normal. MRI showed prominent atrophy of both frontal and temporal lobes. The patient died 4 years following symptom onset. An autopsy was not performed.

One year following her death, a third sibling (aged 54 years, male) became psychotic and left his job as an engineer, ultimately becoming homeless. He presented to a peripheral hospital with aspiration pneumonia 1 year later, where he was placed on ventilator support until his death 4 years following the first episode of psychosis. When examined 1 year prior to death, he had diffuse atrophy and fasciculations, pathologically brisk reflexes, and electrophysiologic studies that showed widespread acute and chronic denervation. An autopsy was not performed.

On reviewing historical records dating back to the early 1900s, we found a range of neurodegenerative disorders, including ALS, ALS-FTD (as both the first and third case show), primary lateral sclerosis (PLS) with FTD (as suggested by the normal electrophysiologic studies of case 2), progressive muscular atrophy, and Alzheimer disease (**Fig. 2**). Genetic testing on archival frontal cortex of our index case was positive for a pathologic expansion of the C9*orf*72 gene.

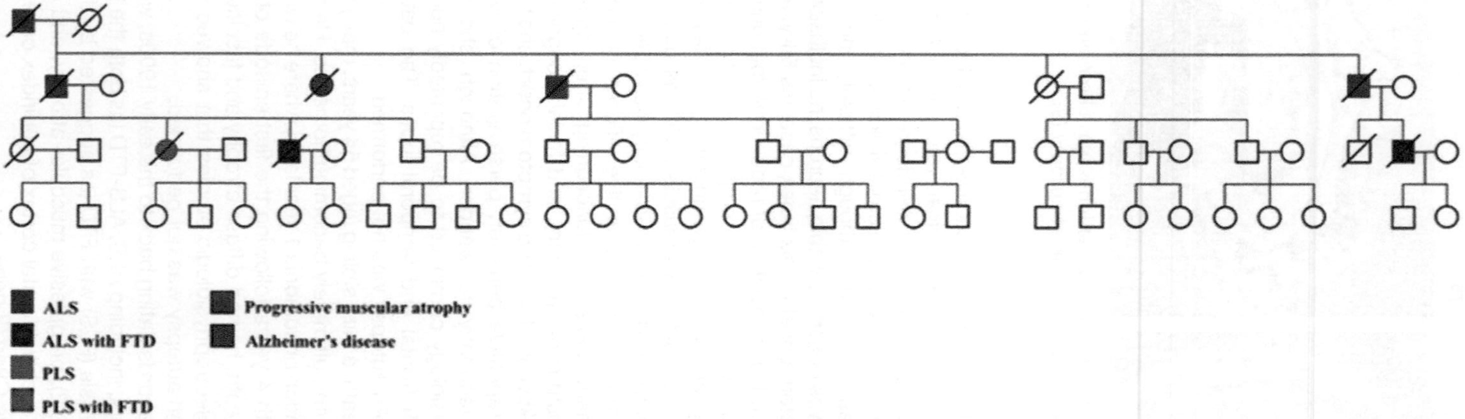


**Fig. 2.** Pedigree shows an autosomal dominant pattern of inheritance of ALS, ALS-FTD, PLS-FTD, progressive muscular atrophy, and Alzheimer disease (progressive muscular atrophy and Alzheimer disease documented through historical records). Based on genetic studies of the index case, the basis of this pedigree is a pathologic expansion of C9*orf*72. At the time of writing, no member of the fourth generation had yet been affected.

## COGNITIVE DEFICITS IN AMYOTROPHIC LATERAL SCLEROSIS

This pedigree highlights not only the spectrum of frontotemporal dysfunction that can coexist with ALS but also its occurrence within a family. However, the diagnosis of frontotemporal dysfunction is often less obvious and, as such, diagnostic criteria have been developed based on formal behavioral and cognitive testing.[2] The diagnostic criteria for mild cognitive impairment in ALS (ALSci) requires deficient neuropsychological test performance on 2 distinct measures of executive functioning. Scores on 2 or more measures should indicate impairment based on age-adjusted and education-adjusted normative data, with scores falling at or below the fifth percentile. Deficits should not be better explained by motor/speech weakness, other medical/psychiatric conditions, or poor effort.

Executive functioning encompasses several cognitive capacities typically mediated by the frontal lobes. These abilities can include set shifting, cognitive flexibility, multitasking, decision making, self-monitoring, error monitoring, judgment, fluency, retrieval, and discrimination. Phonemic verbal fluency is the hallmark of executive dysfunction in ALS, and is seen early in the disease.[19,20] Also known as letter fluency, phonemic verbal fluency correlates with dorsolateral prefrontal cortex dysfunction, may be more severe in patients with bulbar palsy, and correlates with ocular fixation abnormalities.[21] Multiple studies have confirmed deficits in phonemic fluency, making this an accepted indicator of cognitive dysfunction in ALS.

Research of frontal lobe disorders has now progressed past fluency deficits to explore social and emotional processing deficits and decision making. Decision making requires several cognitive capacities, including mental set shifting, weighing options, and flexible thinking. The multifactorial nature of such abilities makes the categorization of deficits complex. In a study of nondemented patients with ALS, subjects failed to learn an advantageous decision-making strategy on a modified gambling task.[22] The poor performance, compared with controls, did not suggest a tendency toward risk taking, but rather an inability to either learn or apply the best approach.

Executive dysfunction and language deficits were previously considered separate and unrelated deficits in ALS. Language deficits received less attention, despite being noted in pivotal studies and even highlighted.[15,23] For example, Ringholz and colleagues[15] found that cognitive impairment correlated with clinical measures of word finding and phrase length. The clinical relevance of language deficits in ALS have been minimized because of the perceived confounds of dysarthria and motor dysfunction. The challenge of assessing language in patients with advanced bulbar disease also compounded the avoidance of routine language testing, and added to the skepticism about the veracity of such deficits. However, differentiation between speech and language is possible in order to characterize changes in this domain in that language dysfunction is at least as common as executive dysfunction and can either co-occur with executive deficits or exist independently.[24]

Subsequent studies have explored language deficits in more detail. Significant semantic impairment occurs in up to 36% of nondemented patients with ALS, with 29% of this cohort having impairment on 2 or more semantic subtests, suggesting that the deficits were not incidental.[25] Patients with ALS were significantly worse than controls, even when verbal tasks were excluded, but patients with ALS were less impaired than patients with ALS-FTD. Right anterior temporal lobe atrophy was associated with semantic deficits in nondemented patients with ALS, whereas patients with ALS-FTD showed bilateral temporal lobe atrophy. Grammatical errors have been shown to be dissociated from motor difficulty, forced vital capacity, and executive dysfunction, suggesting a continuum between ALS and FTD, specifically nonfluent/agrammatic primary progressive aphasia.[26] Syntactic comprehension deficits are present in 28% to 72% of patients with ALS.[18] Deficits in comprehension are not muddled by impaired speech production, therefore providing compelling evidence for more widespread language dysfunction in nondemented patients with ALS. Because the consensus criteria for the diagnosis of frontotemporal syndromes in ALS do not include language dysfunction as a domain of cognitive impairment in ALS, these criteria will be revised to address the relevance of language deficits as well as to provide assessment recommendations specific to language.[2]

Multiple studies suggest that memory deficits are prominent in patients with ALS.[15,27] A recent study suggested that 23% of nondemented patients were impaired in prose recall, and this impairment correlated with gray matter hippocampal atrophy.[27] Despite the identification of neuroanatomic correlates, it is unclear whether impaired memory scores reflect underlying language dysfunction, attentional deficits, or other capacities. However, prognostic studies do not suggest that memory deficits affect survival.[6]

Even when motor speed is controlled for, relative deficits in cognitive processing speed and retrieval are noted in ALS, thus affecting timed test results. Dysarthric patients are more impaired than nondysarthric patients with ALS on untimed tests.[16]

ALS studies of nondemented patients suggest that visuospatial skills are relatively preserved, although some studies document mild deficits.[16] Parietal involvement is not expected in the ALS-FTD spectrum of disease. However, it has been suggested that language is critical for reasoning and problem solving, even on visually mediated tasks.[28] In the study by Baldo and colleagues,[28] performance on a commonly used nonverbal task (Raven Progressive Matrices) correlated with parietal lobe functions as well as left middle and superior temporal gyri. Therefore, visuospatial dysfunction in ALS could be mediated by language dysfunction.

## MILD BEHAVIORAL IMPAIRMENT IN AMYOTROPHIC LATERAL SCLEROSIS

The disease of ALS-FTD is, by definition, one with an insidious onset. Intuitively, the disease must start with mild behavioral abnormalities that evolve into transparent and disabling deficits over time. Detection of change is difficult because many abnormal behaviors mimic symptoms of psychological disorders, personality disorders, and stress reactions. Loss of insight, reduced empathy, self-centeredness, mild impulsivity, and changes in social comportment are examples of behavioral change that could overlap in several neurologic and psychiatric conditions, including ALS and ALS-FTD.

Mioshi and colleagues[29] (2014) studied a large ALS cohort and suggested that mild behavior change predates motor dysfunction in classic ALS, but does not affect survival. In a different cohort of patients who tested cognitively and behaviorally normal (so-called pure ALS), patients with ALS remained significantly different from controls in 3 behavioral domains: abnormal behavior, eating habits, and lack of motivation.[17] Mild behavioral abnormalities can co-occur with cognitive impairment in ALS or occur in isolation.[30]

Early behavioral abnormalities in classic FTD are thought to localize to the orbitofrontal cortex. Patients with ALS also show deficits in capacities that localize to this region. For example, patients with ALS recognize fewer facial emotions than controls, which affects social processing.[22] Patients with ALS also have difficulty inferring the mental state of others, and inhibiting egocentric responses, and these social and emotional deficits presumably dissociate from classic executive dysfunction.[22] These findings support reports from caregivers that reflect high rates of self-centeredness in nondemented patients with ALS.[31]

A 2014 study of emotional empathy in nondemented patients with ALS showed defective emotional empathy attribution compared with controls, localizing to reduced gray-white matter density in the anterior cingulate and right inferior frontal gyrus.[32] A 2015 study suggested that theory-of-mind deficits in ALS correlated with dorsomedial and dorsolateral prefrontal cortices and supplemental motor area, even when executive function scores were controlled for.[33] Executive deficits routinely localize to prefrontal regions, and supplemental motor cortex involvement could be explained as the sequelae of motor disease and not social cognition. However, research outside of motor neuron disease indicates medial prefrontal and inferior frontal gyrus involvement in the inhibition of empathy and self-perspective.[34]

Apathy is the most commonly reported behavioral abnormality in ALS.[22,29,35] These results may be dismissed for the interpretation that apathy reflects voluntary energy conservation, or a natural psychological reaction to a terminal illness. There is obvious overlap between depression and apathy, and the assessment of apathy is confounded by respiratory dysfunction, motor weakness, fatigue, and cognitive symptoms. However, a diffusion tensor imaging study examined a cohort of nondemented patients with ALS and detected a significant reduction in fractional anisotropy in the right anterior cingulate, which correlated with caregiver reports of apathy change, which also dissociated from disease progression biomarkers in the motor cortex.[36] Similar findings were replicated by other investigators and were consistent with research on apathy in FTD and other neurodegenerative diseases in which apathy associates with anterior cingulate abnormalities.[37]

## PSYCHIATRIC SYMPTOMS IN AMYOTROPHIC LATERAL SCLEROSIS

High rates of depression are seen in neurologic diseases such as Parkinson disease, multiple sclerosis, and stroke. In FTD without ALS, depression is rare, presumably because of the lack of insight and apathy. Naive observers assume that patients with ALS should be depressed because of the unrelenting nature of the terminal illness, but rates of clinically diagnosable depression are within a range consistent with the general population or healthy controls.[35,38–40] In the study by Rabkin and colleagues[40] (2015), demographic variables, disease duration and forced vital capacity were unrelated to depression, although depressed patients had significantly lower scores on the total ALSFRS-R (Revised ALS Functional Rating Scale) and gross motor subscale. Nineteen percent of the total sample of nearly 400 patients expressed a wish to die, but only one-third of these patients were clinically depressed. In a longitudinal study of patients with late-stage ALS, 9% had symptoms consistent with major depression, and another 10% had symptoms consistent with minor depression.[41] The investigators suggested that depression does not increase along with increased risk of death.

Depression in ALS tends to be seen early in the disease course, close to the time of diagnosis. Patients who experience a longer time interval between the start of symptoms and ALS diagnosis are at increased risk for depression.[42] This finding is not better explained by previous mental health history or other risk factors associated with depression. Depression and anxiety in patients and their caregivers are moderately associated but do not correlate with physical disability or disease duration.[43]

Somatic delusions, paranoid delusions, and other psychotic symptoms are now considered possible markers for the genetic underpinning of ALS and FTD. Thirty-eight percent of patients with the c9orf72 mutation had a history of significant psychotic symptoms predating the onset of either ALS or FTD, compared with less than 4% of patients with FTD without the mutation.[44] Psychiatric clinicians now need to add neurologic disease to their differentials when evaluating middle-aged patients who present without a history of mental illness. Many patients with ALS-FTD are initially and erroneously diagnosed with depression, late-life mania, or an undifferentiated psychotic disorder, and are ineffectively treated. It is hoped that increased awareness about the overlap between psychotic symptoms and ALS will reduce the delay in diagnosis of the motor disorder, which could potentially reduce the risk of depression as well as caregiver distress.[42]

## DETECTION OF AMYOTROPHIC LATERAL SCLEROSIS–FRONTOTEMPORAL DEMENTIA, AMYOTROPHIC LATERAL SCLEROSIS WITH COGNITIVE IMPAIRMENT, AND AMYOTROPHIC LATERAL SCLEROSIS WITH BEHAVIORAL IMPAIRMENT

The gold standard for the diagnosis of these conditions is neuropsychological assessment in which confounding variables such as dysarthria, motor weakness, education, ethnicity, and age can be adequately controlled for. Comprehensive assessment is essential in patients who do not speak English as a first language. Without detailed testing, simple screens routinely overestimate impairment in these patients. Older patients with ALS are at greater risk for Alzheimer disease or vascular-mediated dementia rather than FTD. Patients more than 75 years of age, as well as those with limited education or clinical depression, all screen poorly compared with other patients with ALS. These factors are well assessed and controlled for with neuropsychological testing.

This approach is often dismissed as a method that is too costly or time consuming. However, neuropsychologists are able to integrate essential cognitive and behavioral findings to best clarify the diagnosis without necessarily fatiguing the patient with extensive assessment. This approach can determine premorbid intellectual capacities to more accurately determine whether clinically significant change has occurred, and whether or not it is consistent with ALS. The time reserved for neuropsychological assessment also provides a means for comprehensive history taking and interview of collateral sources to augment test results. Interviews of family and caregivers is essential when considering an ALS-FTD diagnosis, because many early-stage patients do well on cognitive testing but poorly in social situations. Without the time dedicated to inquiry about social comportment and personality change, behavioral abnormalities may be missed.

As language deficits become more accepted in ALS as a form of cognitive impairment, a means of determining baseline fluency, spelling, and vocabulary capacities will be essential in order to estimate disease-driven change. Screening tools alone cannot control for preexisting verbal learning disorders or other factors that may influence language testing results.

Testing can confirm a diagnosis of dementia, but can also reassure families when dementia is not present. This diagnostic procedure can also be an effective interventional tool, providing education to family members about how to manage cognitive deficits or behavioral dysfunction. For example, by clarifying that a patient is apathetic rather than depressed, or that disinhibition does not reflect anger but brain dysfunction, family members and caregivers can accurately address their situation.

The alternative to gold standard testing is screening. Screens like the Mini-Mental State Examination are not recommended for use in ALS unless a patient is elderly (more than 75 years old) and presents with deficits suggestive of Alzheimer disease, like memory loss and poor orientation. Screening tests such as the Montreal Cognitive

Assessment can be useful early in the disease course when patients can complete both verbal and motor tasks. However, ALS-specific screens are ideal (**Table 1**).

Early recommendations for screening in ALS included verbal fluency testing, like phonemic and semantic fluency, or written verbal fluency, using a calculation to control for weakness. As with any cognitive screen, results are less accurate in patients with extreme levels of educational attainment; this is true for those with advanced education (ie, >20 years) and those with limited education (<8 years). Results of screening are typically expressed in a global score, and because they should be brief, by definition, it is difficult to determine the cause of poor scores. Although organicity is assumed, variables like effort or inattention cannot be ruled out. In contrast, comprehensive neuropsychological testing can control for these confounds and provide diagnosis. Screening typically does not delineate an exact pattern of deficits, which is now known to be relevant for prognostication. For example, deficits on screens of executive dysfunction may result from variable attention and not true cognitive impairment on a brief measure. Alternatively, performance that suggests a memory deficit may result from hearing impairment, insufficient effort, or other factors. Prognostic studies suggest that both the pattern and severity of impairment may be relevant.[6] As a result, screening is ideal to triage resources but not for diagnostic purposes.

Decision-making capacity is a significant issue for families when a demented patient with ALS remains the primary decision maker in the family. Patients may not relinquish this role because of impoverished insight, poor judgment, or inflexibility. Family members may not force the issue because of cultural factors or the desire to allow the patient to save face. This situation becomes a serious concern for clinicians when life-sustaining or emergent interventions present themselves and the patient lacks sufficient capacity. This issue will remain controversial in the care of patients with ALS over time.

## NEUROIMAGING

Neuroimaging is rarely useful as a diagnostic modality for cognitive and behavioral deficits in ALS unless FTD is present and advanced enough to result in frontal and temporal lobe atrophy. PET imaging is used to differentiate FTD from Alzheimer disease, although this and other forms of neuroimaging are not routinely ordered for patients with ALS. Imaging is not feasible after the initial disease stages because of the risk of aspiration, choking, or respiratory distress while supine. In contrast with the studies of static brain images, the study of neural networks is increasingly providing a window into the basis of frontotemporal dysfunction in ALS. Using studies such as resting state functional MRI, which correlates brain regions that are activated concomitantly, 3 major networks (the salience network, the default mode network, and the central executive network) have been highlighted as dysfunctional in ALS.[45,46]

## MOLECULAR, CLINICAL, AND NEUROPATHOLOGIC CORRELATES OF FRONTOTEMPORAL DYSFUNCTION IN AMYOTROPHIC LATERAL SCLEROSIS

Approximately 10% of ALS cases are genetic in origin[47,48] (**Table 2**). With respect to frontotemporal dysfunction, there are few clinical features that are unique to the genes associated with ALS. Moreover, the presence of frontotemporal dysfunction in ALS is typically indistinguishable from that occurring in isolated FTD.[49] This continuum is highlighted by the neuropsychological manifestations of the pathologic expansion of a hexanucleotide repeat (GGGGCC) in *C9orf72* in both familial and sporadic ALS as well as FTD.[50,51] The clinical expression of pathologic expansions of *C9orf72* is heterogeneous, ranging from a rapidly progressive variant with marked

**Table 1**
**ALS-specific screens: options for measuring cognition, behavior, depression, pseudobulbar affect**

| Screen | Administration Time (min) | Cognition Measured | Behavior Measured | Other Symptoms Measured | Comments |
|---|---|---|---|---|---|
| ALS CBS[62] | 5–8 | Yes | Yes | No | Validated, accurate, brief, noncopyrighted. Cutoff scores provided for ALSci, ALSbi, and ALS-FTD. Does not measure psychotic symptoms, assessment of language is limited |
| ALS-BCA[10] | 5–10 | Yes | Yes | No | Validated, brief. Culled from Alzheimer battery, behavioral measure not specific to ALS |
| Written Verbal Fluency Index[11] | 10–12 | Yes | No | No | Controls for motor weakness, correlates with dorsolateral prefrontal cortex dysfunction. No clear norms published for determining degree of impairment, sensitive to education |
| PSSFTS[63,64] | 20–30 | Yes | Yes | No | Not validated against gold standard and no cut scores provided, but decision tree helps with interpretation of results. Requires access to multiple published measures that are not readily available. Time estimate based on published data but may not include time to administer FBI (approximately additional 15 min) |
| ECAS[3,65] | 25 | Yes | Yes | Psychotic symptoms | Thorough assessment of cognition including non-ALS domains (memory, visuospatial functions), assesses psychotic symptoms. Not validated against gold standard but means and standard deviations provided for each subscale |
| Columbia Screen[66] | 30 | Yes | Yes | Depression | Not validated, uses CDR, which could allow for comparison across other dementias |
| UCSF Screening Battery[67] | 35 | Yes | Yes | PBA | Validated against the gold standard, behavioral screen based on established FTD tool (FBI) but reworded for ALS, all subscales freely available |

| | | | | | |
|---|---|---|---|---|---|
| Baylor Short Battery[15] | 45 | Yes | No | No | Validated, ROC analysis. Longer administration time because of assessment of delayed recall, not prepackaged and requires access to multiple copyright protected measures |
| ALS-FTD-Q[68] | 5–10 | No | Yes | No | Cutoff scores for mild and severe behavioral impairments are provided, high construct validity, completed by proxy. Does query about cognitive symptoms but does not test them. Available in 9 languages |
| MiND-B[69] | 2 | No | Yes | No | Brief, ALS specific, based on established measure of FTD. Does not assess cognition. Provides cutoff scores for mild behavioral change but not FTD |
| UCSF Screening Examination[67] | 15 | No | Yes | No | Reworded FTD measure (FBI), no specific cutoffs provided |
| ADI-12[70] | 2 | No | No | Depression | Validated, ALS-specific measure of depression, completed by patient. Freely accessible (no copyright) |
| ELQ[71] | 2–10 | No | No | PBA | Interview of either patient or proxy, includes 3 screening items to short administration time, no validation against clinical diagnosis |
| CNS-LS[72] | 5 | No | No | PBA | Completed by patient, easy to use, no validation against clinical diagnosis |

*Abbreviations:* ADI-12, ALS Depression Inventory; ALS CBS, ALS Cognitive Behavioral Screen; ALS-BCA, ALS Brief Cognitive Assessment; ALS-FTD-Q, ALS-FTD Questionnaire; CDR, Clinical Dementia Rating; CNS-LS, Center for Neurologic Study–Lability Scale; ECAS, Edinburgh Cognitive and Behavioural ALS Screen; ELQ, Emotional Lability Questionnaire; FBI, Frontal Behavioral Inventory; MiND-B, Motor Neuron Disease Behavioural Instrument; PBA, pseudobulbar affect; PSSFTS, Penn State Screen of Frontal and Temporal Dysfunction Syndromes; ROC, receiver operating characteristic; UCSF, University of California San Francisco.

**Table 2**
**ALS-associated genes and their overlap with FTD**

| Protein | Gene | FTD | ALS | ALS-FTD | PLS/Other |
|---|---|---|---|---|---|
| Superoxide dismutase 1[73] | *SOD1* | — | + | — | + (SBMA, PMA) |
| Senataxin[74] | *SETX* | — | + | — | + |
| Spastin[75,76] | *SPAST* | — | + | — | + |
| Fused in sarcoma[77–79] | *FUS* | +[a] | + | + | — |
| Vesicle-associated membrane protein-associated protein B and C[80] | *VAPB* | — | + | — | + (SMA) |
| Angiogenin, ribonuclease, RNase A family[81,82] | *ANG* | — | + | + | + (PBP) |
| TDP-43[83–86] | *TARDBP* | + | + | + | — |
| FIG4 homologue, SAC1 lipid phosphatase domain containing (*Saccharomyces cerevisiae*)[87] | *FIG4* | — | + | — | + |
| Optineurin[88] | *OPTN* | — | + | — | + |
| Ataxin 2[89] | *ATXN 2* | — | + | — | + (SCA2) |
| Valosin-containing protein[90–92] | *VCP* | + | + | + | + |
| Ubiquilin 2[93,94] | *UBQLN2* | + | + | + | — |
| Sigma nonopioid intracellular receptor 1[95,96] | *SIGMAR1* | — | + | – | — |
| Profilin 1[97,98] | *PFN1* | + | + | — | — |
| Chromosome 9 open reading frame 72[50,51] | *C9orf72* | + | + | + | — |
| Charged multivesicular body protein 2B[99] | *CHMP2B* | + | + | — | — |
| Unc-13 homologue A (*Caenorhabditis elegans*)[100] | *UNC13A* | + | + | + | — |
| D-Amino-acid oxidase[101] | *DAO* | — | + | — | |
| Dynactin 1[102,103] | *DCTN1* | — | + | — | + (Perry syndrome) |
| Neurofilament, heavy polypeptide[104] | *NEFH* | — | + | — | — |
| Peripherin[105] | *PRPH* | — | + | — | — |
| Sequestome 1[106] | *SQSTM1* | + | + | + | + (Paget disease of bone) |
| TAF15 RNA polymerase II, TATA box binding protein (TDP)–associated factor, 68 kDa[107] | *TAF15* | — | + | — | — |
| Spastic paraplegia 11[108] | *SPG11* | — | + | — | + (HSP) |
| Elongator acetyltransferase complex subunit 3[109] | *ELP3* | — | + | — | — |

*Abbreviations:* FIG4, factor-induced gene 4; HSP, hereditary spastic paraplegia; PBP, progressive bulbar palsy; SBMA, spinal bulbar muscular atrophy; SCA2, spinocerebellar ataxia type 2; SMA, spinal muscular atrophy.

[a] Disorder only with no known associated mutations.

*Adapted from* Moszczynski AJ, Strong MJ. Cortical manifestations in amyotrophic lateral sclerosis. In: Cechetto D, Weishaupt N, editors. The cerebral cortex in neurodegenerative and neuropsychiatric disorders: experimental approaches to clinical issues. New York: Elsevier Press; 2015; with permission.

neuropsychological abnormalities to an atypically slow progression that may last decades.[52–54]

Considerable controversy exists with respect to the extent of alterations in the microtubule-associated protein tau in the frontotemporal syndromes of ALS, distinct from that observed to occur in the western Pacific variant of ALS. However, in ALSci, we have described prominent glial and neuronal tau immunoreactive NCIs disproportionate from that expected to occur with aging and distinct from that observed with primary age-related tauopathy.[55–59] Tau isolated from ALSci is aberrantly phosphorylated at threonine 175 (pThr175-tau), a modification that induces pathologic intracellular inclusions in vitro.[60,61]

## CURRENT CONTROVERSIES

### *Longitudinal Assessment*

ALS trials are compromised by rapid disease progression and attrition. Few incidence studies have been conducted, and the natural history of ALSci, ALSbi, and ALS-FTD remain poorly characterized. In FTD research, MRI is a primary method for tracking progression. This valuable tool is rendered useless once patients with ALS cannot lie supine, which for patients with bulbar onset occurs early. Therefore, longitudinal MRI data in ALS tend to over-represent patients with limb onset, and provide a partial answer about extramotor progression from a neuroanatomic standpoint. Neuropsychological tests and/or screens need to be modifiable over time to adjust to progressive motor weakness and loss of speech. In addition, patients may seek less care outside the home over time, making follow-up in the clinic less likely.

### *Behavioral Assessment*

Evaluation of behavioral change in ALS relies heavily on collateral reports, primarily from spouses, family members, and caregivers. This reliance is partially based on the assumption that patients may lack insight. Those who excessively complain about marked behavioral problems may be showing a mood disorder rather than frontally mediated behavioral change. Despite the value of proxy interviews, caregiver distress correlates highly with their reports of patient distress and mood disturbance. Therefore, to what extent do behavioral interviews measure caregiver distress?

ALS-specific behavioral questionnaires and interviews are intended to differentiate behaviors that may be explained by weakness or fatigue, but this distinction may not be sustained in the mind of medically naive or stressed informants. Informants have relationships with the patient that predate ALS and may be confounded by marital stress, parental discord, substance abuse, financial strains, or other stressors. Collateral reports can be complicated by subjective feelings about the patient, but are nonetheless the basis for the diagnosis of ALSbi or a prognosis-changing diagnosis of ALS-FTD; this is another reason why screening alone is not ideal in any case in which there is concern about extramotor disease, especially dementia. Neuromuscular clinicians without knowledge of personality disorders or other behavioral disorders that mimic ALS-FTD are at risk for overpathologizing behaviors that may be lifelong or reflect normal adjustment, marital discord, or a mood disorder.

## REFERENCES

1. Strong MJ, Grace GM, Orange JB, et al. Cognition, language and speech in amyotrophic lateral sclerosis: A review. J Clin Exp Neuropsych 1996;18(2): 291–303.

2. Strong MJ, Grace GM, Freedman M, et al. Consensus criteria for the diagnosis of frontotemporal cognitive and behavioural syndromes in amyotrophic lateral sclerosis. Amyotroph Lateral Scler 2009;10(3):131–46.
3. Abrahams S, Newton J, Niven E, et al. Screening for cognition and behaviour changes in ALS. Amyotroph Lateral Scler Frontotemporal Degener 2014; 15(1–2):9–14.
4. Lomen-Hoerth C, Strong MJ. Cognition in amyotrophic lateral sclerosis. In: Mitsumoto H, Przedborksi S, Gordon P, et al, editors. Amyotrophic lateral sclerosis. London: Marcel Dekker; 2006. p. 115–38.
5. Consonni M, Iannaccone S, Cerami C, et al. The cognitive and behavioural profile of amyotrophic lateral sclerosis: application of the consensus criteria. Behav Neurol 2013;27(2):143–53.
6. Elamin M, Phukan J, Bede P, et al. Executive dysfunction is a negative prognostic indicator in patients with ALS without dementia. Neurology 2011;76(14): 1263–9.
7. Montuschi A, Iazzolino B, Calvo A, et al. Cognitive correlates in amyotrophic lateral sclerosis: a population-based study in Italy. J Neurol Neurosurg Psychiatry 2015;86(2):168–73.
8. Oh SI, Park A, Kim HJ, et al. Spectrum of cognitive impairment in Korean ALS patients without known genetic mutations. PLoS One 2014;9(2):e87163.
9. Olney RK, Murphy J, Forshew D, et al. The effects of executive and behavioral dysfunction on the course of ALS. Neurology 2005;65:1774–7.
10. Hu WT, Shelnutt M, Wilson A, et al. Behavior matters–cognitive predictors of survival in amyotrophic lateral sclerosis. PLoS One 2013;8(2):e57584.
11. Abrahams S, Leigh PN, Goldstein LH. Cognitive change in ALS. A prospective study. Neurology 2005;64:1222–6.
12. Elamin M, Bede P, Byrne S, et al. Cognitive changes predict functional decline in ALS: a population-based longitudinal study. Neurology 2013;80(17):1590–7.
13. Strong MJ, Grace GM, Orange JB, et al. A prospective study of cognitive impairment in ALS. Neurology 1999;53:1665–70.
14. Schreiber H, Gaigalat T, Wiedemuth-Catrinescu U, et al. Cognitive function in bulbar- and spinal-onset amyotrophic lateral sclerosis. J Neurol 2005;252: 772–81.
15. Ringholz GM, Appel SH, Bradshaw M, et al. Prevalence and patterns of cognitive impairment in sporadic ALS. Neurology 2005;65:586–90.
16. Sterling LE, Jawaid A, Salamone AR, et al. Association between dysarthria and cognitive impairment in ALS: A prospective study. Amyotroph Lateral Scler 2010;11(1–2):46–51.
17. Lillo P, Savage S, Mioshi E, et al. Amyotrophic lateral sclerosis and frontotemporal dementia: A behavioural and cognitive continuum. Amyotroph Lateral Scler 2012;13(1):102–9.
18. Yoshizawa K, Yasuda N, Fukuda M, et al. Syntactic comprehension in patients with amyotrophic lateral sclerosis. Behav Neurol 2014;2014:230578.
19. Abrahams S, Leigh PN, Harvey A, et al. Verbal fluency and executive dysfunction in amyotrophic lateral sclerosis (ALS). Neuropsychologia 2000;38:734–47.
20. Abrahams S, Goldstein LH, Simmons A, et al. Word retrieval in amyotrophic lateral sclerosis: a functional magnetic resonance imaging study. Brain 2004; 127:1507–17.
21. Donaghy C, Pinnock R, Abrahams S, et al. Ocular fixation instabilities in motor neurone disease. A marker of frontal lobe dysfunction? J Neurol 2009;256(3): 420–6.

22. Girardi A, Macpherson SE, Abrahams S. Deficits in emotional and social cognition in amyotrophic lateral sclerosis. Neuropsychology 2011;25(1):53–65.
23. Rakowicz WP, Hodges JR. Dementia and aphasia in motor neuron disease: an underrecognised association? J Neurol Neurosurg Psychiat 1998;65:881–9.
24. Taylor LJ, Brown RG, Tsermentseli S, et al. Is language impairment more common than executive dysfunction in amyotrophic lateral sclerosis? J Neurol Neurosurg Psychiatry 2013;84(5):494–8.
25. Leslie FV, Hsieh S, Caga J, et al. Semantic deficits in amyotrophic lateral sclerosis. Amyotroph Lateral Scler Frontotemporal Degener 2015;16(1–2):46–53.
26. Ash S, Olm C, McMillan CT, et al. Deficits in sentence expression in amyotrophic lateral sclerosis. Amyotroph Lateral Scler Frontotemporal Degener 2015; 16(1–2):31–9.
27. Raaphorst J, de VM, Linssen WH, et al. The cognitive profile of amyotrophic lateral sclerosis: A meta-analysis. Amyotroph Lateral Scler 2010;11(1–2):27–37.
28. Baldo JV, Bunge SA, Wilson SM, et al. Is relational reasoning dependent on language? A voxel-based lesion symptom mapping study. Brain Lang 2010;113(2): 59–64.
29. Mioshi E, Caga J, Lillo P, et al. Neuropsychiatric changes precede classic motor symptoms in ALS and do not affect survival. Neurology 2014;82(2):149–55.
30. Witgert M, Salamone AR, Strutt AM, et al. Frontal-lobe mediated behavioral dysfunction in amyotrophic lateral sclerosis. Eur J Neurol 2010;17(1):103–10.
31. Gibbons ZC, Richardson A, Neary D, et al. Behaviour in amyotrophic lateral sclerosis. Amyotroph Lateral Scler 2008;9:67–74.
32. Cerami C, Dodich A, Canessa N, et al. Emotional empathy in amyotrophic lateral sclerosis: a behavioural and voxel-based morphometry study. Amyotroph Lateral Scler Frontotemporal Degener 2014;15(1–2):21–9.
33. Carluer L, Mondou A, Buhour MS, et al. Neural substrate of cognitive theory of mind impairment in amyotrophic lateral sclerosis. Cortex 2015;65:19–30.
34. Rice K, Redcay E. Spontaneous mentalizing captures variability in the cortical thickness of social brain regions. Soc Cogn Affect Neurosci 2015;10(3):327–34.
35. Grossman AB, Woolley-Levine S, Bradley WG, et al. Detecting neurobehavioural changes in amyotrophic lateral sclerosis. Amyotroph Lateral Scler 2007;8: 56–61.
36. Woolley SC, Zhang Y, Schuff N, et al. Neuroanatomical correlates of apathy in ALS using 4 Tesla diffusion tensor MRI. Amyotroph Lateral Scler 2011;12(1): 52–8.
37. Tsujimoto M, Senda J, Ishihara T, et al. Behavioral changes in early ALS correlate with voxel-based morphometry and diffusion tensor imaging. J Neurol Sci 2011;307(1–2):34–40.
38. Jelsone-Swain L, Persad C, Votruba KL, et al. The relationship between depressive symptoms, disease state, and cognition in amyotrophic lateral sclerosis. Front Psychol 2012;3:542.
39. Atassi N, Cook A, Pineda CM, et al. Depression in amyotrophic lateral sclerosis. Amyotroph Lateral Scler 2011;12(2):109–12.
40. Rabkin JG, Goetz R, Factor-Litvak P, et al. Depression and wish to die in a multicenter cohort of ALS patients. Amyotroph Lateral Scler Frontotemporal Degener 2015;16(3–4):265–73.
41. Rabkin JG, Albert SM, Del Bene ML, et al. Prevalence of depressive disorders and change over time in late-stage ALS. Neurology 2005;65(1):62–7.
42. Caga J, Ramsey E, Hogden A, et al. A longer diagnostic interval is a risk for depression in amyotrophic lateral sclerosis. Palliat Support Care 2014;19:1–6.

43. Chen D, Guo X, Zheng Z, et al. Depression and anxiety in amyotrophic lateral sclerosis: correlations between the distress of patients and caregivers. Muscle Nerve 2015;51(3):353–7.
44. Snowden JS, Rollinson S, Thompson JC, et al. Distinct clinical and pathological characteristics of frontotemporal dementia associated with C9ORF72 mutations. Brain 2012;135(Pt 3):693–708.
45. Trojsi F, Monsurro MR, Esposito F, et al. Widespread structural and functional connectivity changes in amyotrophic lateral sclerosis: insights from advanced neuroimaging research. Neural Plast 2012;2012:473538.
46. Trojsi F, Esposito F, de SM, et al. Functional overlap and divergence between ALS and bvFTD. Neurobiol Aging 2015;36(1):413–23.
47. Al-Chalabi A, Jones A, Troakes C, et al. The genetics and neuropathology of amyotrophic lateral sclerosis. Acta Neuropathol 2012;124(3):339–52.
48. Renton AE, Chio A, Traynor BJ. State of play in amyotrophic lateral sclerosis genetics. Nat Neurosci 2014;17(1):17–23.
49. Wilson CM, Grace GM, Munoz DG, et al. Cognitive impairment in sporadic ALS. A pathological continuum underlying a multisystem disorder. Neurology 2001; 57:651–7.
50. Dejesus-Hernandez M, Mackenzie IR, Boeve BF, et al. Expanded GGGGCC hexanucleotide repeat in noncoding region of C9ORF72 causes chromosome 9p-linked FTD and ALS. Neuron 2011;72(2):245–56.
51. Renton AE, Majounie E, Waite A, et al. A hexanucleotide repeat expansion in C9ORF72 is the cause of chromosome 9p21-linked ALS-FTD. Neuron 2011; 72(2):257–68.
52. Chester C, de CM, Miltenberger G, et al. Rapidly progressive frontotemporal dementia and bulbar amyotrophic lateral sclerosis in Portuguese patients with C9orf72 mutation. Amyotroph Lateral Scler Frontotemporal Degener 2013;14(1):70–2.
53. Kandiah N, Sengdy P, Mackenzie IR, et al. Rapidly progressive dementia in a Chinese patient due to C90RF72 mutation. Can J Neurol Sci 2012;39(5):676–7.
54. Khan BK, Yokoyama JS, Takada LT, et al. Atypical, slowly progressive behavioural variant frontotemporal dementia associated with C9ORF72 hexanucleotide expansion. J Neurol Neurosurg Psychiatry 2012;83(4):358–64.
55. Yang W, Sopper MM, Leystra-Lantz C, et al. Microtubule-associated tau protein positive neuronal and glial inclusions in amyotrophic lateral sclerosis. Neurology 2003;61(12):1766–73.
56. Yang W, Ang L-C, Strong MJ. Tau protein aggregation in the frontal and entorhinal cortices as a function of aging. Dev Brain Res 2005;156:127–38.
57. Yang W, Strong MJ. Widespread neuronal and glial hyperphosphorylated tau deposition in ALS with cognitive impairment. Amyotroph Lateral Scler 2012; 13(2):178–93.
58. Crary JF, Trojanowski JQ, Schneider JA, et al. Primary age-related tauopathy (PART): a common pathology associated with human aging. Acta Neuropathol 2014;128(6):755–66.
59. Jellinger KA, Alafuzoff I, Attems J, et al. PART, a distinct tauopathy, different from classical sporadic Alzheimer disease. Acta Neuropathol 2015;129(5):757–62.
60. Gohar M, Yang W, Strong WL, et al. Tau phosphorylation at $^{175}$Thr leads to fibril formation. Implications for the tauopathy of amyotrophic lateral sclerosis. J Neurochem 2009;108(3):634–43.
61. Moszczynski AJ, Gohar M, Volkening K, et al. Thr175-phosphorylated tau induces pathologic fibril formation via GSK3beta-mediated phosphorylation of Thr231 in vitro. Neurobiol Aging 2015;36(3):1590–9.

62. Woolley SC, York MK, Moore DH, et al. Detecting frontotemporal dysfunction in ALS: utility of the ALS Cognitive Behavioral Screen (ALS-CBS). Amyotroph Lateral Scler 2010;11(3):303–11.
63. Flaherty-Craig C, Eslinger P, Stephens B, et al. A rapid screening battery to identify frontal dysfunction in patients with ALS. Neurology 2006;67:2070–2.
64. Flaherty-Craig C, Brothers A, Dearman B, et al. Penn State screen exam for the detection of frontal and temporal dysfunction syndromes: application to ALS. Amyotroph Lateral Scler 2009;10(2):107–12.
65. Niven E, Newton J, Foley J, et al. Validation of the Edinburgh Cognitive and Behavioural Amyotrophic Lateral Sclerosis Screen (ECAS): a cognitive tool for motor disorders. Amyotroph Lateral Scler Frontotemporal Degener 2015;16(3–4): 172–9.
66. Gordon PH, Wang Y, Doorish C, et al. A screening assessment of cognitive impairment in patients with ALS. Amyotroph Lateral Scler 2007;8:362–5.
67. Murphy J, Ahmed F, Lomen-Hoerth C. The UCSF screening exam effectively screens cognitive and behavioral impairment in patients with ALS. Amyotroph Lateral Scler Frontotemporal Degener 2015;16(1–2):24–30.
68. Raaphorst J, Beeldman E, Schmand B, et al. The ALS-FTD-Q: a new screening tool for behavioral disturbances in ALS. Neurology 2012;79(13):1377–83.
69. Mioshi E, Hsieh S, Caga J, et al. A novel tool to detect behavioural symptoms in ALS. Amyotroph Lateral Scler Frontotemporal Degener 2014;15(3–4):298–304.
70. Hammer EM, Hacker S, Hautzinger M, et al. Validity of the ALS-depression-inventory (ADI-12)–a new screening instrument for depressive disorders in patients with amyotrophic lateral sclerosis. J Affect Disord 2008;109(1–2):213–9.
71. Newsom-Davis IC, Abrahams S, Goldstein LH, et al. The emotional lability questionnaire: a new measure of emotional lability in amyotrophic lateral sclerosis. J Neurol Sci 1999;169(1–2):22–5.
72. Moore SR, Gresham LS, Bromberg MB, et al. A self report measure of affective lability. J Neurol Neurosurg Psychiatry 1997;63(1):89–93.
73. Rosen DR, Siddique T, Patterson D, et al. Mutations in Cu/Zn superoxide dismutase gene are associated with familial amyotrophic lateral sclerosis. Nature 1993; 362:59–62.
74. Chen Y-Z, Bennett CL, Huynh HM, et al. DNA/RNA helicase gene mutations in a form of juvenile amyotrophic lateral sclerosis (ALS4). Am J Hum Genet 2004;74: 1128–35.
75. Wharton SB, McDermott CJ, Grierson AJ, et al. The cellular and molecular pathology of the motor system in hereditary spastic paraparesis due to mutation of the spastin gene. J Neuropathol Exp Neurol 2003;62(11):1166–77.
76. Munch C, Rolfs A, Meyer T. Heterozygous S44L missense change of the spastin gene in amyotrophic lateral sclerosis. Amyotroph Lateral Scler 2008;9(4):251–3.
77. Vance C, Rogelj B, Hortobágyi T, et al. Mutations in FUS, an RNA processing protein, cause familial amyotrophic lateral sclerosis type 6. Science 2009; 323(5918):1208–11.
78. Kwiatkowski TJ Jr, Bosco DA, Leclerc AL, et al. Mutations in the FUS/TLS gene on chromosome 16 cause familial amyotrophic lateral sclerosis. Science 2009; 323(5918):1205–8.
79. Mackenzie IR, Rademakers R, Neumann M. TDP-43 and FUS in amyotrophic lateral sclerosis and frontotemporal dementia. Lancet Neurol 2010;9(10):995–1007.
80. Nishimura AL, Mitne-Neto M, Silva HCA, et al. A mutation in the vesicle-trafficking protein VAPB causes late-onset spinal muscular atrophy and amyotrophic lateral sclerosis. Am J Hum Genet 2004;75:822–31.

81. Greenway MJ, Andersen PM, Russ C, et al. ANG mutations segregate with familial and 'sporadic' amyotrophic lateral sclerosis. Nat Genet 2006;34(4):411–3.
82. van Es MA, Diekstra FP, Baas F, et al. A case of ALS-FTD in a large FALS pedigree with a K17I ANG mutation. Neurology 2009;72:287–8.
83. Arai T, Hasegawa M, Akiyama H, et al. TDP-43 is a component of ubiquitin-positive tau-negative inclusions in frontotemporal lobar degeneration and amyotrophic lateral sclerosis. Biochem Biophys Res Comm 2006;351(3):602–11.
84. Neumann M, Sampathu DM, Kwong LK, et al. Ubiquitinated TDP-43 in frontotemporal lobar degeneration and amyotrophic lateral sclerosis. Science 2006; 314:130–3.
85. Davidson Y, Kelley T, Mackenzie IRA, et al. Ubiquitinated pathological lesions in frontotemporal lobar degeneration contain the TAR DNA-binding protein, TDP-43. Acta Neuropathol 2007;113:521–33.
86. Sreedharan J, Blair IP, Tripathi VB, et al. TDP-43 mutations in familial and sporadic amyotrophic lateral sclerosis. Science 2008;319:1668–72.
87. Chow CY, Landers JE, Bergren SK, et al. Deleterious variants of FIG4, a phosphoinositide phosphatase, in patients with ALS. Am J Hum Genet 2009;84(1): 85–8.
88. Maruyama H, Morino H, Ito H, et al. Mutations of optineurin in amyotrophic lateral sclerosis. Nature 2010;465(7295):223–6.
89. Elden AC, Kim HJ, Hart MP, et al. Ataxin-2 intermediate-length polyglutamine expansions are associated with increased risk for ALS. Nature 2010; 466(7310):1069–75.
90. Forman MS, Mackenzie IR, Cairns NJ, et al. Novel ubiquitin neuropathology in frontotemporal dementia with valosin-containing protein gene mutations. J Neuropathol Exp Neurol 2006;65(6):571–81.
91. Johnson JO, Mandrioli J, Benatar M, et al. Exome sequencing reveals VCP mutations as a cause of familial ALS. Neuron 2010;68(5):857–64.
92. Weihl CC, Pestronk A, Kimonis VE. Valosin-containing protein disease: inclusion body myopathy with Paget's disease of the bone and fronto-temporal dementia. Neuromuscul Disord 2009;19(5):308–15.
93. Gellera C, Tiloca C, Del BR, et al. Ubiquilin 2 mutations in Italian patients with amyotrophic lateral sclerosis and frontotemporal dementia. J Neurol Neurosurg Psychiatry 2013;84(2):183–7.
94. Ugwu F, Rollinson S, Harris J, et al. A UBQLN2 variant of unknown significance in frontotemporal lobar degeneration. Neurobiol Aging 2015;36(1):546.
95. Al-Saif A, Al-Mohanna F, Bohlega S. A mutation in sigma-1 receptor causes juvenile amyotrophic lateral sclerosis. Ann Neurol 2011;70(6):913–9.
96. Belzil VV, Daoud H, Camu W, et al. Genetic analysis of SIGMAR1 as a cause of familial ALS with dementia. Eur J Hum Genet 2013;21(2):237–9.
97. Smith BN, Vance C, Scotter EL, et al. Novel mutations support a role for Profilin 1 in the pathogenesis of ALS. Neurobiol Aging 2015;36(3):1602–27.
98. van BM, Baker MC, Bieniek KF, et al. Profilin-1 mutations are rare in patients with amyotrophic lateral sclerosis and frontotemporal dementia. Amyotroph Lateral Scler Frontotemporal Degener 2013;14(5–6):463–9.
99. Cox LE, Ferraiuolo L, Goodall EF, et al. Mutations in CHMP2B in lower motor neuron predominant amyotrophic lateral sclerosis (ALS). PLoS One 2010;5(3): e9872.
100. Shatunov A, Mok K, Newhouse S, et al. Chromosome 9p21 in sporadic amyotrophic lateral sclerosis in the UK and seven other countries: a genome-wide association study. Lancet Neurol 2010;9(10):986–94.

101. Mitchell J, Paul P, Chen HJ, et al. Familial amyotrophic lateral sclerosis is associated with a mutation in D-amino acid oxidase. Proc Natl Acad Sci U S A 2010; 107(16):7556–61.
102. Munch C, Sedlmeier R, Meyer T, et al. Point mutations of the p150 subunit of dynactin (DCTN1) gene in ALS. Neurology 2004;63(4):724–6.
103. Farrer MJ, Hulihan MM, Kachergus JM, et al. DCTN1 mutations in Perry syndrome. Nat Genet 2009;41(2):163–5.
104. Al-Chalabi A, Andersen PM, Nilsson D, et al. Deletions of the heavy neurofilament subunit tail in amyotrophic lateral sclerosis. Hum Mol Genet 1999;8(2): 157–64.
105. Corrado L, Carlomagno Y, Falasco L, et al. A novel peripherin gene (PRPH) mutation identified in one sporadic amyotrophic lateral sclerosis patient. Neurobiol Aging 2011;32(3):552–6.
106. Le Ber I, Camuzat A, Guerreiro R, et al. SQSTM1 mutations in French patients with frontotemporal dementia or frontotemporal dementia with amyotrophic lateral sclerosis. JAMA Neurol 2013;70(11):1403–10.
107. Hand CK, Khoris J, Salachas F, et al. A novel locus for familial amyotrophic lateral sclerosis on chromosome 18q. Am J Hum Genet 2002;70(1):251–6.
108. Daoud H, Zhou S, Noreau A, et al. Exome sequencing reveals SPG11 mutations causing juvenile ALS. Neurobiol Aging 2012;33(4):839.
109. Simpson CL, Lemmens R, Miskiewicz K, et al. Variants of the elongator protein 3 (ELP3) gene are associated with motor neuron degeneration. Hum Mol Genet 2009;18(3):472–81.

# Familial Amyotrophic Lateral Sclerosis

Kevin Boylan, MD

**KEYWORDS**

- Amyotrophic lateral sclerosis • ALS • Familial ALS • Genetics • Phenotypes
- Genetic testing

**KEY POINTS**

- Amyotrophic lateral sclerosis (ALS) is genetically heterogeneous with more than 50 potential causative or disease-modifying genes identified, but *C9ORF72*, *SOD1*, *TARDPB*, and *FUS* account for greater than 50% of ALS-linked gene variants found in patients with ALS and variants in other genes are uncommon or rare.
- Genetic risk for ALS probably represents combined effects of multiple genes that establish a person's overall genetic susceptibility, acting with environmental and random effects leading to disease onset.
- Clinical features in general do not reliably separate familial from sporadic ALS (SALS) in individual patients owing to phenotypic overlap; family history, including history of frontotemporal dementia (FTD), aids in recognizing that a patient may have familial ALS (FALS).
- ALS-linked gene variants can be identified in about 60%–70% of patients with FALS, a proportion likely to grow, and a pathogenic ALS gene variant may be found in an increasing minority of patients with SALS.

## BACKGROUND

Familial incidence of ALS was described in scattered publications beginning in the mid-1800s but received limited attention in the literature until the report in 1955 by Kurland and Mulder,[1,2] which suggested that ALS may be familial in nearly 10% of cases. The application of molecular genetic techniques to ALS, marked by the report in 1993 of linkage of the superoxide dismutase 1 (*SOD1*) gene in FALS, signaled an increasing focus on genetics in ALS as a means to gain insights into the pathogenesis of the disease, identify therapeutic targets, and facilitate diagnosis.[3] In recent years, a rapidly expanding list of genetic variations linked to ALS and their related clinical and pathologic correlates continues to provide key insights into the causes of ALS and inform therapy development.[4]

---

Disclosures: No relevant disclosures.
Department of Neurology, Mayo Clinic Jacksonville, 4500 San Pablo Road, Jacksonville, FL 32224, USA
*E-mail address:* boylan.kevin@mayo.edu

Neurol Clin 33 (2015) 807–830
http://dx.doi.org/10.1016/j.ncl.2015.07.001 **neurologic.theclinics.com**
0733-8619/15/$ – see front matter 

This review examines genetic correlates of classic ALS demonstrating combined upper and lower motor neuron signs, but some of the genes discussed may be associated with pure lower motor neuron and pure upper motor neuron phenotypes and, in some cases, FTD and parkinsonian features. Technological developments that have facilitated advances in ALS gene discovery are briefly discussed, and efforts to translate growing knowledge of ALS genetics into patient care are noted. In line with recommendations of the International Human Genome Society, DNA sequence alterations associated with disease are referred to in terms such as genetic sequence variants or sequence variants rather than mutations, recognizing that pathogenicity of some ALS-associated gene variants is less well established than for others.[5]

## RECENT TECHNOLOGICAL DEVELOPMENTS AND AMYOTROPHIC LATERAL SCLEROSIS GENE DISCOVERY

Advances in molecular genetic technology and the capacity for handling extensive data sets generated by large-scale DNA sequencing have had significant impact on the discovery of new gene mutations linked to ALS.[4,6,7] In addition to first-generation methods such as genetic linkage analysis and candidate gene analysis relying on linked DNA markers in ALS pedigrees, newer approaches including genome-wide association studies (GWAS) and next-generation sequencing techniques such as whole exome sequencing and whole genome sequencing have allowed the search for ALS-linked genes to be conducted in large sample sets derived mainly from patients with no family history of ALS and in families from which few DNA samples may be available.[6–8] GWAS optimally requires large case control sample sets, generally at least several thousand samples, and is based on the concept that variants of a given gene commonly associated with ALS may be present in a sufficient number of patients to be detectable if enough patients are studied.[6] Next-generation technology leverages high-throughput, large-scale parallel DNA sequencing of essentially all expressed coding sequences (whole exome sequencing) or the entire genome (whole genome sequencing) in conjunction with software and computing capacity able to sort and align short segments of overlapping DNA sequence and efficiently analyze the tremendous amount of sequence data produced. Whole exome or whole genome sequencing produces essentially complete data on all protein-coding genes or on the entire genetic sequence, respectively, allowing identification of wide range of DNA variants potentially associated with ALS.[6–8]

### *Clinical Spectrum of Amyotrophic Lateral Sclerosis Genetics*

Increasing evidence from clinical and basic research suggests that ALS has multiple causes with an important, although varied, genetic component.[4,9] Genetic factors in ALS range from highly penetrant ALS-linked gene variants to sequence variants with seemingly limited impact on disease susceptibility.[6] Phenotypes associated with these sequence variants include classic ALS, primary lateral sclerosis (PLS), and progressive muscular atrophy (PMA).[4,6,8] An important extramotor feature associated with some gene variants linked to ALS is FTD, which may develop with, before, or after onset of motor signs in ALS and as FTD alone.[10,11] Less common clinical features associated with some ALS-linked gene variants include extrapyramidal features and inclusion body myopathy.[4,12] Although FALS is mainly an adult-onset disorder, a few genes associated with ALS may have phenotypes characterized by juvenile onset.[6,8] Although some clinical patterns may tend to occur in association with specific ALS gene variants, in clinical practice, significant overlap among phenotypes limits practical application as a means to ascertain patients likely to carry a specific ALS-linked gene variant.[12]

## GENETIC SUSCEPTIBILITY TO AMYOTROPHIC LATERAL SCLEROSIS

ALS clinical registry data and more recent meta-analyses based on prospective population-based registries suggest that up to 10% of patients with ALS have a family history of ALS in a first- or second-degree relative, generally classified as FALS.[8,13] The remaining 90% of patients with no evident family history of ALS are designated as SALS, a potentially misleading designation for several reasons. First, persons with ALS associated with a causative gene variant may lack a family history of ALS as a result of reduced penetrance or small family size. In addition, family history may be inaccurate owing to incomplete family history, incorrect diagnoses in ancestors, or death from other causes before the onset of ALS in relatives genetically at risk.[14]

Several studies have investigated the risk of developing ALS in relatives of patients with ALS in efforts to quantitate genetic contributions to ALS susceptibility. An investigation in Sweden of the relative risk of ALS in siblings and children of ALS probands that did not exclude FALS probands found a relative risk of 9.7 (95% confidence interval [CI], 7.2–12.8), and 2 other studies, one in the United Kingdom that considered only patients with SALS and the other in the United States that included patients with FALS and SALS, reported an approximately 1% risk of ALS among first-degree relatives of a patient with ALS.[15–17] Furthermore, estimates of the heritability of ALS, a measure of the extent of phenotypic variability that is attributable to genetic variation, provide additional evidence that genetic factors play a significant role in sporadic as well as familial ALS. In a study of identical twins that included twins with or without a history of ALS in other relatives, heritability was estimated to be about 76% (95% CI, 60–86) for twins with a family history of ALS and approximately 61% (95% CI, 38–78) for twins with no other family history of ALS.[18]

It has been suggested that genetic contributions to ALS may represent the inheritance of risk variants of multiple genes, acting interdependently to cause ALS.[19] The hypothesis that ALS may be oligogenic implies that at least 2 pathogenic ALS gene variants are required to initiate disease. Several studies have shown that a subset of patients with FALS and SALS carry at least 1 known ALS-linked gene variant in conjunction with a second potentially pathogenic variant and offer support for the oligogenic concept of ALS genetics, but these data have been questioned on the basis that the second gene variant may represent a benign variant, potential cohort selection bias, and small sample size, and further validation was recommended.[6,8] Regardless of the extent to which an oligogenic mechanism is proved in ALS pathogenesis, available data suggest that genetic risk for ALS probably represents combined effects of multiple genes that establish a person's overall genetic susceptibility, acting in conjunction with environmental and random effects leading to disease onset.[8,12]

## FAMILIAL INHERITANCE PATTERNS IN AMYOTROPHIC LATERAL SCLEROSIS

Inheritance of most forms of FALS is autosomal dominant, although autosomal recessive and X-linked dominant FALS also occur. Different modes of inheritance may be associated with the same gene depending on the specific sequence variant involved.[12] In practice, there has been some agreement that ALS is considered familial if at least one first- or second-degree relative is reported to have ALS.[20] However, the presentation of ALS and FTD in first-degree relatives in some families, and observed co-occurrence of ALS with FTD in some patients with ALS, was considered in a recently proposed algorithm for the diagnosis of FALS (**Table 1**).[14] Within that framework, a patient with seemingly sporadic ALS with a family history of FTD in a first-degree relative would be considered to have possible FALS.[14] Validity of this concept

**Table 1**
**Criteria for the diagnosis of familial amyotrophic lateral sclerosis**

| Classification/Level of Certainty | Family History |
|---|---|
| Definite | ≥2 First- or second-degree relatives with ALS<br>≥1 Relative with ALS and gene-positive cosegregation |
| Probable | 1 First- or second-degree relative with ALS |
| Possible | Distant relative (third degree or beyond) with ALS<br>Patient with sporadic ALS and no family history of ALS, but positive for an FALS gene<br>≥1 First- or second-degree relative with confirmed frontotemporal dementia |

Definitions: First-degree relatives: parents, children, and siblings; second-degree relatives: grandparent, aunts/uncles.

*Adapted from* Byrne S, Bede P, Elamin M, et al. Proposed criteria for familial amyotrophic lateral sclerosis. Amyotroph Lateral Scler 2011;12(3):158.

is supported by the discovery that an abnormal expansion of a hexanucleotide repeat (GGGGCC) in chromosome 9 open reading frame 72 (*C9ORF72*), a gene of unknown function further discussed later, is the most common gene variant linked to ALS and is also commonly associated with ALS-FTD and pure FTD.[21,22] Although there remains no formally agreed upon definition of FALS in the literature, the proposed working definition based on a history of ALS in a first-degree or second-degree relative, or potentially in the case of a history of FTD in a first-degree relative, seems adequately supported (see **Table 1**).

## GENE VARIANTS LINKED TO AMYOTROPHIC LATERAL SCLEROSIS PATHOGENESIS

A growing number of gene variants associated with mendelian inheritance of ALS have been reported (**Table 2**). In outbred populations, approximately 60% to 70% of FALS is accounted for by known ALS-linked genes.[8] However, reports of families in which linkage to known loci has been excluded indicate further genetic heterogeneity.[23–25] With some geographic variation, the *C9ORF72* hexanucleotide repeat expansion accounts for approximately 40% of FALS in North America and Europe, whereas *SOD1* variants linked to disease are found in about 12%, transactive response DNA binding protein 43 (*TARDPB*) and fused in sarcoma (*FUS*) gene variants account for a few percentage each, and other less common or rare gene variants are found in the remainder.[8] As mentioned, these figures may vary depending on the population being considered; for example, sequence variants such as the *C9ORF72* hexanucleotide repeat expansion in patients with ALS in Finland and *TARDBP* in patients with ALS in Sardinia are significantly more frequent as causes of FALS than in the United States or other parts of Europe, and *SOD1* variants are rare among patients with ALS in the Netherlands.[22,26,27]

Although associations between the foregoing gene variants and FALS are well established, each is also found infrequently in patients with SALS. The possibility of incomplete information regarding the family history may be the basis for some of these observations, but documented nonpenetrance is established for the *C9ORF72* repeat expansion and for some *SOD1*, *TARDBP*, and *FUS* variants.[28–33] De novo occurrence of sequence variants associated with ALS seems to be uncommon but has been documented in a single report of an *SOD1* variant and in multiple reports of *FUS* variants.[34–36] The main message from these observations is that absence of a family

**Table 2**
**Genes linked to ALS pathogenesis**

| Gene | Protein | Function | Inheritance | Phenotypes | %FALS[b] | %SALS[b] |
|---|---|---|---|---|---|---|
| ALS2[a,110] | Alsin | Rho guanine nucleotide exchange factor | AR | Juvenile ALS, Juvenile PLS, HSP | — | — |
| ANG; ALS9[111,112] | Angiogenin | Ribonuclease; angiogenesis | AD/Sporadic | ALS, PD | — | — |
| ATXN2; ALS13[113,114] | Ataxin-2 | RNA processing | Not established | ALS, SCA2, parkinsonism | — | — |
| CHCHD10[115,116] | Coiled-coil-helix-coiled-coil-helix domain containing 10 | Mitochondrial protein | AD | FTD, cerebellar ataxia, myopathy | — | — |
| CHMP2B; ALS17[117] | Chromatin modifying protein 2B | Recycling/degradation of cell surface receptors | AD | ALS, ALS-FTD, FTD | — | — |
| C9ORF72[21,22,118,119] | Chromosome 9 open reading frame 72 | Unknown | AD | ALS, ALS-FTD, FTD, parkinsonism (rare), psychosis | 40 | 7 |
| DAO[120] | D-Amino acid oxidase | Peroxisomal enzyme; potential role in glutamatergic neurotransmission | AD | ALS | — | — |
| DCTN1[121–123] | Dynactin | Axonal transport | AD | PMA, FTD, HMN VIIB, Perry syndrome | — | — |
| FIG4; ALS11[124] | SAC1 lipid phosphatase domain containing (*S cerevisiae*) | Polyphosphoinositide phosphatase | AD, AR | ALS, PLS, CMT4J, Yunis-Varon syndrome | — | — |
| FUS; ALS6[33,68] | Fused in sarcoma | RNA-binding protein, DNA repair, exon splicing | AD | ALS, juvenile ALS, FTD | 4 | 1 |

(*continued on next page*)

Table 2
(*continued*)

| Gene | Protein | Function | Inheritance | Phenotypes | %FALS[b] | %SALS[b] |
|---|---|---|---|---|---|---|
| HNRNPA1; ALS20[85] | Heterogenous nuclear ribonucleoprotein A1 | mRNA processing, transport and metabolism | AD | ALS, FTD, IBMPFD | — | — |
| HNRNPA2B1[85] | Heterogenous nuclear ribonucleoprotein A2B1 | mRNA processing, transport and metabolism | AD | ALS, FTD, IBMPFD | — | — |
| MATR3; ALS21[84] | Matrin 3 | Nuclear matrix protein, may stabilize mRNA species | AD | ALS, distal myopathy 2, ALS plus myopathy | — | — |
| OPTN; ALS12[125] | Optineurin | Membrane and vesicle trafficking, transcription activation | AD, AR | ALS, progressive open angle glaucoma | <1 | <1 |
| PFN1; ALS18[126] | Profilin 1 | Actin binding protein, actin polymerization | AD | ALS | <1 | <1 |
| SETX; ALS4[127] | Senataxin | RNA/DNA helicase | AD | Onset < age 25 y; SETX mutation causes spinocerebellar ataxia 1/ataxia-ocular apraxia 2 | — | — |
| SIGMAR1; ALS16[128–130] | Sigma nonopioid intracellular receptor 1 | Endoplasmic reticulum chaperone protein; proteosome inhibition, mitochondrial stress | AR | ALS, FTD | — | — |
| SOD1; ALS1[3,54,55] | Superoxide dismutase 1 | Oxidative stress | AD, AR, de novo | ALS, FTD (rare), PMA | 12 | 2 |

| | | | | | | |
|---|---|---|---|---|---|---|
| SPG11[131,132] | Spatacsin | DNA damage repair | AR | Juvenile ALS, HSP (SPG11) | — | — |
| SQSTM1[133,134] | Sequestosome 1 | Scaffold protein, NFKB signaling | AD | ALS, FTD | 1 | <1 |
| TARDBP; ALS10[62–64] | TAR DNA binding protein 43 | Transcriptional repressor, splicing regulation | AD, AR, de novo | ALS, FTD, PD | 4 | 1 |
| TBK1[91,92] | TANK-binding kinase 1 | Mediates growth factor activation of NFKB | AD | ALS | — | — |
| TUBA4A; ALS22[135] | Tubulin $\alpha$1 | Structural component of cytoskeleton; GTP binding | AD | Spinal onset ALS, ALS-FTD, FTD | — | — |
| UBQLN2; ALS15[83,90] | Ubiquilin 2 | Ubiquitination, protein degradation | XLD | ALS, FTD | <1 | <1 |
| VAPB; ALS8[136] | Vesicle-associated membrane associated-protein B | Vesicular trafficking | AD | ALS, PMA | — | — |
| VCP; ALS14[93] | Valosin-containing protein | ATP-binding protein, vesicle transport and fusion | AD | ALS, ALS-FTD, FTD, IBMPFD | 1 | 1 |

*Abbreviations:* AD, autosomal dominant; AR, autosomal recessive; CMT, Charcot-Marie-Tooth; HMN, hereditary motor neuropathy; HSP, hereditary spastic paraplegia; IBMPFD, inclusion body myopathy with early-onset Paget disease and frontotemporal dementia; NFKB, nuclear factor kappa-light chain-enhancer of activated B cells; PD, Parkinson disease; SCA, spinocerebellar ataxia; SPG, spastic paraplegia; TANK, TRAF (tumor necrosis factor receptor-associated factor) family member-associated NFKB Activator; XLD, X-linked dominant.

[a] The Human Genome Organization Nomenclature Committee has approved numerical designations for 22 ALS-linked genes or genetic loci to date, ALS1 through ALS22. These designations are not used as a primary numbering system here given that numbers have not been assigned for multiple ALS genes and the gene is not identified for 3 numerically designated forms. ALS3, ALS5, and ALS7 represent ALS-linked gene loci on chromosomes 18q21, 15q15.1-q21.1, and 20p13. Causative genes are not yet established for these loci.

[b] Percentages of FALS and SALS cases are shown where data seem sufficient to support an estimate. Frequency estimates are not listed where data on the frequencies of disease-associated variants are limited, and in most such instances frequency may be low or rare.

history of ALS may not rule out the presence of a gene variant associated with FALS, although the likelihood is modest, approximately 7% in the case of the *C9ORF72* repeat expansion, 1% to 2% for *SOD1* variants, and approximately 1% for *TARDBP*, *FUS*, and *VCP* variants.[8]

Four ALS causative genes linked to more than 50% of patients with FALS are discussed briefly in order based on relative frequency of association with ALS. These genes are also the most likely to be involved in patients with SALS found to carry a recognized ALS-linked gene variant.

### *Chromosome 9 Open Reading Frame 72*

A GGGGCC hexanucleotide repeat in the first intron of a gene that encodes a protein of unknown function on chromosome 9, *C9ORF72,* is the most common gene variant associated with FALS, found in 40% of FALS and about 6% to 8% of patients with SALS, with ethnic variation as noted earlier.[37] C9FTD/ALS phenotypes include classic ALS (infrequently PMA or PLS), ALS/FTD, and FTD, as well as dopa nonresponsive parkinsonian and Huntington disease phenotypes.[38–41] FTD or less severe frontotemporal cognitive impairment in patients with C9FTD/ALS may arise with, before, or after onset of motor signs in up to 50% of patients.[42] Inheritance is autosomal dominant with incomplete penetrance; median age of onset is 58 years, ranging from the fourth through ninth decades.[37] Genetic anticipation, the onset of C9FTD/ALS at an earlier age in affected offspring than in affected parents, was suggested by some reports but is not confirmed.[38,43,44] Normal repeat length is 2 to 10 $G_4C_2$ units; expansions larger than 20 units are reported with c9FTD/ALS but minimum repeat length linked to disease is not established.[21,22,44] Molecular pathogenesis of C9FTD/ALS may include haploinsufficiency of *C9ORF72* proteins and neurotoxicity from RNA-based gain of function mechanisms, although data increasingly support the latter as the primary component.[45,46] Support for the diagnosis of C9FTD/ALS can be obtained at autopsy owing to the presence in brain of distinctive neuronal inclusions reactive for p62, ubiquitin, and dipeptide repeat protein species bidirectionally transcribed from the repeat expansion, referred to as C9RAN proteins.[47,48] These changes occur on a background of ubiquitin- and TAR DNA-binding protein 43 (TDP-43)-positive inclusions in neurons and glia of affected brain regions, similar to that in SALS.[49–51] DNA testing for the repeat expansion is generally based on a polymerase chain reaction (PCR) screening test that does not reliably quantitate repeat number beyond about 50 repeats.[21,22] Southern blot, the gold standard for confirmation of the presence of abnormal *C9ORF72* repeat expansions, is technically demanding and may not allow precise determination of repeat length in patients with long repeats but should be performed if PCR screening results are ambiguous.[21,44] An additional issue is that repeat length varies across and within tissues, and estimates of repeat length in blood may not reflect repeat length in brain.[52]

### *Superoxide Dismutase 1*

Sequence variants in the Cu/Zn superoxide dismutase gene (*SOD1*) on chromosome 21q12.1 were the first causative gene variants identified in ALS.[3] Native *SOD1* protein catalyzes reduction of superoxide to hydrogen peroxide; molecular pathogenesis of SOD1 ALS is not established, but several lines of evidence point to a toxic gain-of-function mechanism.[12] Disease-linked variants are mainly point mutations and account for approximately 12% of patients with FALS and 1% to 2% of SALS, with ethnic variation in prevalence.[3,8] More than 160 pathogenic *SOD1* variants are known, with significant geographic variation reported for some variants.[12] Inheritance with all but one of these is autosomal dominant. The *SOD1* D91A variant, found mainly in patients with ALS in Sweden and Finland, is associated with a slowly progressive motor with autosomal recessive inheritance.[53] Phenotypes of *SOD1* ALS include classic ALS and PMA, often with asymmetrical lower limb onset; when upper motor neuron signs are found, lower motor neuron signs tend to predominate.[54] Age of onset in most reported patients with *SOD1* ALS is approximately 47 $\pm$ 12.5 years, with greater variability in disease duration than for age of onset.[54,55] However, age at onset and severity may vary significantly depending on the variant involved, and within families for some variants such as *SOD1* I114T, and penetrance may be less than 100%.[30,55–57] Frontotemporal cognitive impairment is rare in *SOD1* ALS.[12] Pathologic hallmarks of *SOD1* ALS in postmortem brain and spinal cord include intracellular neuronal and astrocytic protein aggregates marked by ubiquinated neuronal and astrocytic inclusions reactive for SOD1 in motor and nonmotor systems.[54] DNA testing for *SOD1* variants is available through clinical laboratories to establish a genetic diagnosis of *SOD1* ALS.[58]

### *Transactive Response DNA Binding Protein 43*

Identification of *TARDBP* variants in patients with ALS followed the discovery in 2006 that neuronal cytoplasmic inclusions immunoreactive for ubiquitin, a pathologic hallmark in the large majority of cases of FALS and SALS, are also immunoreactive for TDP-43.[59] Recognition at that time that about half of patients with pathologically proven frontotemporal lobar degeneration (the pathologic basis for the clinical syndrome FTD) have similar TDP-43 immunoreactive inclusions established a pathologic link between ALS and FTD and led to the concept that ALS, ALS-FTD, and FTD represent a clinical and pathologic spectrum referred to as TDP-43 proteinopathies.[60] Gene variants in *TARDBP*, which encodes the 43-kD TDP-43, are found in approximately 4% of FALS and 1% of SALS, with some regional variation.[8,29,32] TDP-43 regulates gene expression and RNA splicing.[60] Available evidence suggests that dysregulation of gene expression, including RNA splicing, attributed to pathogenic *TARDPB* variants, in conjunction with a toxic gain-of-function of mutant TDP-43 protein, contributes to neurodegeneration, but the causal mechanism is not established.[61] More than 30 sequence variants have been associated with *TARDBP* ALS, most in the C-terminal glycine-rich domain; inheritance in all is autosomal dominant.[60] Clinical phenotypes linked to pathogenic *TARDPB* variants include classic ALS and rarely Parkinson disease or FTD.[62–66] Upper limb onset is reported to be more common in *TARDBP* ALS and survival somewhat longer than in SALS generally, but in clinical practice these differences have limited utility in identifying patients with *TARDBP* ALS.[64] Pathology of *TARDPB* ALS is similar to that of most cases of SALS, demonstrating neuronal cytoplasmic inclusions immunoreactive for TDP-43 throughout the brain but particularly in motor cortex, spinal cord, basal ganglia, and thalamus.[60] DNA testing for ALS-linked *TARDPB* variants is available through clinical laboratories.[58]

### *Fused in Sarcoma*

Variants in the gene fused in sarcoma (*FUS*) are linked to autosomal dominant ALS in about 4% of patients with FALS and 1% of patients with SALS.[8,33,67,68] FUS seems to regulate DNA and RNA metabolism and be involved in RNA transcription, splicing, and processing; gene sequence variants that alter these functions may contribute to neurodegeneration, but the molecular pathogenesis of *FUS*-related neurodegeneration is not fully defined.[69] Pathogenic *FUS* variants include point mutations and other structural defects and are notable for several reports confirming de novo mutations associated with ALS.[35,36,70–73] Inheritance is autosomal dominant aside from a single family with apparent autosomal recessive inheritance.[68] ALS phenotypes include adult-onset ALS, ALS/FTD, and juvenile ALS, and rarely pure FTD.[69] Lower motor neuron signs may predominate in some patients with FUS ALS, but in clinical practice these features may have limited utility in identifying patients with FUS ALS.[74,75] A single family with a *FUS* ALS-plus syndrome with ocular, autonomic, and cerebellar features also has been reported.[76] Disease progression in juvenile *FUS* ALS tends to be rapid, without development of FTD.[77,78] Pathologic hallmarks of adult-onset *FUS* ALS in postmortem brain and spinal cord include abnormal protein aggregates immunoreactive for FUS, mainly in the cytoplasm and also in nuclei of neurons and glia.[33,79] Juvenile-onset *FUS* ALS demonstrates distinctive pathology marked by neuronal basophilic inclusions immunoreactive for FUS protein; similar pathology has been reported in adult-onset *FUS* FTD but rarely for *FUS* ALS.[77,78,80,81] DNA testing to identify *FUS* variants is available through clinical laboratories.[58]

### *Other Risk Genes and Insights from Genetics on the Pathogenesis of Amyotrophic Lateral Sclerosis*

The list of additional genes with sequence variants associated with ALS and related phenotypes continues to grow, aided by technological advances in large-scale genetic screening in patients with FALS and SALS, particularly whole exome analysis in recent studies (see **Table 2**).[6,7] Although most of these genes contribute to a small proportion of FALS and/or SALS, they and more common FALS genes have offered insights regarding ALS pathogenesis. Shared functional characteristics of protein products of these genes and related postmortem pathology have directed attention to specific molecular pathways in ALS pathogenesis and in turn have supported development of molecular models of ALS pathogenesis and development of new therapeutic strategies.[61,82,83]

Pathogenic *TARDPB* and *FUS* variants found in ALS and recognized functional and structural similarities between TDP-43 and FUS protein focused attention on potentially disordered RNA processing and splicing in ALS generally.[33,62,63,68] The relevance of defective RNA processing to ALS pathogenesis was more recently reinforced by the discovery of pathogenic *MATR3* and *nhRNPA1* variants in patients with ALS, as both genes seem to have a role in normal RNA processing.[84,85] Although the specific function of C9ORF72 protein is not established, molecular and pathologic evidence in C9FTD/ALS offers further support for the concept that disordered RNA processing contributes to ALS.[45,46,86–89]

The discovery that mutations in the ubiquilin-2 gene (*UBQLN2*, which encodes ubiquilin-2) are a rare cause of X-linked dominant ALS and ALS/FTD in males, with reduced penetrance in females, reinforced the concept that disruption of protein degradation pathways may be important in ALS.[90] Abnormal protein aggregates in affected brain regions in most cases of FALS and SALS are immunoreactive at postmortem for ubiquilin-2, and functional analysis suggests that *UBQLN2* mutations resulting in ALS and ALS/FTD are pathogenic because disruption of autophagic protein degradation.[83,90] Relevance of autophagy in ALS is further supported by associations between sequence variants in the genes encoding valosin-containing protein (*VCP*), optineurin (*OPTN*), and TANK-binding kinase 1 (*TBK1*) in ALS.[91–94] Protein products of these genes are involved in normal protein autophagy.[91]

Genes pathogenically associated with ALS and FTD have also been linked to conditions involving other organ systems such as bone and muscle, giving rise to the designation multisystem proteinopathy as a group of genetic disorders demonstrating a wide phenotypic spectrum. In addition to *VCP* and *OPTN*, sequestosome 1/P62 (*SQSTM1/p62*) and heterogeneous ribonucleoprotein A2B1 and A1 (*HNRNPA2B1* and *HNRNPA1*) are genes in this category that have been linked to Paget disease of bone, inclusion body myopathy, and ALS.[85,93,95] Disease-linked variants in these genes are uncommon in ALS, but they have implicated toxic conformational changes in RNA-binding proteins with prionlike domains, such as TDP-43 and FUS, in neurodegeneration.[85,96]

### *Amyotrophic Lateral Sclerosis Susceptibility Genes Associated with Lower Risk and Potential Disease-Modifying Genes*

Apart from the aforementioned genes, an expanding number of additional genes have been implicated in the pathogenesis of ALS, based on varied levels of supporting data and in some cases uncertainty whether reported variants represent modifiers of clinical disease rather than direct causative factors (**Table 3**).[4,6,7] These variants tend to be uncommon, with limited data supporting linkage with ALS; more detailed discussion is beyond the scope of this review, but further information is available in recent reviews.[4,6,7] Further studies are needed to clarify the level of ALS risk associated with these genes and, in some cases, confirm that the reported variant is associated with ALS rather than being a benign variant.[6]

## EPIGENETICS OF AMYOTROPHIC LATERAL SCLEROSIS

Epigenetic factors may influence gene expression and disease states through dynamic cellular and physiologic processes that activate and deactivate parts of the genome. DNA methylation is a well-studied example shown to be involved in neurodegeneration and could potentially play a role in phenotypic expression of FALS as well as SALS.[97] Genomic DNA methylation patterns in ALS examined for alterations that could represent disease-specific epigenetic alterations in ALS have suggested that such changes may influence gene expression, but this requires confirmation.[98,99] More recent studies focusing on ALS associated with the *C9ORF72* repeat expansion offer evidence that, in this form of FALS, histone methylation seems to reduce the expression of the mutant allele, and DNA methylation may be associated with less severe clinical phenotypes in the form of longer survival and reduced mutation-specific pathology in affected brain regions.[100–102] More studies are needed to confirm these results and investigate the potential role of epigenetic factors in other forms of FALS and in SALS. Analysis of epigenetic factors could refine genetic testing in ALS if detection and interpretation of epigenetic characteristics becomes a routine component of a patient's genetic risk profile.

## AMYOTROPHIC LATERAL SCLEROSIS GENE TESTING IN CLINICAL PRACTICE

**Clinical Vignette**

*A 59-year-old woman with a confirmed diagnosis of ALS has mild bulbar features but is mainly disabled by upper limb and less pronounced lower extremity weakness. Symptoms began 14 months earlier, and upper and lower motor neuron signs are now present. There is mild pseudobulbar affect but no features suggestive of neuropsychiatric dysfunction; mild depression responded well to antidepressant medication. The patient questions whether her children are at risk for ALS.*

*There is no known family history of ALS. Her father died at 76 years of a myocardial infarction with no history of neurologic disorders. Her mother died of complications of dementia at age 63 years, characterized as Alzheimer disease with a clinical course of approximately 4 years, becoming mute and bedridden toward the end of her disease course with significant weight loss. The patient's only sibling is an older brother who is well. A maternal aunt developed dementia and died at approximately age 70 years, but no details otherwise are available; the aunt had a son thought to be alive, but the patient has no information otherwise. The maternal grandparents are believed to have lived past age 70 years without neurologic problems.*

*The family history illustrates issues that can arise in evaluating the possibility that ALS in a given patient may be associated with an ALS risk gene. The family history is said to be negative with regard to ALS, but the dementia in the patient's mother had a shorter clinical course than is typical for Alzheimer disease, raising the possibility that the patient's mother may actually have had FTD, perhaps even accompanied by undiagnosed motor neuron disease. Dementia in the maternal aunt could reflect a familial predisposition to dementia, but limited information prevents meaningful conclusions. Family history may be clarified by review of family medical records or autopsy reports, but these may be unavailable.*

*If no further family history becomes available, a case can be made to discuss with the patient the possibility that her disorder could be associated with a C9ORF72 repeat expansion, particularly given that FTD is a recognized phenotype of the C9ORF72 repeat expansion. Dementia is also reported in association with other ALS-linked genes, including FUS and TDP-43, although these are less common. Dementia linked to SOD1 variants, the second most common ALS-linked gene after C9ORF72, is rare. Confirmation of FTD in the patient's mother or the aunt would meet criteria for possible FALS according to criteria suggested by Byrne and colleagues[14] (see* ***Table 1****). A more common situation is the question of whether to offer DNA testing if further investigation suggests that neither the patient's mother nor the aunt is likely to have had FTD in the patient thought to have SALS.*

### *Considerations in the Clinical Application of DNA Testing in Amyotrophic Lateral Sclerosis*

A challenge for the clinician on establishing that a patient has ALS is the question of whether to offer the patient DNA testing to investigate the possibility that the patient carries an ALS-linked gene variant. Although confirmation that the patient carries a sequence variant associated with ALS offers no proven gene-specific treatment options, research in this area may provide the patient with options for participation in future research trials involving gene-targeted therapy. Antisense oligonucleotide and small-molecule therapy have undergone early stage testing, and similar experimental treatment approaches are anticipated to become available in human studies in coming years.[88,103–106]

Clinical features of ALS in general do not provide a reliable basis for separating of FALS from SALS in individual patients given the extent of phenotypic overlap.[12] Clinical characteristics that may offer some insight as to the potential for involvement of one or other specific genes in FALS were discussed earlier. Family history provides critical information when available, and criteria noted in **Table 1** offer a reasonable basis for clinical decision making, recognizing that fully validated criteria are not available.[14,20] In a patient lacking a family history of ALS, the relevance of a family history of dementia in a first- or second-degree relative may be uncertain, as genetic risk applies primarily for FTD and it may be difficult to specifically confirm whether or not the cognitive disorder in the relative in question was FTD as opposed to dementia on some other basis.[14] A further confound is that an amnestic syndrome diagnosable as Alzheimer disease is reported infrequently in patients with a *C9ORF72* repeat expansion.[107]

The foregoing discussion regarding DNA testing refers to patients with suspected FALS, but in view of data suggesting that approximately 10% of patients with SALS may carry a major ALS susceptibility gene variant, there are grounds to make people with SALS aware of this possibility to allow the patient to make an informed decision regarding DNA testing.[8] Although there may be exceptions depending on the experience and training of the clinician, in most situations patients with ALS seeking further information regarding the rationale for DNA testing and review of test results should be referred to a genetic counselor.[108]

An additional issue once the decision to order DNA testing has been made is which test or tests to order. Clinical tests for ALS-linked genes are available, including

**Table 3**
**Genes associated with potential causative or disease-modifying effects in ALS**

| Gene | Protein | Function |
|---|---|---|
| APOE[137] | Apolipoprotein E | Lipoprotein metabolism, immune regulation |
| ARHGEF28[138,139] | Rho guanine nucleotide exchange factor 28 | Regulates integrin and growth factor signaling pathways |
| CHGB[140] | Chromogranin B | Neuroendocrine secretory granule protein |
| CHRNA3[141] | Neuronal acetylcholine receptor subunit α3 | Nicotinic acetylcholine receptor subunit |
| CHRNA4[142] | Neuronal acetylcholine receptor subunit α4 | Nicotinic acetylcholine receptor subunit |
| CHRNB4[141] | Neuronal acetylcholine receptor subunit β4 | Nicotinic acetylcholine receptor subunit |
| CX3CR1[143] | CX3C chemokine receptor 1 | Chemokine receptor |
| DPP6[144–146] | Dipeptidyl peptidase 6 | Alters expression/properties of voltage-gated K+ channels |
| DPYSL3[147] | Dihydropyrimidinase-like 3 | Class 3 semaphorin signaling, cytoskeletal remodeling |
| ELP3[148] | Elongator acetyltransferase complex subunit 3 | Transcript elongation |
| EPHA3[149] | EPH receptor A3 | Neighboring cell signaling, axonal segregation during development |
| EPHA4[149] | EPH receptor A4 | Neighboring cell signaling, repair after nerve injury, angiogenesis |
| ERBB4; ALS19[150] | V-erb-B2 avian erythroblastic leukemia viral oncogene homolog 4 | Tyrosine protein kinase involved in cell signaling; potential effects on antiapoptosis and gene expression |
| ERLIN2[151] | Endoplasmic reticulum lipid raft-associated protein 2 | Endoplasmic reticulum-associated degradation of IP3 receptors |
| EWSR1[152] | EWS RNA-binding protein 1 | Gene expression, cell signaling, RNA processing and transport |
| GRN[153,154] | Progranulin | Regulation of cell growth |
| FGGY[145] | FGGY carbohydrate kinase domain containing | Phosphorylation of carbohydrates |
| HFE[155,156] | Hemochromatosis | Iron absorption |
| ITPR2[157] | Inositol 1,4,5-trisphosphate receptor | Mobilization of intracellular Ca2+ stores |
| KIFAP3[158] | Kinesin-associated protein 3 | Small G-protein |
| MAOB[159] | Monoamine oxidase B | Mitochondrial metabolism of neuroactive and vasoactive amines |
| MAPT[160] | Microtubule-associated protein tau | Supports microtubule assembly and stability |
| NEFH[161,162] | Neurofilament heavy polypeptide | Intracellular axonal and dendritic transport, axonal structure |
| PON1, 2,3[163] | Paraoxonase | Hydrolysis of organophosphates |

(*continued on next page*)

| Table 3 (continued) | | |
|---|---|---|
| **Gene** | **Protein** | **Function** |
| PPARGC1A[164] | Peroxisome proliferator-activated receptor gamma, coactivator 1α | Transcriptional coactivator, regulates genes involved in energy metabolism |
| PRPH[165] | Peripherin | Cytoskeletal protein |
| SMN1[166] | Survival of motor neuron 1 | mRNA processing |
| SPAST[167–169] | Spastin | Microtubule function |
| SS18L1[170,171] | Synovial sarcoma translocation gene on chromosome 18-like 1 | Neuronal chromatin-remodeling, neurite outgrowth |
| TAF15[96] | TATA box binding protein–associated factor | RNA polymerase II gene transcription |
| TMEM106B[172,173] | Transmembrane protein 106B | Lysosomal trafficking, dendrite morphogenesis and maintenance |
| TREM2[174] | Triggering receptor expressed on myeloid cells 2 | Immune system regulation |
| UNC13A[175,176] | Unc-13 homolog A | Synaptic neurotransmitter release |
| VEGF[177] | Vascular endothelial growth factor | Vasculogenesis and angiogenesis factor |
| ZNF512B[178,179] | Zinc finger protein 512B | Regulation of transcription |

*C9ORF72*, *SOD1*, *FUS*, and *TARDBP*, variants of which are found in more than 50% of patients with FALS.[8] Although DNA tests can involve screening for several genes ordered as a group, a case can be made to consider sequential testing based on published frequency data for individual genes, in which case the *C9ORF72* repeat expansion is the most frequent, followed by *SOD1* and then *FUS* and *TARDPB* variants. Clinical DNA test options are anticipated to increase as new ALS genes are identified. Furthermore, as the cost of whole exome and whole genome testing declines, it is likely that these methods may supplant test panels composed of a limited number of disease-linked genes. The likelihood that genetic susceptibility to ALS is polygenic and increasing knowledge of gene variants that modify clinical phenotype will also motivate the use of next-generation screening techniques, to support more efficient and cost-effective evaluation of the genetic risk profile of individual patients.

## SUMMARY

Although genetic mechanisms in ALS pathogenesis seem to play a major role in the development of ALS in a minority of patients, studies suggest that genetic factors at some level are important components of disease risk in most patients with ALS.[8] However, identification of gene variants associated with ALS, regardless of the prevalence or magnitude of associated risk, has informed concepts of the pathogenesis of ALS, aided the identification of therapeutic targets, facilitated research to develop new ALS biomarkers, and supported the establishment of clinical diagnostic tests for ALS-linked genes. It has been suggested that a deeper understanding of the genetic landscape of ALS is key to recognition of environmental risk factors in ALS given the likelihood that sensitivity to environmental risks is influenced by a person's genetic background.[109]

New treatment strategies aimed at blocking expression of ALS gene mutations have successfully completed early phase safety testing in the case of *SOD1* antisense oligonucleotide therapy, and efforts are underway to introduce small molecule and gene therapy targeting expression of the *C9ORF72* repeat expansion.[88,104–106] Results of studies applying increasingly powerful next-generation sequencing methodology to the discovery of new ALS risk genes and work to identify and characterize epigenetic factors contributing to ALS pathogenesis are anticipated. These efforts are likely to contribute significantly to ALS therapy development and continue to move ALS into the realm of individualized medicine.

## REFERENCES


1. Kurland LT, Mulder DW. Epidemiologic investigations of amyotrophic lateral sclerosis. 2. Familial aggregations indicative of dominant inheritance. I. Neurology 1955;5(3):182–96.
2. Kurland LT, Mulder DW. Epidemiologic investigations of amyotrophic lateral sclerosis. 2. Familial aggregations indicative of dominant inheritance. II. Neurology 1955;5(4):249–68.
3. Rosen DR, Siddique T, Patterson D, et al. Mutations in Cu/Zn superoxide dismutase gene are associated with familial amyotrophic lateral sclerosis. Nature 1993; 362(6415):59–62.
4. Su XW, Broach JR, Connor JR, et al. Genetic heterogeneity of amyotrophic lateral sclerosis: implications for clinical practice and research. Muscle Nerve 2014;49(6):786–803 [Review].
5. den Dunnen JT, Antonarakis SE. Mutation nomenclature extensions and suggestions to describe complex mutations: a discussion. Hum Mutat 2000;15(1):7–12.
6. Leblond CS, Kaneb HM, Dion PA, et al. Dissection of genetic factors associated with amyotrophic lateral sclerosis. Exp Neurol 2014;262 Pt B:91–101 [Review].
7. Marangi G, Traynor BJ. Genetic causes of amyotrophic lateral sclerosis: New genetic analysis methodologies entailing new opportunities and challenges. Brain Res 2014;1607:75–93.
8. Renton AE, Chio A, Traynor BJ. State of play in amyotrophic lateral sclerosis genetics. Nat Neurosci 2014;17(1):17–23.
9. Kenna KP, McLaughlin RL, Byrne S, et al. Delineating the genetic heterogeneity of ALS using targeted high-throughput sequencing. J Med Genet 2013;50(11): 776–83 [Research Support, Non-U.S. Gov't].
10. Abrahams S, Leigh PN, Goldstein LH. Cognitive change in ALS: a prospective study. Neurology 2005;64(7):1222–6.
11. Bennion Callister J, Pickering-Brown SM. Pathogenesis/genetics of frontotemporal dementia and how it relates to ALS. Exp Neurol 2014;262 Pt B:84–90 [Review].
12. Andersen PM, Al-Chalabi A. Clinical genetics of amyotrophic lateral sclerosis: what do we really know? Nat Rev Neurol 2011;7(11):603–15.
13. Harms MB, Baloh RH. Clinical neurogenetics: amyotrophic lateral sclerosis. Neurol Clin 2013;31(4):929–50.
14. Byrne S, Bede P, Elamin M, et al. Proposed criteria for familial amyotrophic lateral sclerosis. Amyotroph Lateral Scler 2011;12(3):157–9.
15. Fang F, Kamel F, Lichtenstein P, et al. Familial aggregation of amyotrophic lateral sclerosis. Ann Neurol 2009;66(1):94–9.
16. Hanby MF, Scott KM, Scotton W, et al. The risk to relatives of patients with sporadic amyotrophic lateral sclerosis. Brain 2011;134(Pt 12):3454–7.
17. Wingo TS, Cutler DJ, Yarab N, et al. The heritability of amyotrophic lateral sclerosis in a clinically ascertained United States research registry. PLoS One 2011; 6(11):e27985 [Research Support, U.S. Gov't, Non-P.H.S.].

18. Al-Chalabi A, Fang F, Hanby MF, et al. An estimate of amyotrophic lateral sclerosis heritability using twin data. J Neurol Neurosurg Psychiatry 2010;81(12):1324–6 [Meta-Analysis Research Support, Non-U.S. Gov't].
19. van Blitterswijk M, van Es MA, Hennekam EA, et al. Evidence for an oligogenic basis of amyotrophic lateral sclerosis. Hum Mol Genet 2012;21(17):3776–84.
20. Byrne S, Elamin M, Bede P, et al. Absence of consensus in diagnostic criteria for familial neurodegenerative diseases. J Neurol Neurosurg Psychiatry 2012;83(4):365–7.
21. Dejesus-Hernandez M, Mackenzie IR, Boeve BF, et al. Expanded GGGGCC hexanucleotide repeat in noncoding region of C9ORF72 causes chromosome 9p-linked FTD and ALS. Neuron 2011;72(2):245–56.
22. Renton AE, Majounie E, Waite A, et al. A hexanucleotide repeat expansion in C9ORF72 is the cause of chromosome 9p21-linked ALS-FTD. Neuron 2011;72(2):257–68.
23. Hand CK, Khoris J, Salachas F, et al. A novel locus for familial amyotrophic lateral sclerosis, on chromosome 18q. Am J Hum Genet 2002;70(1):251–6.
24. Hosler BA, Siddique T, Sapp PC, et al. Linkage of familial amyotrophic lateral sclerosis with frontotemporal dementia to chromosome 9q21-q22. Jama 2000;284(13):1664–9.
25. Sapp PC, Hosler BA, McKenna-Yasek D, et al. Identification of two novel loci for dominantly inherited familial amyotrophic lateral sclerosis. Am J Hum Genet 2003;73(2):397–403.
26. Borghero G, Pugliatti M, Marrosu F, et al. Genetic architecture of ALS in Sardinia. Neurobiol Aging 2014;35(12):2882.e7–12.
27. van Es MA, Dahlberg C, Birve A, et al. Large-scale SOD1 mutation screening provides evidence for genetic heterogeneity in amyotrophic lateral sclerosis. J Neurol Neurosurg Psychiatry 2010;81(5):562–6.
28. Gamez J, Caponnetto C, Ferrera L, et al. I112M SOD1 mutation causes ALS with rapid progression and reduced penetrance in four Mediterranean families. Amyotroph Lateral Scler 2011;12(1):70–5.
29. Kabashi E, Valdmanis PN, Dion P, et al. TARDBP mutations in individuals with sporadic and familial amyotrophic lateral sclerosis. Nat Genet 2008;40(5):572–4.
30. Lopate G, Baloh RH, Al-Lozi MT, et al. Familial ALS with extreme phenotypic variability due to the I113T SOD1 mutation. Amyotroph Lateral Scler 2010;11(1–2):232–6.
31. Robberecht W, Aguirre T, Van den Bosch L, et al. D90A heterozygosity in the SOD1 gene is associated with familial and apparently sporadic amyotrophic lateral sclerosis. Neurology 1996;47(5):1336–9.
32. Sreedharan J, Blair IP, Tripathi VB, et al. TDP-43 mutations in familial and sporadic amyotrophic lateral sclerosis. Science 2008;319(5870):1668–72.
33. Vance C, Rogelj B, Hortobagyi T, et al. Mutations in FUS, an RNA processing protein, cause familial amyotrophic lateral sclerosis type 6. Science 2009;323(5918):1208–11.
34. Alexander MD, Traynor BJ, Miller N, et al. "True" sporadic ALS associated with a novel SOD-1 mutation. Ann Neurol 2002;52(5):680–3.
35. Chio A, Calvo A, Moglia C, et al. A de novo missense mutation of the FUS gene in a "true" sporadic ALS case. Neurobiol Aging 2011;32(3):553.e23–6.
36. Dejesus-Hernandez M, Kocerha J, Finch N, et al. De novo truncating FUS gene mutation as a cause of sporadic amyotrophic lateral sclerosis. Hum Mutat 2010;31(5):E1377–89.

37. Majounie E, Renton AE, Mok K, et al. Frequency of the C9orf72 hexanucleotide repeat expansion in patients with amyotrophic lateral sclerosis and frontotemporal dementia: a cross-sectional study. Lancet Neurol 2012;11(4):323–30.
38. Boeve BF, Boylan KB, Graff-Radford NR, et al. Characterization of frontotemporal dementia and/or amyotrophic lateral sclerosis associated with the GGGGCC repeat expansion in C9ORF72. Brain 2012;135(Pt 3):765–83.
39. Hensman Moss DJ, Poulter M, Beck J, et al. C9orf72 expansions are the most common genetic cause of Huntington disease phenocopies. Neurology 2014; 82(4):292–9.
40. O'Dowd S, Curtin D, Waite AJ, et al. C9ORF72 expansion in amyotrophic lateral sclerosis/frontotemporal dementia also causes parkinsonism. Mov Disord 2012; 27(8):1072–4.
41. van Rheenen W, van Blitterswijk M, Huisman MH, et al. Hexanucleotide repeat expansions in C9ORF72 in the spectrum of motor neuron diseases. Neurology 2012;79(9):878–82.
42. Byrne S, Elamin M, Bede P, et al. Cognitive and clinical characteristics of patients with amyotrophic lateral sclerosis carrying a C9orf72 repeat expansion: a population-based cohort study. Lancet Neurol 2012;11(3):232–40.
43. Chio A, Borghero G, Restagno G, et al. Clinical characteristics of patients with familial amyotrophic lateral sclerosis carrying the pathogenic GGGGCC hexanucleotide repeat expansion of C9ORF72. Brain 2012;135(Pt 3):784–93.
44. Rohrer JD, Isaacs AM, Mizielinska S, et al. C9orf72 expansions in frontotemporal dementia and amyotrophic lateral sclerosis. Lancet Neurol 2015;14(3):291–301 [Review].
45. Gendron TF, Belzil VV, Zhang YJ, et al. Mechanisms of toxicity in C9FTLD/ALS. Acta Neuropathol 2014;127(3):359–76.
46. Mizielinska S, Isaacs AM. C9orf72 amyotrophic lateral sclerosis and frontotemporal dementia: gain or loss of function? Curr Opin Neurol 2014;27(5): 515–23.
47. Mackenzie IR, Arzberger T, Kremmer E, et al. Dipeptide repeat protein pathology in C9ORF72 mutation cases: clinico-pathological correlations. Acta Neuropathol 2013;126(6):859–79 [Research Support, Non-U.S. Gov't].
48. Gendron TF, Bieniek KF, Zhang YJ, et al. Antisense transcripts of the expanded C9ORF72 hexanucleotide repeat form nuclear RNA foci and undergo repeat-associated non-ATG translation in c9FTD/ALS. Acta Neuropathol 2013;126(6): 829–44.
49. Brettschneider J, Del Tredici K, Toledo JB, et al. Stages of pTDP-43 pathology in amyotrophic lateral sclerosis. Ann Neurol 2013;74(1):20–38 [Research Support, N.I.H., Extramural Research Support, Non-U.S. Gov't].
50. Cooper-Knock J, Hewitt C, Highley JR, et al. Clinico-pathological features in amyotrophic lateral sclerosis with expansions in C9ORF72. Brain 2012;135(Pt 3):751–64.
51. Murray ME, Dejesus-Hernandez M, Rutherford NJ, et al. Clinical and neuropathologic heterogeneity of c9FTD/ALS associated with hexanucleotide repeat expansion in C9ORF72. Acta Neuropathol 2011;122(6):673–90.
52. van Blitterswijk M, DeJesus-Hernandez M, Niemantsverdriet E, et al. Association between repeat sizes and clinical and pathological characteristics in carriers of C9ORF72 repeat expansions (Xpansize-72): a cross-sectional cohort study. Lancet Neurol 2013;12(10):978–88.
53. Andersen PM, Forsgren L, Binzer M, et al. Autosomal recessive adult-onset amyotrophic lateral sclerosis associated with homozygosity for Asp90Ala

CuZn-superoxide dismutase mutation. A clinical and genealogical study of 36 patients. Brain 1996;119(Pt 4):1153–72.
54. Andersen PM. Amyotrophic lateral sclerosis associated with mutations in the CuZn superoxide dismutase gene. Curr Neurol Neurosci Rep 2006;6(1): 37–46.
55. Cudkowicz ME, McKenna-Yasek D, Sapp PE, et al. Epidemiology of mutations in superoxide dismutase in amyotrophic lateral sclerosis. Ann Neurol 1997;41(2): 210–21.
56. Cudkowicz ME, McKenna-Yasek D, Chen C, et al. Limited corticospinal tract involvement in amyotrophic lateral sclerosis subjects with the A4V mutation in the copper/zinc superoxide dismutase gene. Ann Neurol 1998;43(6):703–10.
57. Felbecker A, Camu W, Valdmanis PN, et al. Four familial ALS pedigrees discordant for two SOD1 mutations: are all SOD1 mutations pathogenic? J Neurol Neurosurg Psychiatry 2010;81(5):572–7.
58. Gene_Tests. Web site with information on facilities that offer DNA testing for ALS linked gene variants. Available at: https://www.genetests.org/. Accessed August 5, 2015.
59. Neumann M, Sampathu DM, Kwong LK, et al. Ubiquitinated TDP-43 in frontotemporal lobar degeneration and amyotrophic lateral sclerosis. Science 2006; 314(5796):130–3.
60. Chen-Plotkin AS, Lee VM, Trojanowski JQ. TAR DNA-binding protein 43 in neurodegenerative disease. Nat Rev Neurol 2010;6(4):211–20.
61. Scotter EL, Chen HJ, Shaw CE. TDP-43 proteinopathy and ALS: insights into disease mechanisms and therapeutic targets. Neurotherapeutics 2015;12(2): 352–63.
62. Benajiba L, Le Ber I, Camuzat A, et al. TARDBP mutations in motoneuron disease with frontotemporal lobar degeneration. Ann Neurol 2009;65(4):470–3.
63. Borroni B, Bonvicini C, Alberici A, et al. Mutation within TARDBP leads to frontotemporal dementia without motor neuron disease. Hum Mutat 2009;30(11):E974–83.
64. Corcia P, Valdmanis P, Millecamps S, et al. Phenotype and genotype analysis in amyotrophic lateral sclerosis with TARDBP gene mutations. Neurology 2012; 78(19):1519–26.
65. Quadri M, Cossu G, Saddi V, et al. Broadening the phenotype of TARDBP mutations: the TARDBP Ala382Thr mutation and Parkinson's disease in Sardinia. Neurogenetics 2011;12(3):203–9.
66. Rayaprolu S, Fujioka S, Traynor S, et al. TARDBP mutations in Parkinson's disease. Parkinsonism Relat Disord 2013;19(3):312–5.
67. Hewitt C, Kirby J, Highley JR, et al. Novel FUS/TLS mutations and pathology in familial and sporadic amyotrophic lateral sclerosis. Arch Neurol 2010;67(4): 455–61.
68. Kwiatkowski TJ Jr, Bosco DA, Leclerc AL, et al. Mutations in the FUS/TLS gene on chromosome 16 cause familial amyotrophic lateral sclerosis. Science 2009; 323(5918):1205–8.
69. Deng H, Gao K, Jankovic J. The role of FUS gene variants in neurodegenerative diseases. Nat Rev Neurol 2014;10(6):337–48.
70. Calvo A, Moglia C, Canosa A, et al. De novo nonsense mutation of the FUS gene in an apparently familial amyotrophic lateral sclerosis case. Neurobiol Aging 2014;35(6):1513.e7–11.
71. Kim YE, Oh KW, Kwon MJ, et al. De novo FUS mutations in 2 Korean patients with sporadic amyotrophic lateral sclerosis. Neurobiol Aging 2015;36(3): 1604.e17–9.

72. Robertson J, Bilbao J, Zinman L, et al. A novel double mutation in FUS gene causing sporadic ALS. Neurobiol Aging 2011;32(3):553.e27–30.
73. Zou ZY, Cui LY, Sun Q, et al. De novo FUS gene mutations are associated with juvenile-onset sporadic amyotrophic lateral sclerosis in China. Neurobiol Aging 2013;34(4):1312.e1–8.
74. Blair IP, Williams KL, Warraich ST, et al. FUS mutations in amyotrophic lateral sclerosis: clinical, pathological, neurophysiological and genetic analysis. J Neurol Neurosurg Psychiatry 2010;81(6):639–45.
75. Millecamps S, Salachas F, Cazeneuve C, et al. SOD1, ANG, VAPB, TARDBP, and FUS mutations in familial amyotrophic lateral sclerosis: genotype-phenotype correlations. J Med Genet 2010;47(8):554–60.
76. Tateishi T, Hokonohara T, Yamasaki R, et al. Multiple system degeneration with basophilic inclusions in Japanese ALS patients with FUS mutation. Acta Neuropathol 2010;119(3):355–64.
77. Baumer D, Hilton D, Paine SM, et al. Juvenile ALS with basophilic inclusions is a FUS proteinopathy with FUS mutations. Neurology 2010;75(7):611–8.
78. Huang EJ, Zhang J, Geser F, et al. Extensive FUS-immunoreactive pathology in juvenile amyotrophic lateral sclerosis with basophilic inclusions. Brain Pathol 2010;20(6):1069–76.
79. Neumann M, Rademakers R, Roeber S, et al. A new subtype of frontotemporal lobar degeneration with FUS pathology. Brain 2009;132(Pt 11):2922–31.
80. Matsuoka T, Fujii N, Kondo A, et al. An autopsied case of sporadic adult-onset amyotrophic lateral sclerosis with FUS-positive basophilic inclusions. Neuropathology 2011;31(1):71–6.
81. Munoz DG, Neumann M, Kusaka H, et al. FUS pathology in basophilic inclusion body disease. Acta Neuropathol 2009;118(5):617–27.
82. Bettencourt C, Houlden H. Exome sequencing uncovers hidden pathways in familial and sporadic ALS. Nat Neurosci 2015;18(5):611–3.
83. Fecto F, Siddique T. UBQLN2/P62 cellular recycling pathways in amyotrophic lateral sclerosis and frontotemporal dementia. Muscle Nerve 2012;45(2):157–62.
84. Johnson JO, Pioro EP, Boehringer A, et al. Mutations in the Matrin 3 gene cause familial amyotrophic lateral sclerosis. Nat Neurosci 2014;17(5):664–6.
85. Kim HJ, Kim NC, Wang YD, et al. Mutations in prion-like domains in hnRNPA2B1 and hnRNPA1 cause multisystem proteinopathy and ALS. Nature 2013;495(7442):467–73.
86. Cooper-Knock J, Walsh MJ, Higginbottom A, et al. Sequestration of multiple RNA recognition motif-containing proteins by C9orf72 repeat expansions. Brain 2014;137(Pt 7):2040–51.
87. Donnelly CJ, Zhang PW, Pham JT, et al. RNA toxicity from the ALS/FTD C9ORF72 expansion is mitigated by antisense intervention. Neuron 2013;80(2):415–28.
88. Lagier-Tourenne C, Baughn M, Rigo F, et al. Targeted degradation of sense and antisense C9orf72 RNA foci as therapy for ALS and frontotemporal degeneration. Proc Natl Acad Sci U S A 2013;110(47):E4530–9.
89. Lee YB, Chen HJ, Peres JN, et al. Hexanucleotide repeats in ALS/FTD form length-dependent RNA foci, sequester RNA binding proteins, and are neurotoxic. Cell Rep 2013;5(5):1178–86.
90. Deng HX, Chen W, Hong ST, et al. Mutations in UBQLN2 cause dominant X-linked juvenile and adult-onset ALS and ALS/dementia. Nature 2011;477(7363):211–5.

91. Cirulli ET, Lasseigne BN, Petrovski S, et al. Exome sequencing in amyotrophic lateral sclerosis identifies risk genes and pathways. Science 2015;347(6229):1436–41.
92. Freischmidt A, Wieland T, Richter B, et al. Haploinsufficiency of TBK1 causes familial ALS and fronto-temporal dementia. Nat Neurosci 2015;18(5):631–6.
93. Johnson JO, Mandrioli J, Benatar M, et al. Exome sequencing reveals VCP mutations as a cause of familial ALS. Neuron 2010;68(5):857–64.
94. Murayama S. Clinical and pathological characteristics of FUS/TLS-associated amyotrophic lateral sclerosis (ALS). Rinsho Shinkeigaku 2010;50(11):948–50 [in Japanese].
95. Benatar M, Wuu J, Fernandez C, et al. Motor neuron involvement in multisystem proteinopathy: implications for ALS. Neurology 2013;80(20):1874–80.
96. Couthouis J, Hart MP, Shorter J, et al. Feature article: A yeast functional screen predicts new candidate ALS disease genes. Proc Natl Acad Sci U S A 2011; 108(52):20881–90.
97. Martin LJ, Wong M. Aberrant regulation of DNA methylation in amyotrophic lateral sclerosis: a new target of disease mechanisms. Neurotherapeutics 2013;10(4):722–33.
98. Figueroa-Romero C, Hur J, Bender DE, et al. Identification of epigenetically altered genes in sporadic amyotrophic lateral sclerosis. PLoS ONE 2012; 7(12):e52672.
99. Morahan JM, Yu B, Trent RJ, et al. A genome-wide analysis of brain DNA methylation identifies new candidate genes for sporadic amyotrophic lateral sclerosis. Amyotroph Lateral Scler 2009;10(5–6):418–29.
100. Belzil VV, Bauer PO, Prudencio M, et al. Reduced C9orf72 gene expression in c9FTD/ALS is caused by histone trimethylation, an epigenetic event detectable in blood. Acta Neuropathol 2013;126(6):895–905.
101. Liu EY, Russ J, Wu K, et al. C9orf72 hypermethylation protects against repeat expansion-associated pathology in ALS/FTD. Acta Neuropathol 2014;128(4): 525–41.
102. Russ J, Liu EY, Wu K, et al. Hypermethylation of repeat expanded C9orf72 is a clinical and molecular disease modifier. Acta Neuropathol 2015;129(1):39–52.
103. Kalmar B, Lu CH, Greensmith L. The role of heat shock proteins in amyotrophic lateral sclerosis: the therapeutic potential of arimoclomol. Pharmacol Ther 2014; 141(1):40–54.
104. Miller TM, Pestronk A, David W, et al. An antisense oligonucleotide against SOD1 delivered intrathecally for patients with SOD1 familial amyotrophic lateral sclerosis: a phase 1, randomised, first-in-man study. Lancet Neurol 2013;12(5):435–42.
105. Sareen D, O'Rourke JG, Meera P, et al. Targeting RNA foci in iPSC-derived motor neurons from ALS patients with a C9ORF72 repeat expansion. Sci Transl Med 2013;5(208):208ra149.
106. Su Z, Zhang Y, Gendron TF, et al. Discovery of a biomarker and lead small molecules to target r(GGGGCC)-associated defects in c9FTD/ALS. Neuron 2014; 83(5):1043–50.
107. Majounie E, Abramzon Y, Renton AE, et al. Repeat expansion in C9ORF72 in Alzheimer's disease. N Engl J Med 2012;366(3):283–4.
108. Chio A, Battistini S, Calvo A, et al. Genetic counselling in ALS: facts, uncertainties and clinical suggestions. J Neurol Neurosurg Psychiatry 2014;85(5): 478–85.
109. Al-Chalabi A, Hardiman O. The epidemiology of ALS: a conspiracy of genes, environment and time. Nat Rev Neurol 2013;9(11):617–28 [Research Support, Non-U.S. Gov't Review].

110. Hadano S, Hand CK, Osuga H, et al. A gene encoding a putative GTPase regulator is mutated in familial amyotrophic lateral sclerosis 2. Nat Genet 2001;29(2):166–73.
111. Greenway MJ, Andersen PM, Russ C, et al. ANG mutations segregate with familial and 'sporadic' amyotrophic lateral sclerosis. Nat Genet 2006;38(4):411–3.
112. van Es MA, Schelhaas HJ, van Vught PW, et al. Angiogenin variants in Parkinson disease and amyotrophic lateral sclerosis. Ann Neurol 2011;70(6):964–73.
113. Daoud H, Belzil V, Martins S, et al. Association of long ATXN2 CAG repeat sizes with increased risk of amyotrophic lateral sclerosis. Arch Neurol 2011;68(6):739–42.
114. Elden AC, Kim HJ, Hart MP, et al. Ataxin-2 intermediate-length polyglutamine expansions are associated with increased risk for ALS. Nature 2010;466(7310):1069–75.
115. Bannwarth S, Ait-El-Mkadem S, Chaussenot A, et al. A mitochondrial origin for frontotemporal dementia and amyotrophic lateral sclerosis through CHCHD10 involvement. Brain 2014;137(Pt 8):2329–45.
116. Johnson JO, Glynn SM, Gibbs JR, et al. Mutations in the CHCHD10 gene are a common cause of familial amyotrophic lateral sclerosis. Brain 2014;137(Pt 12):e311.
117. Parkinson N, Ince PG, Smith MO, et al. ALS phenotypes with mutations in CHMP2B (charged multivesicular body protein 2B). Neurology 2006;67(6):1074–7.
118. Lesage S, Le Ber I, Condroyer C, et al. C9orf72 repeat expansions are a rare genetic cause of parkinsonism. Brain 2013;136(Pt 2):385–91.
119. Snowden JS, Rollinson S, Thompson JC, et al. Distinct clinical and pathological characteristics of frontotemporal dementia associated with C9ORF72 mutations. Brain 2012;135(Pt 3):693–708.
120. Mitchell J, Paul P, Chen HJ, et al. Familial amyotrophic lateral sclerosis is associated with a mutation in D-amino acid oxidase. Proc Natl Acad Sci U S A 2010;107(16):7556–61.
121. Münch C, Rosenbohm A, Sperfeld A-D, et al. Heterozygous R1101K mutation of the *DCTN1* gene in a family with ALS and FTD. Ann Neurol 2005;58(5):777–80.
122. Munch C, Sedlmeier R, Meyer T, et al. Point mutations of the p150 subunit of dynactin (DCTN1) gene in ALS. Neurology 2004;63(4):724–6.
123. Vilarino-Guell C, Wider C, Soto-Ortolaza AI, et al. Characterization of DCTN1 genetic variability in neurodegeneration. Neurology 2009;72(23):2024–8.
124. Chow CY, Landers JE, Bergren SK, et al. Deleterious variants of FIG4, a phosphoinositide phosphatase, in patients with ALS. Am J Hum Genet 2009;84(1):85–8.
125. Maruyama H, Morino H, Ito H, et al. Mutations of optineurin in amyotrophic lateral sclerosis. Nature 2010;465(7295):223–6.
126. Wu CH, Fallini C, Ticozzi N, et al. Mutations in the profilin 1 gene cause familial amyotrophic lateral sclerosis. Nature 2012;488(7412):499–503.
127. Chen YZ, Bennett CL, Huynh HM, et al. DNA/RNA helicase gene mutations in a form of juvenile amyotrophic lateral sclerosis (ALS4). Am J Hum Genet 2004;74(6):1128–35.
128. Al-Saif A, Al-Mohanna F, Bohlega S. A mutation in sigma-1 receptor causes juvenile amyotrophic lateral sclerosis. Ann Neurol 2011;70(6):913–9.
129. Belzil VV, Daoud H, Camu W, et al. Genetic analysis of SIGMAR1 as a cause of familial ALS with dementia. Eur J Hum Genet 2013;21(2):237–9.
130. Fukunaga K, Shinoda Y, Tagashira H. The role of SIGMAR1 gene mutation and mitochondrial dysfunction in amyotrophic lateral sclerosis. J Pharmacol Sci 2015;127(1):36–41.

131. Daoud H, Zhou S, Noreau A, et al. Exome sequencing reveals SPG11 mutations causing juvenile ALS. Neurobiol Aging 2012;33(4):839.e5–9.
132. Orlacchio A, Babalini C, Borreca A, et al. SPATACSIN mutations cause autosomal recessive juvenile amyotrophic lateral sclerosis. Brain 2010;133(Pt 2): 591–8.
133. Fecto F, Yan J, Vemula SP, et al. SQSTM1 mutations in familial and sporadic amyotrophic lateral sclerosis. Arch Neurol 2011;68(11):1440–6.
134. Yang Y, Tang L, Zhang N, et al. Six SQSTM1 mutations in a Chinese amyotrophic lateral sclerosis cohort. Amyotroph Lateral Scler Frontotemporal Degener 2015; 24:1–7.
135. Smith BN, Ticozzi N, Fallini C, et al. Exome-wide rare variant analysis identifies TUBA4A mutations associated with familial ALS. Neuron 2014;84(2): 324–31.
136. Nishimura AL, Mitne-Neto M, Silva HC, et al. A mutation in the vesicle-trafficking protein VAPB causes late-onset spinal muscular atrophy and amyotrophic lateral sclerosis. Am J Hum Genet 2004;75(5):822–31.
137. Zetterberg H, Jacobsson J, Rosengren L, et al. Association of APOE with age at onset of sporadic amyotrophic lateral sclerosis. J Neurol Sci 2008;273(1–2): 67–9.
138. Droppelmann CA, Wang J, Campos-Melo D, et al. Detection of a novel frameshift mutation and regions with homozygosis within ARHGEF28 gene in familial amyotrophic lateral sclerosis. Amyotroph Lateral Scler Frontotemporal Degener 2013;14(5–6):444–51.
139. Ma Y, Tang L, Chen L, et al. ARHGEF28 gene exon 6/intron 6 junction mutations in Chinese amyotrophic lateral sclerosis cohort. Amyotroph Lateral Scler Frontotemporal Degener 2014;15(3–4):309–11.
140. Gros-Louis F, Andersen PM, Dupre N, et al. Chromogranin B P413L variant as risk factor and modifier of disease onset for amyotrophic lateral sclerosis. Proc Natl Acad Sci U S A 2009;106(51):21777–82.
141. Sabatelli M, Eusebi F, Al-Chalabi A, et al. Rare missense variants of neuronal nicotinic acetylcholine receptor altering receptor function are associated with sporadic amyotrophic lateral sclerosis. Hum Mol Genet 2009;18(20): 3997–4006.
142. Sabatelli M, Lattante S, Conte A, et al. Replication of association of CHRNA4 rare variants with sporadic amyotrophic lateral sclerosis: the Italian multicentre study. Amyotroph Lateral Scler 2012;13(6):580–4.
143. Lopez-Lopez A, Gamez J, Syriani E, et al. CX3CR1 is a modifying gene of survival and progression in amyotrophic lateral sclerosis. PLoS ONE 2014;9(5): e96528.
144. Li XG, Zhang JH, Xie MQ, et al. Association between DPP6 polymorphism and the risk of sporadic amyotrophic lateral sclerosis in Chinese patients. Chin Med J (Engl) 2009;122(24):2989–92.
145. Daoud H, Valdmanis PN, Dion PA, et al. Analysis of DPP6 and FGGY as candidate genes for amyotrophic lateral sclerosis. Amyotroph Lateral Scler 2010; 11(4):389–91.
146. van Es MA, van Vught PW, Blauw HM, et al. Genetic variation in DPP6 is associated with susceptibility to amyotrophic lateral sclerosis. Nat Genet 2008;40(1): 29–31.
147. Blasco H, Bernard-Marissal N, Vourc'h P, et al. A rare motor neuron deleterious missense mutation in the DPYSL3 (CRMP4) gene is associated with ALS. Hum Mutat 2013;34(7):953–60.

148. Simpson CL, Lemmens R, Miskiewicz K, et al. Variants of the elongator protein 3 (ELP3) gene are associated with motor neuron degeneration. Hum Mol Genet 2009;18(3):472–81.
149. Van Hoecke A, Schoonaert L, Lemmens R, et al. EPHA4 is a disease modifier of amyotrophic lateral sclerosis in animal models and in humans. Nat Med 2012; 18(9):1418–22.
150. Takahashi Y, Fukuda Y, Yoshimura J, et al. ERBB4 mutations that disrupt the neuregulin-ErbB4 pathway cause amyotrophic lateral sclerosis type 19. Am J Hum Genet 2013;93(5):900–5.
151. Al-Saif A, Bohlega S, Al-Mohanna F. Loss of ERLIN2 function leads to juvenile primary lateral sclerosis. Ann Neurol 2012;72(4):510–6.
152. Couthouis J, Hart MP, Erion R, et al. Evaluating the role of the FUS/TLS-related gene EWSR1 in amyotrophic lateral sclerosis. Hum Mol Genet 2012;21(13): 2899–911.
153. Cannon A, Fujioka S, Rutherford NJ, et al. Clinicopathologic variability of the GRN A9D mutation, including amyotrophic lateral sclerosis. Neurology 2013; 80(19):1771–7.
154. Sleegers K, Brouwers N, Maurer-Stroh S, et al. Progranulin genetic variability contributes to amyotrophic lateral sclerosis. Neurology 2008;71(4):253–9.
155. Goodall EF, Greenway MJ, van Marion I, et al. Association of the H63D polymorphism in the hemochromatosis gene with sporadic ALS. Neurology 2005;65(6): 934–7.
156. He X, Lu X, Hu J, et al. H63D polymorphism in the hemochromatosis gene is associated with sporadic amyotrophic lateral sclerosis in China. Eur J Neurol 2011;18(2):359–61.
157. van Es MA, Van Vught PW, Blauw HM, et al. ITPR2 as a susceptibility gene in sporadic amyotrophic lateral sclerosis: a genome-wide association study. Lancet Neurol 2007;6(10):869–77.
158. Landers JE, Melki J, Meininger V, et al. Reduced expression of the kinesin-associated protein 3 (KIFAP3) gene increases survival in sporadic amyotrophic lateral sclerosis. Proc Natl Acad Sci U S A 2009;106(22):9004–9.
159. Orru S, Mascia V, Casula M, et al. Association of monoamine oxidase B alleles with age at onset in amyotrophic lateral sclerosis. Neuromuscul Disord 1999; 9(8):593–7.
160. Fang P, Xu W, Wu C, et al. MAPT as a predisposing gene for sporadic amyotrophic lateral sclerosis in the Chinese Han population. Neural Regen Res 2013; 8(33):3116–23.
161. Al-Chalabi A, Andersen PM, Nilsson P, et al. Deletions of the heavy neurofilament subunit tail in amyotrophic lateral sclerosis. Hum Mol Genet 1999;8(2): 157–64.
162. Figlewicz DA, Krizus A, Martinoli MG, et al. Variants of the heavy neurofilament subunit are associated with the development of amyotrophic lateral sclerosis. Hum Mol Genet 1994;3(10):1757–61.
163. Wills AM, Cronin S, Slowik A, et al. A large-scale international meta-analysis of paraoxonase gene polymorphisms in sporadic ALS. Neurology 2009;73(1): 16–24.
164. Eschbach J, Schwalenstocker B, Soyal SM, et al. PGC-1alpha is a male-specific disease modifier of human and experimental amyotrophic lateral sclerosis. Hum Mol Genet 2013;22(17):3477–84.
165. Leung CL, He CZ, Kaufmann P, et al. A pathogenic peripherin gene mutation in a patient with amyotrophic lateral sclerosis. Brain Pathol 2004;14(3):290–6.

166. Corcia P, Mayeux-Portas V, Khoris J, et al. Abnormal SMN1 gene copy number is a susceptibility factor for amyotrophic lateral sclerosis. Ann Neurol 2002;51(2): 243–6.
167. Brugman F, Wokke JH, Scheffer H, et al. Spastin mutations in sporadic adult-onset upper motor neuron syndromes. Ann Neurol 2005;58(6):865–9.
168. Meyer T, Schwan A, Dullinger JS, et al. Early-onset ALS with long-term survival associated with spastin gene mutation. Neurology 2005;65(1):141–3.
169. Munch C, Rolfs A, Meyer T. Heterozygous S44L missense change of the spastin gene in amyotrophic lateral sclerosis. Amyotroph Lateral Scler 2008;9(4):251–3.
170. Chesi A, Staahl BT, Jovicic A, et al. Exome sequencing to identify de novo mutations in sporadic ALS trios. Nat Neurosci 2013;16(7):851–5.
171. Teyssou E, Vandenberghe N, Moigneu C, et al. Genetic analysis of SS18L1 in French amyotrophic lateral sclerosis. Neurobiol Aging 2014;35(5):1213.e9–12.
172. Gallagher MD, Suh E, Grossman M, et al. TMEM106B is a genetic modifier of frontotemporal lobar degeneration with C9orf72 hexanucleotide repeat expansions. Acta Neuropathol 2014;127(3):407–18.
173. Vass R, Ashbridge E, Geser F, et al. Risk genotypes at TMEM106B are associated with cognitive impairment in amyotrophic lateral sclerosis. Acta Neuropathol 2011;121(3):373–80.
174. Cady J, Koval ED, Benitez BA, et al. TREM2 variant p.R47H as a risk factor for sporadic amyotrophic lateral sclerosis. JAMA Neurol 2014;71(4):449–53.
175. Chio A, Mora G, Restagno G, et al. UNC13A influences survival in Italian amyotrophic lateral sclerosis patients: a population-based study. Neurobiol Aging 2013;34(1):357.e1–5.
176. Diekstra FP, van Vught PW, van Rheenen W, et al. UNC13A is a modifier of survival in amyotrophic lateral sclerosis. Neurobiol Aging 2012;33(3):630.e3–8.
177. Lambrechts D, Poesen K, Fernandez-Santiago R, et al. Meta-analysis of vascular endothelial growth factor variations in amyotrophic lateral sclerosis: increased susceptibility in male carriers of the -2578AA genotype. J Med Genet 2009;46(12):840–6.
178. Iida A, Takahashi A, Kubo M, et al. A functional variant in ZNF512B is associated with susceptibility to amyotrophic lateral sclerosis in Japanese. Hum Mol Genet 2011;20(18):3684–92.
179. Tetsuka S, Morita M, Iida A, et al. ZNF512B gene is a prognostic factor in patients with amyotrophic lateral sclerosis. J Neurol Sci 2013;324(1–2):163–6.

# Spinal Muscular Atrophy

Stephen J. Kolb, MD, PhD[a,b,*], John T. Kissel, MD[a]

**KEYWORDS**

• Spinal muscular atrophy • Motor neuron • Survival motor neuron gene • *SMN1* • *SMN2*

**KEY POINTS**

- Spinal muscular atrophy (SMA) is the most common genetic cause of infant mortality and is characterized by proximal muscular weakness.
- Humans have 2 nearly identical inverted SMN genes (*SMN1* and *SMN2*) on chromosome 5q13 and homozygous deletion of the SMN1 gene results in SMA.
- The *SMN2* gene produces mostly a shortened, unstable SMN messenger RNA (mRNA) and, through alternative splicing, a relatively small amount of full-length, functional SMN mRNA.
- The *SMN2* gene copy number is a good prognostic biomarker of SMA clinical severity.
- Clinical management of SMA is supportive; however, current and planned clinical trials designed to increase SMN expression levels in motor neurons hold great promise.

## INCIDENCE

The incidence of SMA is 1 in 11,000 live births.[1]

## PREVALENCE

The prevalence of the carrier state is approximately 1 in 54.[1]

## SEVERITY

The clinical severity of spinal muscular atrophy (SMA) correlates inversely with *SMN2* gene copy number and varies from an extreme weakness and paraplegia of infancy to a mild proximal weakness of adulthood.

---

S.J. Kolb has received compensation for consulting from Biogen, F. Hoffman-La Roche, Jeffries LLC, and the Deerfield Institute. He is supported by NIH Grant K08NS067282; U01NS079163.
[a] Department of Neurology, The Ohio State University Wexner Medical Center, Columbus, OH, USA; [b] Department of Biological Chemistry and Pharmacology, The Ohio State University Wexner Medical Center, Columbus, OH 43210-1228, USA
* Corresponding author. Department of Neurology, The Ohio State University Wexner Medical Center, Hamilton Hall, Room 337B, 1645 Neil Avenue, Columbus, OH 43210-1228.
*E-mail address:* stephen.kolb@osumc.edu

Neurol Clin 33 (2015) 831–846
http://dx.doi.org/10.1016/j.ncl.2015.07.004 neurologic.theclinics.com
0733-8619/15/$ – see front matter 

## NATURAL HISTORY

The natural history of SMA is complex and variable. For this reason, clinical subgroups have been defined based upon best motor function attainment during development. Type 1 SMA infants never sit independently. Type 2 SMA children sit at some point during their childhood, but never walk independently. Type 3 SMA children and adults are able to walk independently at some point in their childhood.

## INTRODUCTION

The term "spinal muscular atrophy (SMA)" refers to a group of genetic disorders all characterized by degeneration of anterior horn cells and resultant muscle atrophy and weakness. The most common SMA, accounting for more than 95% of cases, is an autosomal-recessive disorder that results from a homozygous deletion or mutation in the 5q13 survival of motor neuron (*SMN1*) gene. In a large, multiethnic study to test the feasibility of high-throughput genetic testing for SMA carriers, the overall carrier frequency was 1 in 54 with an incidence of 1 in 11,000 live births.[1] The severity of SMA is highly variable and the clinical features can be classified into 4 main phenotypes on the basis of age of onset and maximum motor function achieved.[2] There is no cure for SMA; however, an understanding of the molecular genetics of SMA has led to the development of preclinical models and numerous potential therapeutic approaches.[3–5] There is great excitement in the SMA field because these therapeutic approaches have recently entered early phase clinical trials.

Paired with the excitement of an active therapeutic pipeline has been a focus on understanding the natural history of this disorder as well as early diagnosis and clinical intervention. This has led to the development of clinical standards of care.[6,7] The natural history of the most severe form of SMA (type 1) has been the subject of particular attention and is characterized by a rapid loss of motor and respiratory function in the first year of life.[8] Studies have shown that survival beyond 1 year in these infants can be improved to 70% or more with proactive use of noninvasive ventilatory support and enteral feeding.[9–11] In contrast, studies on the natural history of the milder forms of SMA (types 2 and 3) have shown little decrease in motor and respiratory function during the course of a single year.[12,13]

This article focuses on the clinical manifestations of SMA and how it relates to the molecular genetics and pathogenesis of the disease. We discuss genetic testing and review the clinical management of SMA with particular attention to aspects of care and methods of assessment that can be used in clinical practice and as clinical trial outcome measures. We also review current therapeutic approaches and highlight current controversies in clinical management, newborn screening, and clinical trial design.

## CLINICAL FEATURES

The predominant clinical features of SMA are muscle weakness and atrophy. Weakness is usually symmetric, with proximal muscles more affected than distal groups as in NP7.[14] Over the last 125 years, reports detailing the clinical manifestations and wide range of clinical severity have all recognized and emphasized the seminal pathology as anterior horn cell degeneration, as well as the pertinent clinical features of symmetric, proximal predominant extremity weakness that also affects axial, intercostal, and bulbar musculature.[15] The multiple described phenotypes were eventually formalized into a classification scheme at an International Consortium on Spinal Muscular Atrophy sponsored by the Muscular Dystrophy Association in 1991.[16] This classification highlighted 3 SMA types based on the highest level of motor function (ie, sitting or standing) and age of onset. Subsequent modifications divided the type 3 category by age of onset, added a type 4 for adult-onset cases, and included a type 0 for patients with prenatal onset and death within weeks.[17,18] Although there are degrees of severity even within an individual type, and as many as 25% of patients elude precise classification, this scheme remains relevant in the genetic era and provides useful clinical and prognostic information (**Table 1**).

### *Spinal Muscular Atrophy Type 0*

SMA type 0 is used to describe neonates who present with severe weakness and hypotonia with a history of decreased fetal movements. In this case, the weakness is probably of prenatal onset. On examination, infants with type 0 may have areflexia, facial diplegia, atrial septal defects, and joint contractures. Respiratory failure is a major concern early on. Life expectancy is reduced and most are unable to survive beyond 6 months of age (see **Table 1**).[19,20]

### *Spinal Muscular Atrophy Type 1*

Infants with type 1 SMA, also known as Werdnig–Hoffman disease, present with hypotonia, poor head control, and reduced or absent tendon reflexes before 6 months of age. By definition, they never achieve the ability to sit unassisted (**Fig. 1**, see **Table 1**). The profound hypotonia can manifest as a "frog-leg" posture when lying and poor to absent head control. The weakness in intercostal muscles, with relative sparing of the diaphragm, produces a bell-shaped chest and a pattern of paradoxic breathing sometimes referred to as "belly breathing." Infants with type 1 SMA develop tongue and swallowing weakness and tongue fasciculations are often present. Facial weakness does develop, although this does not usually manifest early in the course of the disease. As the tongue and pharyngeal muscles weaken, these infants are at risk of aspiration and failure to thrive. Infants with type 1 SMA usually develop respiratory failure before 2 years of life.[8,21,22] Despite the profound weakness, cognition is normal in infants with type 1 SMA are often alert, attentive, and bright at the time of diagnosis.

### *Spinal Muscular Atrophy Type 2*

Children with type 2 SMA are able to sit unassisted at some point during their development; however, they are never able to walk independently (**Fig. 2**; see **Table 1**). This intermediate form of SMA tends to manifest as progressive proximal leg weakness that is greater than weakness in the arms. There is hypotonia and areflexia on examination. Many of the comorbidities in this patient population are related to the

**Table 1**
**Spinal muscular atrophy classification**

| Type | Age of Onset | Highest Function | Natural Age of Death | SMN2 # |
|---|---|---|---|---|
| 0 | Prenatal | Respiratory support | <1 mo | 1 |
| 1 | 0–6 mo | Never sit | <2 y | 2 |
| 2 | <18 mo | Never stand | >2 y | 3,4 |
| 3 | >18 mo | Stand alone | Adult | — |
| 3a | 18 mo–3 y | Stand alone | Adult | 3,4 |
| 3b | >3 y | Stand alone | Adult | 4 |
| 4 | >21 y | Stand alone | Adult | 4–8 |

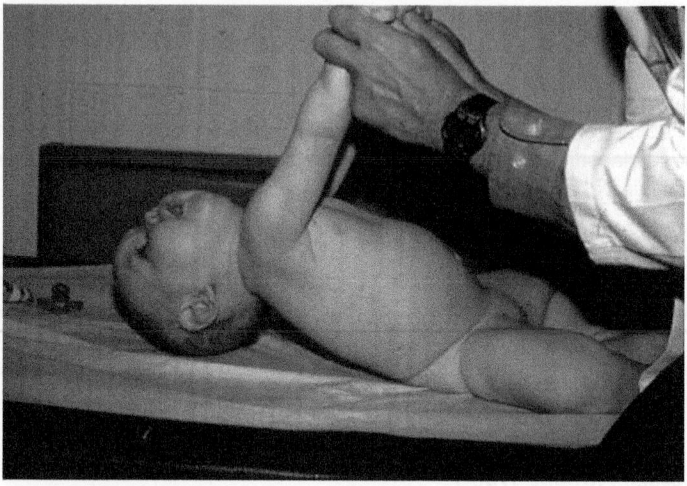

**Fig. 1.** Spinal muscular atrophy type 1.

orthopedic complications of bone and joint development in the setting of muscular weakness, and progressive scoliosis, joint contractures, and ankylosis of the mandible may develop. The combination of scoliosis and intercostal muscle weakness can also result in significant restrictive lung disease. In these children, cognition is normal.[23]

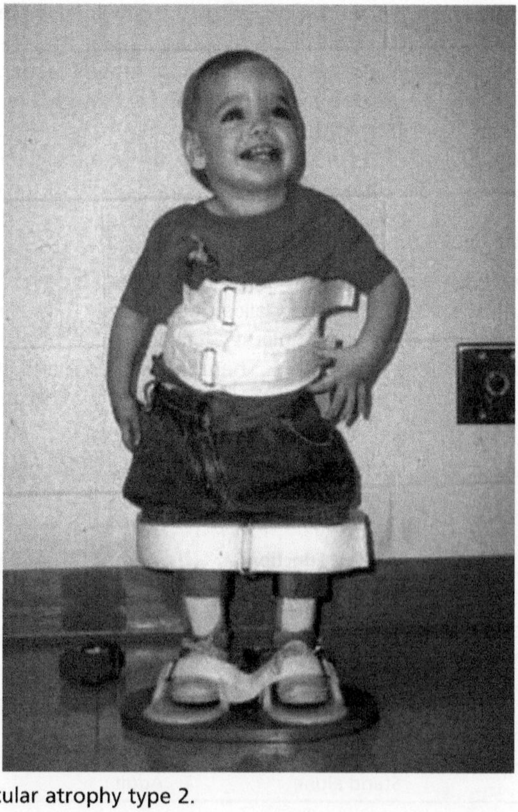

**Fig. 2.** Spinal muscular atrophy type 2.

### Spinal Muscular Atrophy Type 3

Children and adults with type 3 SMA, also referred to as Kugelberg–Welander disease, are able to walk unassisted at some point during their lifetime (**Fig. 3**, see **Table 1**). They present with progressive proximal weakness of the legs more than the arms. The leg weakness may necessitate the need of a wheelchair at some point. Unlike, those with type 2 SMA, these individuals are mostly spared the comorbidities of scoliosis and have little or no respiratory muscle weakness. Cognition and life expectancy are not altered in this group.[18,24]

### Spinal Muscular Atrophy Type 4

At the mild end of the continuum are individuals classified as having SMA type 4. They represent less than 5% of SMA cases and have the mildest form of the disease. These individuals are ambulatory and they are similar to type 3; however, onset is in adulthood, often considered to present at age 30 or older, but can be of juvenile onset.[22,25]

**Case Vignette**

*This 37-year-old police officer presented with a chief complaint of leg weakness. He dated his symptoms back 12 months when he noticed difficulty going up stairs and getting out of deep chairs. To more detailed questioning, he recalled that 10 years previously while in the police academy he had had to push off his knees with his arms to stand up after shooting practice from a kneeling position. He complained of muscle cramps and occasional "twitches" in his legs, but denied arm or bulbar weakness or sensory problems. He had been evaluated at an outside hospital where an electromyogram revealed "diffuse denervation" a diagnosis of amyotrophic lateral sclerosis was made, he was told to "get his affairs in order."*

*Examination revealed intact cranial nerves, symmetric 4+ weakness in the shoulder abductors, symmetric 2 grade weakness in the hip flexors and extensors, and 4– knee flexors and extensor strength. Distal groups were grade 5 in both the arms and legs, and sensation and reflexes were normal. Repeat electromyogram confirmed diffuse denervation and SMN genetic testing revealed a homozygous deletion in SMN1 gene with 5 copies of SMN2.*

*Comment. In this patient with SMA type 4, the symmetric weakness, preferential involvement of hip flexors, and lack of upper motor neuron signs all suggested that amyotrophic lateral sclerosis was not the correct diagnosis. The 5 copies of SMN2 account for the mild phenotype. Eight years after diagnosis, the patient is still working as a police officer doing desk duties.*

## MOLECULAR GENETICS

Before the discovery of the genetic etiology, SMA presented a riddle with regard to severity: how can 1 gene defect result in such a wide range of clinical severity? The solution to this riddle began with the discovery by the Melki laboratory in 1995 that 95% of cases of SMA, irrespective of type, are caused by a homozygous deletion in the *SMN1* gene on chromosome 5q13.[26] In humans, 2 forms of the *SMN* gene exist on each allele: a telomeric form (*SMN1*) and a centromeric form (*SMN2*; **Fig. 4**). Transcription of the *SMN1* gene produces full-length messenger RNA (mRNA) transcripts that encode the SMN protein. The *SMN2* gene is identical to the *SMN1* gene with the exception of a C to T substitution in an exonic splicing enhancer that results in the exclusion of exon 7 during transcription. The resultant, truncated protein is not functional and is degraded rapidly. Critically, the exclusion of exon 7 from *SMN2* mRNAs is not complete, and so a small fraction of the total mRNA transcripts (approximately 10%–15%) arising from the *SMN2* gene do contain exon 7, which encodes the normal SMN protein (see **Fig. 4**).

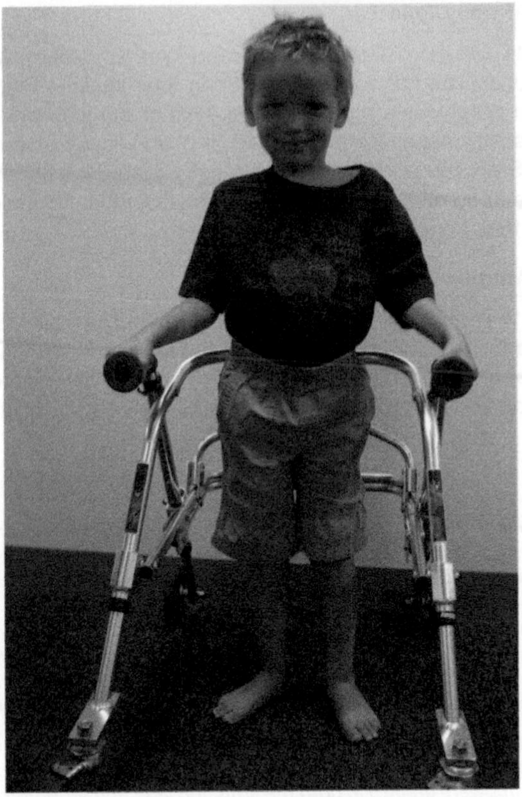

**Fig. 3.** Spinal muscular atrophy type 3.

All patients with SMA lack a functioning *SMN1* gene and are thus dependent on their *SMN2* gene, however inefficient, to produce the SMN protein necessary for survival. Thus, SMA is caused by a deficiency of the SMN protein that, for reasons still unknown, results in selective motor neuron loss. The riddle of severity was solved by the variability of *SMN2* gene copy number that was found in SMA patients.[27] Several subsequent genotype/phenotype analyses confirmed a positive correlation between *SMN2* copy number and milder phenotype.[28] Although *SMN2* copy number is now known to be the primary determinant of SMA severity, it is clearly not the only phenotypic modifier. Prior and colleagues[29] described 3 adult patients with mild 3b phenotypes and only 2 copies of *SMN2*, a seemingly incongruous finding that was explained by the fact that these individuals had a c.859 G > C exon 7 mutation that created an exon splice enhancing element resulting in increased full-length SMN protein production and a milder phenotype. Other modifiers have been described and more are expected as the understanding of the molecular pathogenesis of SMA is refined. Thus, the SMA phenotype cannot always be deduced solely from the *SMN2* copy number determination, a fact crucial when performing genetic counseling with patients and families. Because clinically validated genetic testing is available, it is feasible to someday add the SMA gene test to newborn screening panels.[30,31] For this to occur, however, clear evidence of an effective therapy for SMA and improved ability to understand genetic modifiers of disease severity is required.

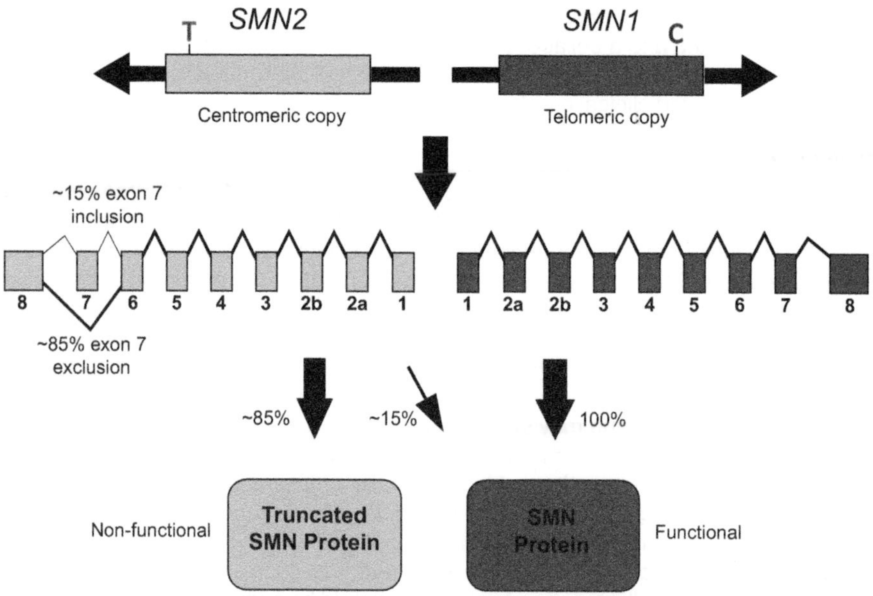


**Fig. 4.** Schematic of *SMN* gene. Schematic diagram of the human *SMN1* and *SMN2* genes and the resultant pre-mRNAs. Patients with SMA have deletions or mutations in both copies of *SMN1*. The *SMN2* gene is expressed; however, the majority of the resultant SMN2 pre-mRNA lacks exon 7 because of a C-to-T transition at position 6 of exon 7. The truncated SMN protein is unstable and nonfunctional. A small proportion of full-length mRNA containing exon 7 is produced by the SMN2 pre-mRNA, resulting in full-length SMN protein that is functional. mRNA, messenger RNA; SMA, spinal muscular atrophy.

### *Molecular Pathology*

Although a detailed discussion of the pathogenesis of SMA is beyond the scope of this review, a few comments are in order. SMN is found throughout the cytoplasm and nucleus where it functions as part of a multiprotein complex, the SMN complex, that plays an essential role in spliceosomal small nuclear ribonuclear protein biogenesis and pre-mRNA splicing.[32] Small nuclear ribonuclear protein biogenesis is altered in the cells of SMA mice. The SMN protein has also been detected in the axons of motor neurons. These observations have led to a central question: although the SMN protein influences RNA processing functions in all cells, does the protein have an additional, unique function in motor neurons?[33,34] One parsimonious explanation may be that the downstream consequences of altered RNA processing that result from insufficient expression of SMN are not favorable for motor neuron development, survival, or both. In this sense, because the motor neuron transcriptome is unique, a global alteration in splicing, for example, could have a unique effect on the transcriptome of motor neurons. The relevant function(s) of the SMN protein in SMA is an area of active research that holds promise to add to our understanding of basic motor neuron biology, which may prove relevant in other disorders affecting the lower motor neuron.

## CLINICAL MANAGEMENT

Over the past decade, there has been a marked improvement in the ability of clinicians to manage the multiple respiratory, nutritional, orthopedic, rehabilitative, emotional, and social problems that develop in the majority of these patients. A notable achievement in this regard was the development of a comprehensive standard of care document by Wang and a collaborating panel of experts that was published in 2007[6] and is currently being updated. This document established guidelines for managing the multiple expected clinical problems that develop in patients with SMA as they age.

### *Pulmonary*

The ultimate cause of death in infants and children with types 1 and 2 SMA is usually respiratory failure. It is critical that a therapeutic relationship with an experienced pulmonary specialist familiar with pediatric neuromuscular disorders be established at the time of initial diagnosis. There is early involvement of the expiratory muscles of ventilation with relative sparing of the diaphragm.[35,36] In infants with type 1 SMA, the early implementation of noninvasive ventilatory support has been show to improve survival and quality of life.[10,37] Bilevel positive airway pressure, when applied with appropriate pressure settings and mask placement, is well-tolerated, does not affect hemodynamic balance, and may increase chemosensitivity and improve daytime hypercapnic ventilatory drive.[38–40] Patients with this degree of respiratory weakness also have a weak cough that puts them at increased risk of aspiration and hypoxemia secondary to mucus plugging as well as increased risk of recurrent pulmonary infections. Infants at risk for mucus plugging should be monitored with overnight oximetry during acute illnesses and assisted airway clearance methods, such as manual suctioning, is recommended. Generally, the use of antibiotics should be applied to these infants during any acute illness because of the risk for pneumonia and associated pulmonary complications.[6,37,41]

The goal of pulmonary intervention in type 1 infants is to improve quality of life and not necessarily to prolong life. For example, noninvasive ventilation can prevent and may reverse changes in chest wall compliance and lung development.[42] Ultimately, however, a decision must be made about what to do once noninvasive ventilatory support is not sufficient. The use of a tracheostomy and permanent ventilatory support can be implemented successfully in individuals with SMA.[43] However, a commitment to lifelong, full-time ventilatory support is an individual choice for the child's family that must be discussed in a multidisciplinary setting, ideally involving a palliative care team.[37]

The management of respiratory function in type 2 or nonambulatory SMA children (ie, type 3 children who with progression of illness eventually lose ambulation) is similar to that of type 1 infants; however, the complications are less severe. Physical examination and assessment of cough effectiveness and respiratory muscle function should be monitored routinely. For children who are older than 5 years of age, forced vital capacity can be monitored routinely and noninvasive ventilatory support can be managed long term. Nocturnal hypoventilation should also be treated with noninvasive ventilation.[39]

### *Gastrointestinal and Nutritional*

Gastrointestinal complications are common in individuals with SMA, and it is not clear if this is owing to immobility and nutritional deficiencies or whether there is a primary defect is gastrointestinal mobility.[44,45] Infants with type 1 SMA often have prolonged feeding times and tire quickly. This reduction in feeding can be the first sign of progressive weakness and can lead to failure to thrive and aspiration.[41] Gastrointestinal dysfunction includes difficulty feeding and swallowing owing to bulbar dysfunction and manifests as tongue weakness, difficulty opening the mouth, and poor head control. Other associated problems include gastrointestinal reflux, delayed gastric emptying, and constipation.[41] These complications are also seen in individuals who, for other reasons, cannot sit or stand, and are less commonly seen in ambulant individuals with SMA.

The management of aspiration associated with feeding and dysphagia includes changing food consistency to include semisolid and thickened liquids. However, in infants with type 1 SMA, early gastrostomy and laparoscopic Nissen fundoplication (if gastrointestinal reflux is present) is recommended because of the importance of maintaining proper nutrition and to reduce the risk of infection secondary to aspiration.[46–48] The operation can be performed soon after diagnosis when the infant is healthy so that the infant will not become hungry as oral feeding decreases.

Malnutrition, secondary to decreased oral intake, can also be an insidious problem for some type 2 SMA children and adolescents.[49] Malnutrition and periods of fasting should be avoided, because these behaviors may contribute to decreases in muscle mass and subsequent impaired function. In clinical practice, height and weight plots in individuals with SMA can be deceiving owing to reduced lean body mass.[50] In fact, high-functioning, nonambulatory individuals with SMA are prone to adiposity, despite their low resting energy expenditure and are at risk of becoming overweight.[51,52] To manage these complications, each child should be evaluated individually during routine visits by a dietitian with the goal of maintaining the growth curve and to avoid inadequate or excessive intake. Because of the tendency for decreased bone mineral density with advancing age, adequate intake of vitamin D and calcium should be provided.[53]

### *Orthopedic and Musculoskeletal Complications*

Weakness and impaired mobility predispose to numerous musculoskeletal issues. Early recognition and appropriate management are helpful in maintaining function, preventing deterioration in vital capacity, and improving quality of life. In nonambulatory individuals with SMA, contractures are common and regular stretching and bracing programs to preserve flexibility and prevent contractures are the main goals of therapy.[54,55] Manual and motorized wheelchairs may be initiated as early as 18 to 24 months of age. Children who are able to bear some weight and have some trunk control may use a standing frame or mobile stander with ankle–foot orthoses. Physical therapy can help to maximize endurance, fitness, and safety by incorporating activities, such as swimming, aquatic therapy, and adaptive sports. Neuromuscular fatigue seems to contribute to functional limitations in individuals with SMA.[56] Wheelchairs and modifications in the environment and at home should be considered to allow for safe accessibility and to optimize independence.

Scoliosis occurs in almost all nonambulant individuals with SMA.[57] When untreated, scoliosis causes chest cage deformities with subsequent respiratory restriction. Spinal fusion and bracing are the treatments of choice for scoliosis; however, there is no clear consensus for their efficacy.[58–61]

## THERAPEUTIC DEVELOPMENT

Before the 1990s, there were relatively few clinical trials in SMA because there was no clear molecular target. Those studies that were undertaken usually involved pharmacologic agents that were repurposed and had shown encouraging results in other diseases characterized by muscle weakness, such as amyotrophic lateral sclerosis or muscular dystrophy. Within 5 years of the discovery of the *SMN* gene, however, animal models of SMA were developed that mimic many of the pathologic and electrophysiologic changes seen in patients and have formed the cornerstone for all therapeutic developments that followed. Burghes and colleagues[62] found that mice with 2 copies of human *SMN2* on a null $smn^{-/-}$ background are viable with a severe SMA-like phenotype, loss of motor neurons, and lifespan of 5 days, whereas mice with 8 copies of *SMN2* on the same background are normal. This and subsequent murine models, as well as the development of SMA models in zebrafish, *Drosophila*, and pig have provided "proof of principle" that increasing expression of the full-length SMN protein is protective. These models also established superb preclinical model systems for screening potential therapies, and permitted in-depth molecular and biochemical studies of disease pathogenesis.[63,64]

The elucidation of the genetic and molecular basis of SMA described suggested several possible therapeutic approaches based on the general principle of increasing the expression of the SMN protein. These strategies include pharmacologic or gene-based therapies to increase *SMN2* expression (leading to more full-length SMN mRNA), antisense oligonucleotide (ASO)-based therapies to favor incorporation of exon 7 into *SMN2*-derived mRNA transcripts, and viral-mediated therapies to replace the entire *SMN1* gene. The development of these approaches is now proceeding at a rapid rate, with human clinical trials using RNA-based oligonucleotide and gene therapy approaches currently underway.

### *Small Molecule Therapy*

The past decade has witnessed several large SMA drug development projects coordinated by the National Institute of Neurological Disorders and Stroke (NINDS), private foundations and the pharmaceutical, and biotechnology industries. These projects have focused on developing cell-based, high-throughput assays to screen for candidate small molecules that can increase SMN protein levels. Compounds that increase SMN levels in these assays have been tested in SMA animal models. Through this approach, a diverse set of compounds has been identified that include histone deacetylase inhibitors, aminoglycosides, and quinazolone derivatives. Histone deacetylase inhibitors such as valproic acid, sodium butyrate, phenylbutyrate, and trichstatin A activate the *SMN2* promoter resulting in increased full-length SMN protein. Despite favorable results in mouse models, clinical trials with several of these agents, most notably phenylbutyrate, valproic acid, and hydroxyurea, have been disappointing, with no substantial clinical benefit demonstrated. Multiple issues related to dosing, duration of therapy, and timing of therapy (ie, when in the course of the disease therapy is instituted), may have confounded these earlier studies; however, there are now many new small molecules that have been discovered and developed specifically for their ability to affect the splicing of the *SMN2* gene to increase the amount of full-length SMN mRNA transcript. The development and testing of these compounds in clinical trials is an active area that holds promise for disease-modifying activity.

### *RNA-Based Therapy*

Alteration of *SMN2* splicing to favor inclusion of exon 7 into the final mRNA transcript and increased expression of the full-length SMN protein is a second promising strategy to treat SMA. These approaches target interactions between cis-acting sequence motifs found in the introns and exons of *SMN2* pre-mRNA and the various trans-acting splicing factors involved in the regulation of exon 7 splicing. ASOs are therapeutic RNA molecules designed to bind to their complementary sequences within a targeted intron or exon that can either enhance or disrupt the targeted splicing event. Initial efforts to increase the inclusion of exon 7 from *SMN2* pre-mRNA used an ASO designed to inhibit a 3′ spice site of exon 8.[65] Since then, additional splice site regulators have been identified and refinements have been made to the chemical stability of ASOs. One such additional splice site regulator is the intron 7 intronic splicing silencer N1 in the *SMN2* gene.[66] ASO-induced blocking of the intronic splicing silencer N1 strongly enhances exon 7 inclusion in cultured fibroblasts and results in increased SMN1 protein. In vivo efficacy testing of these ASOs resulted in efficient inclusion of exon 7 and increased full-length SMN protein levels in mice.[67] In this first preclinical ASO study, systemic administration failed to penetrate the blood–brain barrier; however, this obstacle was overcome quickly by several groups, resulting in increased full-length SMN mRNA and protein in mouse spinal cord when delivered by intracerebroventricular injection.[68,69]

There are now a number of variations on the theme of RNA-based therapies for SMA that are in various stages of preclinical development. For example, a Morpholino-based ASO that targets an intronic repressor, Element1, also improves survival in a mouse model of SMA.[70] Bifunctional RNAs are ASOs that are either linked covalently to a peptide or to a sequence recognized by specific splicing modulators to enhance the stability and/or activity of the therapeutic RNA. Lorson and colleagues[71] engineered a bifunctional RNA containing an ASO directed to the intron7–exon 8 junction that also contained a sequence that recruited hnRNP-A1, a splicing factor that prevents exon 8 inclusion, resulting in more exon 7 inclusion. Intracerebroventricular injections of this bifunctional RNA therapeutic molecule and other bifunctional RNAs raised full-length SMN levels in brain.[71,72] *Trans*-splicing RNAs (tsRNA) are an additional RNA-based strategy that has been applied to SMA mouse models. Therapeutic *tsRNA* for SMA is a synthetic RNA molecule that interacts with the endogenous *SMN2* pre-mRNA, resulting in a hybrid mRNA that has the endogenous mutation spliced out, thus resulting in more full-length SMN mRNA and protein. Preclinical studies with therapeutic tsRNA in SMA mouse models have also been successfully applied.[73,74]

### *Gene Therapy*

Perhaps the most direct approach to SMA therapy is to correct the fundamental cause of the disorder by replacing the missing *SMN1* gene. The successful rescue of a mouse model of severe SMA using a self-complementary adeno-associated viral vector, serotype 9 (scAAV9) by Foust and colleagues[75] was a landmark first step in this direction. In this study, mouse pups were treated on postnatal day 1 with a single intravenous injection of $5 \times 10^{11}$ viral scAAV9 particles carrying the *SMN1* gene. This resulted in *SMN1* expression in 60% of spinal cord motor neurons and complete rescue of motor function and strength, muscle physiology, and life span, so that the treated mice had a normal life span of greater than 400 days, compared with a life span of approximately 16 days in the untreated animals. This approach has been reproduced by other groups using both AAV8 and AAV9 constructs to deliver *SMN1* to motor neurons.[76–78] An important caveat to this approach is that injections done in the mice have their maximal effect on postnatal day 1; the effect falls off rapidly with advancing age, so that injections on day 5 had only a partial effect and injections on postnatal day 10 had no effect. This may mean that therapies designed to increase SMN expression, whether via gene therapy approach or otherwise, in humans will have to be coordinated with early disease detection and immediate institution of therapy, hopefully before clinically significant symptomatology develops. This observation suggests that there may be a critical period in development where sufficient SMN protein is essential for the future health of motor neurons, and further study of this aspect of motor neuron biology may yield great insight into the determinants of motor neuron viability. In a recent report of a porcine model of SMA, investigators were able to demonstrate that gene therapy delivered when piglets were symptomatic was beneficial.[63]

## SUMMARY

SMA is a motor neuron disease of infancy, childhood, and adulthood and the genetics and pathophysiology has received extensive study over the last 20 years. This increased focus has led to an improvement of our understanding of the natural history of the many subtypes of SMA and to the development and distribution of standard of care recommendations. The dramatic preclinical results in SMA models systems have also led to incredible cooperation between clinicians, scientists, government, industry, and volunteer organizations on an international scale to develop the guidelines needed for clinical trial readiness.

The SMA community stands at the threshold of an exciting era of opportunity to translate the unusual success in treating SMA mouse models into effective therapy for SMA patients. Owing to the remarkable progress made over the past 2 decades in understanding the molecular pathogenesis of this disease, investigators are now able to effectively screen potential therapies *in vitro*, test them in accurate animal models, and then move promising agents forward to clinical trials in patients identified in an early or possibly presymptomatic stage of disease. It will be a challenging responsibility to prioritize and advance the most promising therapies forward to clinical trials in an efficient, timely, and safe manner under the guidance of the US Food and Drug Administration and other regulatory agencies. Testing any therapy will involve developing outcome measures, biomarkers, and an infrastructure to conduct meaningful clinical trials, while simultaneously providing optimal supportive care as these new therapies are being developed.

## REFERENCES

1. Sugarman EA, Nagan N, Zhu H, et al. Pan-ethnic carrier screening and prenatal diagnosis for spinal muscular atrophy: clinical laboratory analysis of >72,400 specimens. Eur J Hum Genet 2012;20(1):27–32.
2. Munsat TL, Davies KE. International SMA consortium meeting. (26-28 June 1992, Bonn, Germany). Neuromuscul Disord 1992;2(5–6):423–8.
3. Kolb SJ, Kissel JT. Spinal muscular atrophy: a timely review. Arch Neurol 2011; 68(8):979–84.
4. Arnold WD, Burghes AH. Spinal muscular atrophy: development and implementation of potential treatments. Ann Neurol 2013;74(3):348–62.
5. Lorson CL, Rindt H, Shababi M. Spinal muscular atrophy: mechanisms and therapeutic strategies. Hum Mol Genet 2010;19(R1):R111–8.
6. Wang CH, Finkel RS, Bertini ES, et al. Consensus statement for standard of care in spinal muscular atrophy. J Child Neurol 2007;22(8):1027–49.
7. D'Amico A, Mercuri E, Tiziano FD, et al. Spinal muscular atrophy. Orphanet J Rare Dis 2011;6:71.
8. Finkel RS, McDermott MP, Kaufmann P, et al. Observational study of spinal muscular atrophy type I and implications for clinical trials. Neurology 2014; 83(9):810–7.
9. Finkel RS, Weiner DJ, Mayer OH, et al. Respiratory muscle function in infants with spinal muscular atrophy type I. Pediatr Pulmonol 2014;49(12):1234–42.
10. Oskoui M, Levy G, Garland CJ, et al. The changing natural history of spinal muscular atrophy type 1. Neurology 2007;69(20):1931–6.
11. Boitano LJ. Equipment options for cough augmentation, ventilation, and noninvasive interfaces in neuromuscular respiratory management. Pediatrics 2009; 123(Suppl 4):S226–30.
12. Swoboda KJ, Prior TW, Scott CB, et al. Natural history of denervation in SMA: relation to age, SMN2 copy number, and function. Ann Neurol 2005;57(5):704–12.

13. Kaufmann P, McDermott MP, Darras BT, et al. Observational study of spinal muscular atrophy type 2 and 3: functional outcomes over 1 year. Arch Neurol 2011;68(6):779–86.
14. Statland JM, Barohn RJ, McVey AL, et al. Patterns of weakness, classification of motor neuron disease & clinical diagnosis of sporadic ALS. Neurol Clin 2015, in press.
15. Dubowitz V. Ramblings in the history of spinal muscular atrophy. Neuromuscul Disord 2009;19(1):69–73.
16. Munsat TL. Workshop Report: International SMA collaboration. Neuromuscul Disord 1991;1:81–3.
17. Russman BS. Spinal muscular atrophy: clinical classification and disease heterogeneity. J Child Neurol 2007;22(8):946–51.
18. Zerres K, Davies KE. 59th ENMC international workshop: spinal muscular atrophies: recent progress and revised diagnostic criteria 17-19 April 1998, Soestduinen, The Netherlands. Neuromuscul Disord 1999;9(4):272–8.
19. Dubowitz V. Very severe spinal muscular atrophy (SMA type 0): an expanding clinical phenotype. Eur J Paediatr Neurol 1999;3(2):49–51.
20. MacLeod MJ, Taylor JE, Lunt PW, et al. Prenatal onset spinal muscular atrophy. Eur J Paediatr Neurol 1999;3(2):65–72.
21. Thomas NH, Dubowitz V. The natural history of type I (severe) spinal muscular atrophy. Neuromuscul Disord 1994;4(5–6):497–502.
22. Zerres K, Rudnik-Schoneborn S. Natural history in proximal spinal muscular atrophy. Clinical analysis of 445 patients and suggestions for a modification of existing classifications. Arch Neurol 1995;52(5):518–23.
23. von Gontard A, Zerres K, Backes M, et al. Intelligence and cognitive function in children and adolescents with spinal muscular atrophy. Neuromuscul Disord 2002;12(2):130–6.
24. Zerres K, Rudnik-Schöneborn S, Forrest E, et al. A collaborative study on the natural history of childhood and juvenile onset proximal spinal muscular atrophy (type II and III SMA): 569 patients. J Neurol Sci 1997;146(1):67–72.
25. Piepers S, van den Berg LH, Brugman F, et al. A natural history study of late onset spinal muscular atrophy types 3b and 4. J Neurol 2008;255(9):1400–4.
26. Lefebvre S, Bürglen L, Reboullet S, et al. Identification and characterization of a spinal muscular atrophy-determining gene. Cell 1995;80(1):155–65.
27. Lefebvre S, Burlet P, Liu Q, et al. Correlation between severity and SMN protein level in spinal muscular atrophy. Nat Genet 1997;16(3):265–9.
28. Mailman MD, Heinz JW, Papp AC, et al. Molecular analysis of spinal muscular atrophy and modification of the phenotype by SMN2. Genet Med 2002;4(1):20–6.
29. Prior TW, Krainer AR, Hua Y, et al. A positive modifier of spinal muscular atrophy in the SMN2 gene. Am J Hum Genet 2009;85(3):408–13.
30. Taylor JL, Lee FK, Yazdanpanah GK, et al. Newborn blood spot screening test using multiplexed real-time PCR to simultaneously screen for spinal muscular atrophy and severe combined immunodeficiency. Clin Chem 2015;61(2):412–9.
31. Prior TW, Snyder PJ, Rink BD, et al. Newborn and carrier screening for spinal muscular atrophy. Am J Med Genet A 2010;152A(7):1608–16.
32. Kolb SJ, Battle DJ, Dreyfuss G. Molecular Functions of the SMN Complex. J Child Neurol 2007;22(8):990–4.
33. Burghes AH, Beattie CE. Spinal muscular atrophy: why do low levels of survival motor neuron protein make motor neurons sick? Nat Rev Neurosci 2009;10(8):597–609.
34. Pellizzoni L. Chaperoning ribonucleoprotein biogenesis in health and disease. EMBO Rep 2007;8(4):340–5.

35. Kuru S, Sakai M, Konagaya M, et al. An autopsy case of spinal muscular atrophy type III (Kugelberg-Welander disease). Neuropathology 2009;29(1):63–7.
36. Araki S, Hayashi M, Tamagawa K, et al. Neuropathological analysis in spinal muscular atrophy type II. Acta Neuropathol 2003;106(5):441–8.
37. Schroth MK. Special considerations in the respiratory management of spinal muscular atrophy. Pediatrics 2009;123(Suppl 4):S245–9.
38. Panitch HB. The pathophysiology of respiratory impairment in pediatric neuromuscular diseases. Pediatrics 2009;123(Suppl 4):S215–8.
39. Markstrom A, Cohen G, Katz-Salamon M. The effect of long term ventilatory support on hemodynamics in children with spinal muscle atrophy (SMA) type II. Sleep Med 2010;11(2):201–4.
40. Nickol AH, Hart N, Hopkinson NS, et al. Mechanisms of improvement of respiratory failure in patients with restrictive thoracic disease treated with non-invasive ventilation. Thorax 2005;60(9):754–60.
41. Iannaccone ST. Modern management of spinal muscular atrophy. J Child Neurol 2007;22(8):974–8.
42. Roper H, Quinlivan R, Workshop P. Implementation of "the consensus statement for the standard of care in spinal muscular atrophy" when applied to infants with severe type 1 SMA in the UK. Arch Dis Child 2010;95(10):845–9.
43. Gilgoff IS, Kahlstrom E, MacLaughlin E, et al. Long-term ventilatory support in spinal muscular atrophy. J Pediatr 1989;115(6):904–9.
44. Karasick D, Karasick S, Mapp E. Gastrointestinal radiologic manifestations of proximal spinal muscular atrophy (Kugelberg-Welander syndrome). J Natl Med Assoc 1982;74(5):475–8.
45. Ionasescu V, Christensen J, Hart M. Intestinal pseudo-obstruction in adult spinal muscular atrophy. Muscle Nerve 1994;17(8):946–8.
46. Durkin ET, Schroth MK, Helin M, et al. Early laparoscopic fundoplication and gastrostomy in infants with spinal muscular atrophy type I. J Pediatr Surg 2008;43(11):2031–7.
47. Yuan N, Wang CH, Trela A, et al. Laparoscopic Nissen fundoplication during gastrostomy tube placement and noninvasive ventilation may improve survival in type I and severe type II spinal muscular atrophy. J Child Neurol 2007;22(6):727–31.
48. Birnkrant DJ, Pope JF, Martin JE, et al. Treatment of type I spinal muscular atrophy with noninvasive ventilation and gastrostomy feeding. Pediatr Neurol 1998;18(5):407–10.
49. Chen YS, Shih HH, Chen TH, et al. Prevalence and risk factors for feeding and swallowing difficulties in spinal muscular atrophy types II and III. J Pediatr 2012;160(3):447–51.e1.
50. Tilton AH, Miller MD, Khoshoo V. Nutrition and swallowing in pediatric neuromuscular patients. Semin Pediatr Neurol 1998;5(2):106–15.
51. Sproule DM, Montes J, Montgomery M, et al. Increased fat mass and high incidence of overweight despite low body mass index in patients with spinal muscular atrophy. Neuromuscul Disord 2009;19(6):391–6.
52. Sproule DM, Montes J, Dunaway S, et al. Adiposity is increased among high-functioning, non-ambulatory patients with spinal muscular atrophy. Neuromuscul Disord 2010;20(7):448–52.
53. Kinali M, Banks LM, Mercuri E, et al. Bone mineral density in a paediatric spinal muscular atrophy population. Neuropediatrics 2004;35(6):325–8.
54. Fujak A, Kopschina C, Gras F, et al. Contractures of the lower extremities in spinal muscular atrophy type II. Descriptive clinical study with retrospective data collection. Ortop Traumatol Rehabil 2011;13(1):27–36.

55. Wang HY, Ju YH, Chen SM, et al. Joint range of motion limitations in children and young adults with spinal muscular atrophy. Arch Phys Med Rehabil 2004;85(10):1689–93.
56. Montes J, McDermott MP, Martens WB, et al. Six-Minute Walk Test demonstrates motor fatigue in spinal muscular atrophy. Neurology 2010;74(10):833–8.
57. Haaker G, Fujak A. Proximal spinal muscular atrophy: current orthopedic perspective. Appl Clin Genet 2013;6(11):113–20.
58. Tangsrud SE, Carlsen KC, Lund-Petersen I, et al. Lung function measurements in young children with spinal muscle atrophy; a cross sectional survey on the effect of position and bracing. Arch Dis Child 2001;84(6):521–4.
59. Granata C, Merlini L, Magni E, et al. Spinal muscular atrophy: natural history and orthopaedic treatment of scoliosis. Spine (Phila Pa 1976) 1989;14(7):760–2.
60. Fujak A, Ingenhorst A, Heuser K, et al. Treatment of scoliosis in intermediate spinal muscular atrophy (SMA type II) in childhood. Ortop Traumatol Rehabil 2005;7(2):175–9.
61. Rodillo E, Marini ML, Heckmatt JZ, et al. Scoliosis in spinal muscular atrophy: review of 63 cases. J Child Neurol 1989;4(2):118–23.
62. Monani UR, Sendtner M, Coovert DD, et al. The human centromeric survival motor neuron gene (SMN2) rescues embryonic lethality in Smn(-/-) mice and results in a mouse with spinal muscular atrophy. Hum Mol Genet 2000;9(3):333–9.
63. Duque SI, Arnold WD, Odermatt P, et al. A large animal model of Spinal Muscular Atrophy and correction of phenotype. Ann Neurol 2015;77(3):399–414.
64. Schmid A, DiDonato CJ. Animal models of spinal muscular atrophy. J Child Neurol 2007;22(8):1004–12.
65. Lim SR, Hertel KJ. Modulation of survival motor neuron pre-mRNA splicing by inhibition of alternative 3' splice site pairing. J Biol Chem 2001;276(48):45476–83.
66. Singh NK, Singh NN, Androphy EJ, et al. Splicing of a critical exon of human Survival Motor Neuron is regulated by a unique silencer element located in the last intron. Mol Cell Biol 2006;26(4):1333–46.
67. Hua Y, Vickers TA, Okunola HL, et al. Antisense masking of an hnRNP A1/A2 intronic splicing silencer corrects SMN2 splicing in transgenic mice. Am J Hum Genet 2008;82(4):834–48.
68. Williams JH, Schray RC, Patterson CA, et al. Oligonucleotide-mediated survival of motor neuron protein expression in CNS improves phenotype in a mouse model of spinal muscular atrophy. J Neurosci 2009;29(24):7633–8.
69. Hua Y, Sahashi K, Hung G, et al. Antisense correction of SMN2 splicing in the CNS rescues necrosis in a type III SMA mouse model. Genes Dev 2010;24(15):1634–44.
70. Osman EY, Miller MR, Robbins KL, et al. Morpholino antisense oligonucleotides targeting intronic repressor Element1 improve phenotype in SMA mouse models. Hum Mol Genet 2014;23(18):4832–45.
71. Dickson A, Osman E, Lorson CL. A negatively acting bifunctional RNA increases survival motor neuron both in vitro and in vivo. Hum Gene Ther 2008;19(11):1307–15.
72. Baughan TD, Dickson A, Osman EY, et al. Delivery of bifunctional RNAs that target an intronic repressor and increase SMN levels in an animal model of spinal muscular atrophy. Hum Mol Genet 2009;18(9):1600–11.
73. Coady TH, Baughan TD, Shababi M, et al. Development of a single vector system that enhances trans-splicing of SMN2 transcripts. PLoS One 2008;3(10):e3468.
74. Coady TH, Lorson CL. Trans-splicing-mediated improvement in a severe mouse model of spinal muscular atrophy. J Neurosci 2010;30(1):126–30.

75. Foust KD, Wang X, McGovern VL, et al. Rescue of the spinal muscular atrophy phenotype in a mouse model by early postnatal delivery of SMN. Nat Biotechnol 2010;28(3):271–4.
76. Passini MA, Bu J, Roskelley EM, et al. CNS-targeted gene therapy improves survival and motor function in a mouse model of spinal muscular atrophy. J Clin Invest 2010;120(4):1253–64.
77. Dominguez E, Marais T, Chatauret N, et al. Intravenous scAAV9 delivery of a codon-optimized SMN1 sequence rescues SMA mice. Hum Mol Genet 2011;20(4):681–93.
78. Valori CF, Ning K, Wyles M, et al. Systemic delivery of scAAV9 expressing SMN prolongs survival in a model of spinal muscular atrophy. Sci Transl Med 2010;2(35):35ra42.

# Spinal and Bulbar Muscular Atrophy

Christopher Grunseich, MD*, Kenneth H. Fischbeck, MD

**KEYWORDS**

• Spinal and bulbar muscular atrophy • Kennedy disease • Motor neuron disease
• Androgen receptor

**KEY POINTS**

- Spinal and bulbar muscular atrophy is a neuromuscular disorder with degeneration of lower motor neurons and muscle resulting in slowly progressive weakness, atrophy, and fasciculations.
- Genetic testing of a CAG trinucleotide repeat in the androgen receptor gene confirms the diagnosis. Laboratory testing of serum creatine kinase and electrophysiology studies are frequently abnormal, and testing of swallow function may help in identifying those at risk of developing aspiration.
- There is currently no effective therapy to prevent progression of the disease, and management is focused on preventing complications and improving mobility and function.

## INTRODUCTION

Spinal and bulbar muscular atrophy (SBMA), also known as Kennedy disease,[1] is caused by progressive degeneration of the lower motor neurons and muscle. A trinucleotide (CAG) repeat expansion in the androgen receptor (AR) gene on the X chromosome is the cause.[2] Repeat lengths of 38 to 68 CAGs have been reported in patients, with 11 to 32 CAGs in normal individuals.[3–5] Affected men typically develop symptoms and findings in the limb and bulbar muscles with weakness, atrophy, and fasciculations. Bulbar weakness indicates NP8/MP7 overlap.[6] The age of onset correlates inversely with the length of the CAG repeat,[7] with earlier age of onset in those with longer repeats. The disease has been widely reported in European, Asian, and American populations.

The authors have nothing to disclose.
Neurogenetics Branch, National Institute of Neurological Disorders and Stroke, NIH, 35 Convent Drive, Bethesda, MD 20892, USA
* Corresponding author.
*E-mail address:* Christopher.grunseich@nih.gov

Neurol Clin 33 (2015) 847–854
http://dx.doi.org/10.1016/j.ncl.2015.07.002
0733-8619/15/$ – see front matter Published by Elsevier Inc.

## MECHANISM

The CAG repeat is expressed as an expanded polyglutamine tract in the AR, and studies in animal models and patients indicate that androgen-dependent gain of function by the receptor results in toxicity of the mutant protein.[8,9] Unlike other polyglutamine diseases in which the native function of the disease protein is unclear, the function of the AR has been well characterized. In the absence of androgen, the receptor is localized in the cytoplasm and bound to heat shock proteins. Testosterone or dihydrotestosterone binding by the receptor results in nuclear translocation and binding to androgen-responsive elements throughout the genome.[10] Translocation of the mutant AR into the nucleus also seems to be necessary for toxicity, as deletion of the nuclear localization signal prevents toxicity in a mouse model.[11] The features of disease result from a loss as well as gain in function of the receptor because patients often have gynecomastia and reduced fertility in addition to weakness and muscle atrophy. The mutated receptor has a propensity to aggregate and form inclusions in tissues where it is expressed.[12] Toxicity of the mutant AR is likely mediated through transcriptional dysregulation,[13] with disruption of mitochondrial function,[14] protein homeostasis,[15] and cellular signaling.[16] The transcriptional coactivator CREB-binding protein (CBP) is sequestered and depleted in SBMA and other polyglutamine diseases.[17] Defects in autophagy, the cellular process responsible for degrading and recycling cellular constituents, have been implicated in the disease.[18] Alteration of autophagy through genetic and pharmacologic mechanisms has been shown to be protective in several models of the disease.[11]

Although the AR is expressed in various tissues throughout the body, the predominant site of toxicity is in the spinal cord and muscles. Brain stem motor nuclei are also susceptible, except for the third, fourth, and sixth cranial nerves. Loss of anterior horn cells in the spinal cord has been described,[19] and a direct role of the mutant AR in muscle degeneration has been demonstrated in animal models of the disease.[20] Several studies have reported that selective expression or correction of the mutant AR in mouse muscle can reproduce or ameliorate the disease manifestations, respectively.[21,22] The relative contributions of the motor neuron and muscle toward the pathogenesis in patients remain to be defined. Affected males can also experience mild sensory loss in the distal extremities from degeneration of dorsal root ganglion cells.

## DISEASE COURSE

The average age of onset is usually in the mid 40s, with a range of 18 to 64 years of age.[4] Clinical features of the disease can vary among affected individuals in the same family. Weakness affects the upper and lower extremities, following NP7 with both proximal and distal muscles.[6] Features of androgen insensitivity, such as sexual dysfunction, gynecomastia, and testicular atrophy, may be apparent before motor involvement. Overall, the most common presenting features are weakness, tremor, and cramping.[3,4] The progression of weakness in the disease is slow, with an approximately 2% decrease in muscle strength by quantitative muscle testing (QMT) per year.[23] Patients may experience a stepwise decrease in performance as critical thresholds needed for function tend to be more readily perceived as function is lost. Patients with SBMA generally have good preservation of mobility until late in the disease, requiring a cane or other assistive device at a median age of 60 years. Those with progressive loss of gait and balance function may eventually require a wheelchair. Bulbar manifestations, including dysarthria and nasal speech, can present early in the disease course and may progress to dysphagia. There are subtle to prominent tongue and facial muscle fasciculations, whereas limb fasciculations are not prominent.

Patients with advanced disease may develop difficulty managing secretions with the risk of aspiration pneumonia.[3] The average life expectancy is reduced as a result of bulbar and respiratory muscle weakness, although many patients have a normal life span. Muscle stretch reflexes are absent or reduced. There are often subclinical vibratory changes in the legs more than the arms coupled with reduction of sensory nerve action potential (SNAP) amplitude on nerve conduction studies.

The CAG repeat size has been found to correlate with clinical features of the disease.[3,4,24] A larger CAG repeat is associated with earlier disease onset and earlier age for requiring the use of a handrail, cane, or wheelchair. The rate of progression of the disease was not significantly influenced by CAG repeat length in a natural history study of 223 subjects.[3] Although patients with larger CAG repeat lengths reach loss-of-function milestones faster, the rate of decline between milestones does not seem to be affected by the CAG repeat size alone.

## DIAGNOSIS

Genetic testing is the preferred method for making a diagnosis, with all patients with SBMA having a CAG repeat expansion of at least 38 CAGs. Variation in the CAG repeat length can be seen among affected members of the same family.[7,25] The serum creatine kinase (CK) level in most patients is usually elevated to 2 to 4 times the upper limit of normal, up to 900 to 1400 U/L.[3,4] Liver enzymes are also often found to be abnormal, with mild elevation in aspartate and alanine aminotransferase levels. Additional investigations are currently ongoing to evaluate liver dysfunction in the disease. In a study of 144 Japanese subjects with SBMA, 12% were found to have a Brugada-type electrocardiogram with a coved or saddle-back-type ST-segment elevation in more than one right precordial lead.[26] Additional studies are needed to determine whether this finding is present in other patient populations.

A family history helps in making the diagnosis, as most patients have other affected relatives. As an X-linked disease, SBMA generally affects men and may be transmitted through asymptomatic women. Cramping and other symptoms have been reported in a minority of female carriers.[27] A genetic diagnosis should ideally be established in an affected family member before testing unaffected family members.

On examination, lower motor neuron signs are typically found, including muscle atrophy, fasciculations, and decreased or absent deep tendon reflexes. The weakness often initially occurs in the lower extremities.[4,24] Distal loss of sensation for various modalities may be noted on examination. More than 90% of patients with SBMA have low SNAP amplitudes on nerve conduction study.[4] The motor unit number estimation (MUNE) is reduced to about 50% of healthy control values in the abductor pollicis brevis muscle.[28] Muscle biopsy may show evidence of both myopathic (central nuclei, myofibrillar disorganization) and neurogenic (fiber type grouping, angulated fibers) changes.[29]

The availability of genetic testing has helped to standardize the diagnosis of SBMA. Many patients are misdiagnosed with amyotrophic lateral sclerosis (ALS) before receiving the correct diagnosis.[4] Unlike SBMA, individuals with ALS have upper motor neuron signs, such as hyperreflexia and spasticity. The disease course in ALS is also more rapidly progressive with greater asymmetry. SNAP amplitudes are lower in SBMA compared with ALS,[30] providing another useful tool in the differential diagnosis of these two diseases. SBMA may also be mistaken for other neuromuscular disorders, such as myasthenia gravis, chronic inflammatory polyneuropathy, polymyositis, and metabolic myopathy. SBMA should be considered in patients thought to have myasthenia who are antibody negative and do not improve on therapy.

## CLINICAL CASE

A 45-year-old man presented with a 9-month history of progressive leg weakness. The weakness is symmetric and has led to impairment of walking and difficulty with balance on uneven surfaces. He has also had recent choking spells and mild paresthesias in the distal lower extremities.

Examination is remarkable for gynecomastia. He has a nasal, airy voice with fibrillations in the tongue, decreased movement of the palate, and reduced posterior pharyngeal wall contraction. Fasciculations are seen in the chin. Mild atrophy in the first dorsal interosseous is appreciated in both hands, with mild weakness in these muscles. Light touch and vibratory sensation are reduced in both lower extremities in a gradient distribution, and reflexes are diminished throughout. No upper motor neuron signs are present. On gait testing he has mild difficulty squatting and with tandem gait.

On laboratory testing he has elevation of CK to 950 U/L. Electrophysiology studies show decreased MUNE, positive sharp waves, and reduced sural sensory nerve amplitudes. Genetic testing for the CAG repeat expansion in the AR gene shows a repeat size of 45 CAG, and further discussion of the family history identifies a male maternal cousin with a similar history.

## MANAGEMENT

Management of SBMA is focused on preventing complications of the disease, such as falls, fractures, aspiration, and reduced mobility. There is currently no effective treatment to prevent progression of the disease. Those at risk for dysphagia should undergo a swallow study to identify risks of aspiration. Deficits in swallow function can be seen as abnormal pharyngeal retention of barium during videofluorography.[31] Exercises and precautionary measures can be recommended to reduce the risk of aspiration. A physical therapy assessment can be helpful in enhancing the mobility of patients by providing assistive devices and recommending targeted exercises for the preservation of gait and mobility.

Exercise has been demonstrated to be beneficial for many forms of neuromuscular disease.[32] The effect of 12 weeks of moderate-intensity aerobic exercise was investigated in a group of 8 subjects with SBMA.[33] Although there was no change in maximal oxygen uptake, an increase in maximum work capacity was detected. In a separate 12-week study of 50 subjects with SBMA, functional exercise was compared with stretching exercise.[34] There was no improvement in the primary outcome measure, the total adult myopathy assessment tool (AMAT) score, although post hoc analysis showed that low-functioning individuals had a relative improvement in the functional AMAT score. Although it is unclear what the long-term effect of exercise may be on the disease progression, short-term periods of exercise seem to be well tolerated. Exercise should be adjusted to the patients' level of function and titrated with input from a physiatrist.

Clinical trials in the disease have focused on reducing AR ligand. Androgen reduction with leuprorelin and castration has been shown to mitigate disease manifestations in transgenic animal models of SBMA.[35,36] Leuprorelin is a luteinizing hormone-releasing hormone analogue that reduces the production of testosterone and its derivative, dihydrotestosterone. In a 48-week phase 2 study, patients with SBMA on leuprorelin did not have significant improvement compared with placebo in the primary outcome measure (the ALS Functional Rating Scale), although there was evidence of increased duration of cricopharyngeal opening on videofluorography.[37] A subsequent phase 3 placebo-controlled study did not show a significant effect on swallow function, although a post hoc subgroup analysis showed a benefit in subjects with less than 10 years disease duration.[38] Another agent, the 5α-reductase inhibitor dutasteride, was evaluated in a 2-year randomized, double-blind, placebo-controlled study of 50 subjects; it did not show an effect on the primary measure of muscle strength (quantitative muscle assessment).[23]

Activation of pathways that mitigate AR toxicity has also been pursued as a therapeutic strategy. Insulin-like growth factor 1 (IGF-1) has direct anabolic effects on muscle and also increases mutant AR clearance through the ubiquitin-proteasome system.[39] Phosphorylation of the AR by Akt enhances this clearance, and activated phospho-Akt can be measured as a biomarker for agents targeting this pathway. In SBMA mice, overexpression and exogenous delivery of IGF-1 rescue behavioral and histopathologic changes in the transgenic mice overexpressing mutant AR. In a recent open-label trial of the β2-agonist clenbuterol in 16 subjects with SBMA, an increase in the 6-minute walk test and forced vital capacity was seen after 12 months of intervention.[40] Future randomized placebo-controlled studies of drugs in this class will be needed to confirm their functional efficacy.

## A DISEASE OF NERVE OR MUSCLE?

SBMA is considered primarily a disease of the motor neuron. Degeneration of motor neurons is seen in the anterior horn of the spinal cord from patients; evidence of motor neuron dysfunction is seen in electrophysiology studies, with a reduction in MUNE.[4] Abnormalities in motor neuron cell models of the disease have also been reported.[41,42] Recently, there has been increasing evidence that muscle also plays a role in the disease process. A knock-in mouse model of SBMA has histologic and molecular signs of muscle pathology before the appearance of pathologic changes in the spinal cord.[20] Transgenic mice that selectively overexpress the normal AR in muscle have also been found to have pathologic findings similar to transgenic mice with overexpression of the mutant AR.[43]

A conditional mouse model of the disease has been helpful in identifying tissue-specific contributions to the disease.[21] In this model, a full-length human AR transgene with 121 CAG repeats was expressed under the control of the endogenous AR promoter. The transcriptional start site of the promoter was flanked by loxP sites, allowing its removal with Cre recombinase, thus effectively knocking out expression of the mutant gene in specific tissues. With this model, muscle-specific knockout of the mutant AR significantly ameliorated the disease phenotype despite continued expression of the mutant AR in the spinal cord. Antisense oligonucleotides (ASOs) have been investigated as potential therapeutic agents to knock down expression of the mutant AR in mice. Disease manifestations in knock-in mice were rescued with subcutaneous delivery of the ASO to decrease expression in the muscle. Intraventricular delivery of the ASO to reduce AR expression in the spinal cord did not affect the disease manifestations in these mice.[22]

In clinical trials, the site of the disease pathogenesis is an important factor in choosing the optimum route of delivery for the intervention being tested. Animal studies indicate that the muscle may be playing an important role in the disease mechanism. Future studies are needed to define how the muscle deterioration is affecting the disease process in patients and to understand the interaction between motor neuron and muscle in SBMA.

## SUMMARY

SBMA is caused by a polyglutamine repeat expansion in the AR, and it is inherited in an X-linked pattern. Neurologic symptoms usually begin in the early to mid 40s, with weakness as a predominant feature of the disease. Manifestations of the disease likely result from both gain and loss of function of the androgen receptor. Although no therapy currently exists to prevent progression of the disease, supportive intervention may improve mobility and prevent complications. Mild to moderate exercise is safe; however, patients who exercise have not been found to significantly improve muscle strength or function. Randomized placebo-controlled clinical trials of androgen reduction therapy have not shown significant effects on primary outcome measures. Expressing the mutant AR in a restricted tissue-specific manner in mice has helped to establish the muscle as a primary site for the disease. Studies are ongoing to identify and evaluate new therapeutic strategies in disease models and patients.

## REFERENCES


1. Kennedy WR, Alter M, Sung JH. Progressive proximal spinal and bulbar muscular atrophy of late onset: a sex-linked recessive trait. Neurology 1968; 18:671–80.
2. La Spada AR, Wilson EM, Lubahn DB, et al. Androgen receptor gene mutations in X-linked spinal and bulbar muscular atrophy. Nature 1991;352:77–9.
3. Atsuta N, Watanabe H, Ito M, et al. Natural history of spinal and bulbar muscular atrophy (SBMA): a study of 223 Japanese patients. Brain 2006;129:1446–55.
4. Rhodes LE, Freeman BK, Auh S, et al. Clinical features of spinal and bulbar muscular atrophy. Brain 2009;132:3242–51.
5. Grunseich C, Kats IR, Bott LC, et al. Early onset and novel features in a spinal and bulbar muscular atrophy patient with a 68 CAG repeat. Neuromuscul Disord 2014;24(11):978–81.
6. Statland JM, Barohn RJ, McVey AL, et al. Patterns of Weakness, Classification of Motor Neuron Disease, and Clinical Diagnosis of Sporadic Amyotrophic Lateral Sclerosis. Neruol Clin 2015, in press.
7. La Spada AR, Roling D, Harding AE, et al. Meiotic stability and genotype-phenotype correlation of the trinucleotide repeat in X-linked spinal and bulbar muscular atrophy. Nat Genet 1992;2:301–4.
8. Katsuno M, Adachi H, Kume A, et al. Testosterone reduction prevents phenotypic expression in a transgenic mouse model of spinal and bulbar muscular atrophy. Neuron 2002;35:843–54.
9. Schmidt BJ, Greenberg CR, Allingham-Hawkins DJ, et al. Expression of X-linked bulbospinal muscular atrophy (Kennedy disease) in two homozygous women. Neurology 2002;59(5):770–2.
10. Shaffer PL, Jivan A, Dollins DE, et al. Structural basis of androgen receptor binding to selective androgen response elements. Proc Natl Acad Sci U S A 2004; 101(14):4758–63.
11. Montie HL, Cho MS, Holder L, et al. Cytoplasmic retention of polyglutamine-expanded androgen receptor ameliorates disease via autophagy in a mouse model of spinal and bulbar muscular atrophy. Hum Mol Genet 2009;18(11): 1937–50.
12. Li M, Miwa S, Kobayashi Y, et al. Nuclear inclusions of the androgen receptor protein in spinal and bulbar muscular atrophy. Ann Neurol 1998;44:249–54.
13. Nedelsky NB, Pennuto M, Smith RB, et al. Native functions of the androgen receptor are essential to pathogenesis in a Drosophila model of spinobulbar muscular atrophy. Neuron 2010;67(6):936–52.
14. Ranganathan S, Harmison GG, Meyertholen K, et al. Mitochondrial abnormalities in spinal and bulbar muscular atrophy. Hum Mol Genet 2009;18:27–42.

15. Pandey UB, Nie Z, Batlevi Y, et al. HDAC6 rescues neurodegeneration and provides an essential link between autophagy and the UPS. Nature 2007;447(7146):859–63.
16. Katsuno M, Adachi H, Minamiyama M, et al. Disrupted transformed growth factor-beta signaling in spinal and bulbar muscular atrophy. J Neurosci 2010;30(16):5702–12.
17. McCampbell A, Taylor JP, Taye AA, et al. CREB-binding protein sequestration by expanded polyglutamine. Hum Mol Genet 2000;9:2197–202.
18. Cortes CJ, Miranda HC, Frankowski H, et al. Polyglutamine-expanded androgen receptor interferes with TFEB to elicit autophagy defects in SBMA. Nat Neurosci 2014;17(9):1180–9.
19. Ogata A, Matsuura T, Tashiro K, et al. Expression of androgen receptor in X-linked spinal and bulbar muscular atrophy and amyotrophic lateral sclerosis. J Neurol Neurosurg Psychiatry 1994;57:1274–5.
20. Yu Z, Dadgar N, Albertelli M, et al. Androgen-dependent pathology demonstrates myopathic contribution to the Kennedy disease phenotype in a mouse knock-in model. J Clin Invest 2006;116:2663–72.
21. Cortes CJ, Ling SC, Guo LT, et al. Muscle expression of mutant androgen receptor accounts for systemic and motor neuron disease phenotypes in spinal and bulbar muscular atrophy. Neuron 2014;82(2):295–307.
22. Lieberman AP, Yu Z, Murray S, et al. Peripheral androgen receptor gene suppression rescues disease in mouse models of spinal and bulbar muscular atrophy. Cell Rep 2014;7(3):774–84.
23. Fernández-Rhodes LE, Kokkinis AD, White MJ, et al. Efficacy and safety of dutasteride in patients with spinal and bulbar muscular atrophy: a randomised placebo-controlled trial. Lancet Neurol 2011;10:140–7.
24. Fratta P, Nirmalananthan N, Masset L, et al. Correlation of clinical and molecular features in spinal bulbar muscular atrophy. Neurology 2014;82(23):2077–84.
25. Watanabe M, Abe K, Aoki M, et al. Mitotic and meiotic stability of the CAG repeat in the X-linked spinal and bulbar muscular atrophy gene. Clin Genet 1996;50(3):133–7.
26. Araki A, Katsuno M, Suzuki K, et al. Brugada syndrome in spinal and bulbar muscular atrophy. Neurology 2014;82(20):1813–21.
27. Ishihara H, Kanda F, Nishio H, et al. Clinical features and skewed X-chromosome inactivation in female carriers of X-linked recessive spinal and bulbar muscular atrophy. J Neurol 2001;248:856–60.
28. Lehky TJ, Chen CJ, Di Prospero NA, et al. Standard and modified statistical MUNE evaluations in spinal-bulbar muscular atrophy. Muscle Nerve 2009;40:809–14.
29. Soraru G, D'Ascenzo C, Polo A, et al. Spinal and bulbar muscular atrophy: skeletal muscle pathology in male patients and heterozygous females. J Neurol Sci 2008;264:100–5.
30. Hama T, Hirayama M, Hara T, et al. Discrimination of spinal and bulbar muscular atrophy from amyotrophic lateral sclerosis using sensory nerve action potentials. Muscle Nerve 2012;45(2):169–74.
31. Grunseich C, Rinaldi C, Fischbeck KH. Spinal and bulbar muscular atrophy: pathogenesis and clinical management. Oral Dis 2014;20(1):6–9.
32. Cup EH, Pieterse AJ, Broek-Pastoor T, et al. Exercise therapy and other types of physical therapy for patients with neuromuscular diseases: a systematic review. Arch Phys Med Rehabil 2007;88(11):1452–64.
33. Preisler N, Andersen G, Thøgersen F, et al. Effect of aerobic training in patients with spinal and bulbar muscular atrophy (Kennedy disease). Neurology 2009;72(4):317–23.

34. Shrader JA, Kats I, Kokkinis A, et al. A randomized controlled trial of exercise in spinal and bulbar muscular atrophy. Ann Clin Transl Neurol 2015;2(7):739–47.
35. Katsuno M, Adachi H, Doyu M, et al. Leuprorelin rescues polyglutamine-dependent phenotypes in a transgenic mouse model of spinal and bulbar muscular atrophy. Nat Med 2003;9:768–73.
36. Chevalier-Larsen ES, O'Brien CJ, Wang H, et al. Castration restores function and neurofilament alterations of aged symptomatic males in a transgenic mouse model of spinal and bulbar muscular atrophy. J Neurosci 2004;24(20):4778–86.
37. Banno H, Katsuno M, Suzuki K, et al. Phase 2 trial of leuprorelin in patients with spinal and bulbar muscular atrophy. Ann Neurol 2009;65(2):140–50.
38. Katsuno M, Banno H, Suzuki K, et al. Efficacy and safety of leuprorelin in patients with spinal and bulbar muscular atrophy (JASMITT study): a multicentre, randomised, double-blind, placebo-controlled trial. Lancet Neurol 2010;9(9):875–84.
39. Palazzolo I, Stack C, Kong L, et al. Overexpression of IGF-1 in muscle attenuates disease in a mouse model of spinal and bulbar muscular atrophy. Neuron 2009;63(3):316–28.
40. Querin G, D'Ascenzo C, Peterle E, et al. Pilot trial of clenbuterol in spinal and bulbar muscular atrophy. Neurology 2013;80(23):2095–8.
41. Orr CR, Montie HL, Liu Y, et al. An interdomain interaction of the androgen receptor is required for its aggregation and toxicity in spinal and bulbar muscular atrophy. J Biol Chem 2010;285(46):35567–77.
42. Grunseich C, Zukosky K, Kats IR, et al. Stem cell-derived motor neurons from spinal and bulbar muscular atrophy patients. Neurobiol Dis 2014;70:12–20.
43. Monks DA, Johansen JA, Mo K, et al. Overexpression of wild-type androgen receptor in muscle recapitulates polyglutamine disease. Proc Natl Acad Sci U S A 2007;104(46):18259–64.

# Neuropathology of Amyotrophic Lateral Sclerosis and Its Variants

Shahram Saberi, MD, Jennifer E. Stauffer, BA, Derek J. Schulte, BS, John Ravits, MD*

**KEYWORDS**

- Amyotrophic lateral sclerosis • Neuropathology • TDP-43
- Motor neuron degeneration • C9orf72

**KEY POINTS**

- ALS has a distinctive and complex neuropathology, from which its name is derived.
- Many developments in ALS research have been driven by key neuropathologic insights, such as the identification of ubiquitinated cytoplasmic inclusions, which led to the identification of TDP-43 in ALS.
- New microscopic, molecular, and computerization techniques are allowing researchers unprecedented visualization of the inner workings of the disease at the tissue, cellular and molecular levels.

## INTRODUCTION

The first case reports of amyotrophic lateral sclerosis (ALS) date back to Charles Bell in 1824.[1] Although a variety of other clinical descriptions followed throughout the 1850s,[2–4] the correlations between key clinical features of progressive muscle atrophy and muscle spasticity and key neuropathologic features of loss of anterior horn cells and sclerosis in the lateral columns of the spinal cord were first made by Charcot in the 1860s,[5] and thus, he named the clinical disease by its distinctive neuropathology.[6] Significant subsequent contributions included the observation of loss of the giant cells of Betz, best summarized by Brodmann in 1909,[7] of eosinophilic inclusions now called Bunina bodies in 1962,[8] the discovery of ubiquitinated cytoplasmic inclusions in 1988,[9,10] and the discovery that the ubiquitinated inclusions comprised primarily TDP-43 in 2006.[11,12] The association between ALS, the clinical disease frontotemporal dementia (FTD), and FTD neuropathology referred to as frontotemporal lobar dementia (FTLD) has taken 3 decades to establish.[13,14] With advances in genetics beginning in

Disclosures: The authors have nothing to disclose.
Department of Neurosciences, ALS Translational Research, University of California (San Diego), 9500 Gilman Drive, MC0624, La Jolla, CA 92093, USA
* Corresponding author.
*E-mail address:* jravits@ucsd.edu

Neurol Clin 33 (2015) 855–876
http://dx.doi.org/10.1016/j.ncl.2015.07.012 neurologic.theclinics.com

1993, distinctive neuropathology is being identified in the genetic forms, the main ones being SOD1,[15] TDP-43,[16] FUS,[17,18] and C9orf72 repeat expansions.[19,20]

## CLASSIC AMYOTROPHIC LATERAL SCLEROSIS NEUROPATHOLOGY

### *Gross*

In most brains with ALS, no gross abnormalities are observed. The spinal cord often shows atrophy of the anterior nerve roots.[21] Some cases show atrophy of the precentral gyrus.[21] In patients with dementia, atrophy of the frontal or temporal cortex may be seen,[21–24] the atrophy being greatest in brains from patients with overlap ALS–frontotemporal dementia. In addition to these gray matter abnormalities, white matter reduction is also observed, particularly, but not exclusively, in the corticospinal tract.[14,25,26]

### *Microscopic*

Microscopic changes include neuronal and axon loss. There is loss of myelinated axons in the lateral and anterior columns of the spinal cord and decreases in size of anterior horn of the spinal cord, best shown by myelin stains such as Luxol fast blue (**Fig. 1**A, B).[21] There is degeneration and loss of the large motor neurons in the anterior horn of the spinal cord, lower cranial motor nuclei of the brainstem, and Betz cells in the motor cortex, best seen with routine stains such as hematoxylin-eosin (H&E) (see **Fig. 1**C, D; **Fig. 2**A–F).[21,27–29] Morphometric studies of the spinal anterior horn have shown a global reduction of all neurons in the anterior horn, not just the large α motor neurons.[30] There is evidence of reduction in neuron size as well as loss and atrophy of nerve fibers. Other pathologic features of ALS include vacuolization, large empty

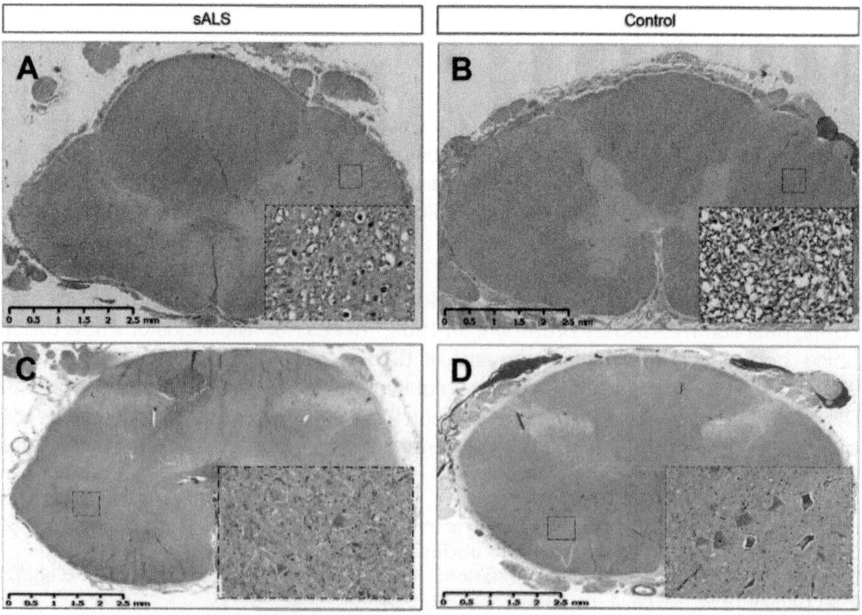


**Fig. 1.** ALS. Lateral sclerosis is shown in the thoracic spinal cord in SALS (*A*) and compared with control (*B*). Inserts show loss of myelin in the white matter tracts under higher power (20X). Loss of motor neurons is shown in the lumbar spinal cord in SALS (*C*) and compared with control (*D*). Inserts (40X) show motor neurons in anterior horns under higher power (40X) (Luxol fast blue with H&E [*A, B*]; H&E [*C, D*]). Low power views are 1X.

spaces near neurons, and spongiosis, microscopic holes, resulting in a spongelike appearance (see **Fig. 2**G, H).

Bunina bodies are small (3–6 μm), round to oval eosinophilic intracellular inclusions in the motor neurons of the spinal cord and brain stem of both patients with sporadic ALS (SALS) and patients with familial ALS (FALS), best seen with H&E (see **Fig. 2**I, J).[31,32] They are most frequently found in the cytoplasm of motor neurons but can occasionally be found in dendrites.[33] Their number per neuron is highly variable, and they can sometimes make chains and clusters. They are rarely seen in Betz cells, neurons of oculomotor nuclei, and Onuf nuclei.[34–36] Immunohistochemically, Bunina bodies are positive for cystatin c (see **Fig. 2**K, L) and transferrin and partially colocalize with peripherin,[37,38] but they are negative for a variety of proteins commonly associated with neurodegeneration, including tau, α, and β tubulin, synaptophysin, amyloid precursor protein, glial fibrillary acidic protein (GFAP), α-synuclein, and p62.[37,39–41] It remains controversial whether or not Bunina bodies are positive for ubiquitin.[10,42] Their biological significance is unknown.

The complexity of glial cells is now well established, and recent studies[43] have shown they are crucial in the biology of ALS neurodegeneration. Reactive astrogliosis surrounds degenerating motor neurons in patients with ALS and ALS animal models.[44–46] Reactive astrocytes show increased immunoreactivity for GFAP and the calcium-binding protein S100β and express inflammatory makers such as cyclooxygenase 2, inducible nitric oxide synthase (NOS), and neuronal NOS. Increase in GFAP-immunoreactive astrocytes is particularly notable in the gray matter of the spinal cord ventral horn, where normally, astrocytes express GFAP at low levels. Cytoplasmic hyaline inclusions and markers of oxidative and nitrative stress accompany astrocyte disease.[47,48]

Activation of microglia is a critical aspect of glial neuropathology.[44] It has been correlated with severity of upper motor neuron (UMN) degeneration in ALS (reviewed in Ref.[49]). Activated microglia, responding to neuronal distress, release a variety of proinflammatory cytokines, leading to a higher degree of inflammation in the brains of patients with ALS. These proinflammatory molecules include but are not limited to tumor necrosis factor α, interleukin 1β, and ionized calcium-binding adapter molecule 2 (see **Fig. 2** M, N). Microglia also release reactive oxygen species such as superoxide and nitric oxide, as well as chemokines (monocyte chemoattractant protein 1, macrophage colony stimulating factor) and neurotrophic factors (insulinlike growth factor 1).[50] It seems neuroinflammation is a 2-edged sword: some of it protects against neurodegeneration and some of it drives it.[43–45]

## MOLECULAR NEUROPATHOLOGY: INCLUSIONS AND PROTEINOPATHIES

### *Ubiquitin*

Some of the most important progress in understanding ALS biology has been driven by key neuropathologic discoveries. This progress began in 1988, when Leigh and colleagues[9,51] and Lowe and colleagues[10] independently discovered ubiquitin-positive skeinlike or dense, round structures in the cytoplasm of anterior horn cells in both FALS and SALS (**Fig. 3**A–D), inclusions that are not detected by H&E and other routine staining methods. Such inclusions were later identified in FTLD and became the cornerstone of distinguishing FTLD with ubiquinated inclusions (FTLD-U) from FTLD with tau (FTLD-tau) and other inclusions.[52–54] In both ALS and FTLD-U, the ubiquitin-positive inclusions have been observed in neurons of the frontal cortex, temporal cortex, hippocampus, and striatum.[31,55–58] Although they are most commonly found in neurons, they have occasionally been seen in glial cells.[59] They are negative

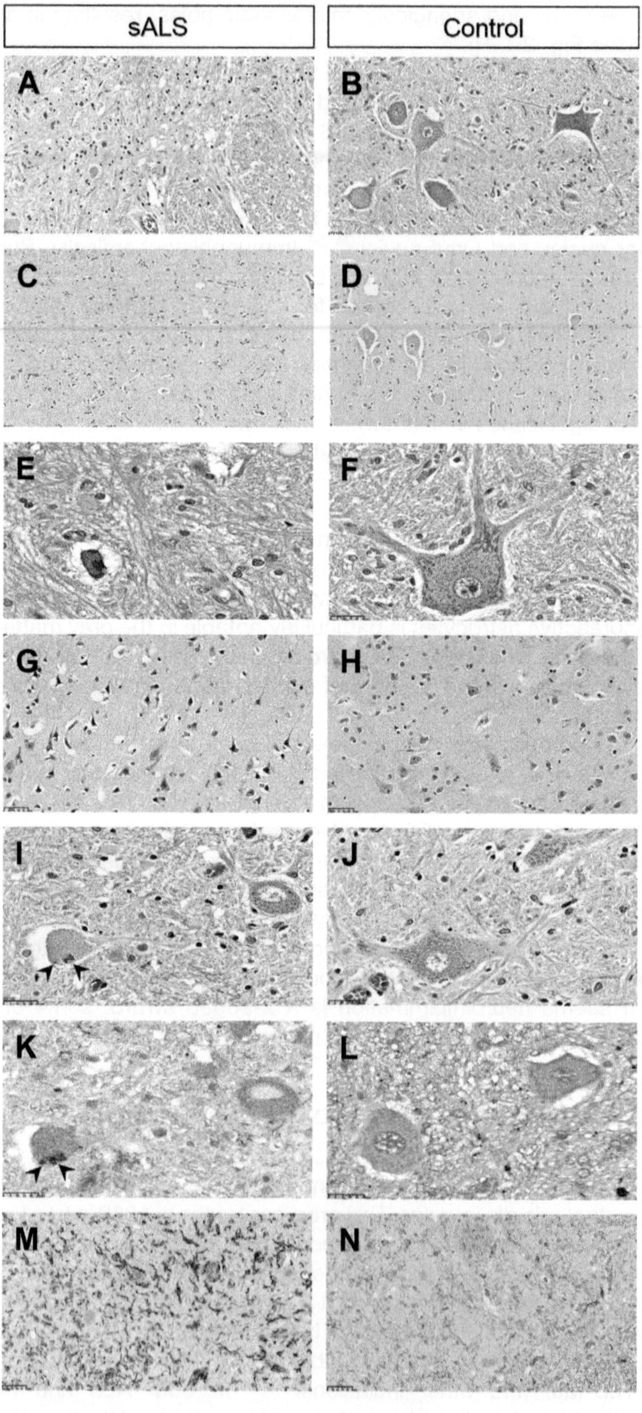
sALS
Control
A
B
C
D
E
F
G
H
I
J
K
L
M
N

for proteins commonly associated with neurodegenerative inclusions, such as tau and α-synuclein.[55,59]

### *TDP-43*

The presence of ubiquitin-positive inclusions suggested a problem with some other protein(s). Eighteen years later, TDP-43 was identified as the main component of ubiquitinated inclusions in both patients with ALS and patients with FTD.[11,12] This finding connected ALS and FTLD-U as TDP-43 proteinopathies (**Table 1**).[60] TDP-43 is a heterogeneous nuclear ribonucleoprotein and has many different cellular functions, including messenger RNA (mRNA) stability,[61,62] mRNA processing,[63,64] mRNA transport and translation,[65,66] and negative regulation of alternative splicing.[67] Under normal conditions, TDP-43 is expressed in many tissues, including the nuclei of neurons and glial cells. In SALS and most FALS as well as FTLD-TDP-43 (now renamed from FTLD-U), there is loss of nuclear TDP-43 and formation of pathologic aggregates in the cytoplasm (see **Fig. 3**E–H).[68] The mechanism behind this redistribution is poorly understood and could be either the translocation of TDP-43 from the nuclei to the cytoplasm or an impaired TDP-43 cytoplasm-to-nucleus shuttling process.[12,69–71] With the use of immunoblot analysis, extracted material from brains of patients with FTD-TDP-43, FTD-ALS, and ALS was found to be phosphorylated TDP-43 band at 45 kDa.[11,72] This finding suggested a posttranslational modification to TDP-43. Antibodies against TDP-43 phosphopeptides stain ubiquitinated TDP-43 positive inclusions in patients with FTD/ALS (see **Fig. 3**I, J).[73,74]

There are different kinds of TDP-43 inclusions, including fine skeins, coarse skeins, and dotlike and dense round inclusions (see **Fig. 3** E, G, I). Fine and coarse inclusions are seen with a similar frequency in lower motor neurons (LMNs) and UMNs, whereas dotlike and round inclusions are seen more frequently in the motor neurons of the anterior horn (see **Fig. 3**E–H).[75] In some cases, there is evidence of TDP-43 proteinopathy such as nuclear clearing or diffuse or granular cytoplasmic TDP-43, despite the absence of frank cytoplasmic inclusions (see **Fig. 3**E).[12,76]

It is now apparent that TDP-43 inclusions are not pathognomonic for ALS or FTLD-TDP-43, because inclusions are also observed in Alzheimer disease,[77–79] Lewy body diseases,[78–81] Guamanian parkinsonism dementia complex,[78,79,82] and posttraumatic encephalopathy and neurodegeneration.[83] TDP-43 is present in the mesiotemporal lobe structure in about 30% of the people 65 years or older, regardless of mental illness status,[84] indicating that the aggregation and misfolding of TDP-43 may be caused by processes normally associated with aging.

## SEQUENTIAL CHANGES AND NEUROPATHOLOGIC STAGING

### *Cellular and Microscopic*

Although it is known that motor neurons degenerate and die in ALS, how this degeneration is initiated and progresses or the exact morphologic stages of cell

**Fig. 2.** Classic ALS neuropathology. Loss of motor neurons and astrogliosis is shown in an anterior horn of the spinal cord (*A*, 20X) and motor cortex (*C*, 10X) of ALS and compared with control spinal cord (*B*, 20X) and motor cortex (*D*, 20X). Shrinkage and contraction of motor neuron in ALS (*E*, 40X) is compared with control (*F*, 40X). Vacuolization and spongiosis in motor cortex is shown in ALS (*G*, 20X) and compared with control (*H*, 20X). Bunina bodies are seen in the cytoplasm of motor neurons of ALS (*I*, 40X, *arrowheads*) and compared with control (*J*, 40X). Bunina bodies are positive for cystatin c in ALS (*K*, 40X, *arrowheads*) and compared with the effect of the stain in control (*L*, 40X). Microglial activation is shown by IBA1 in the anterior horn of the spinal cord in ALS (*M*, 20X) but not control (*N*, 20X). (H&E [*A–J*]).

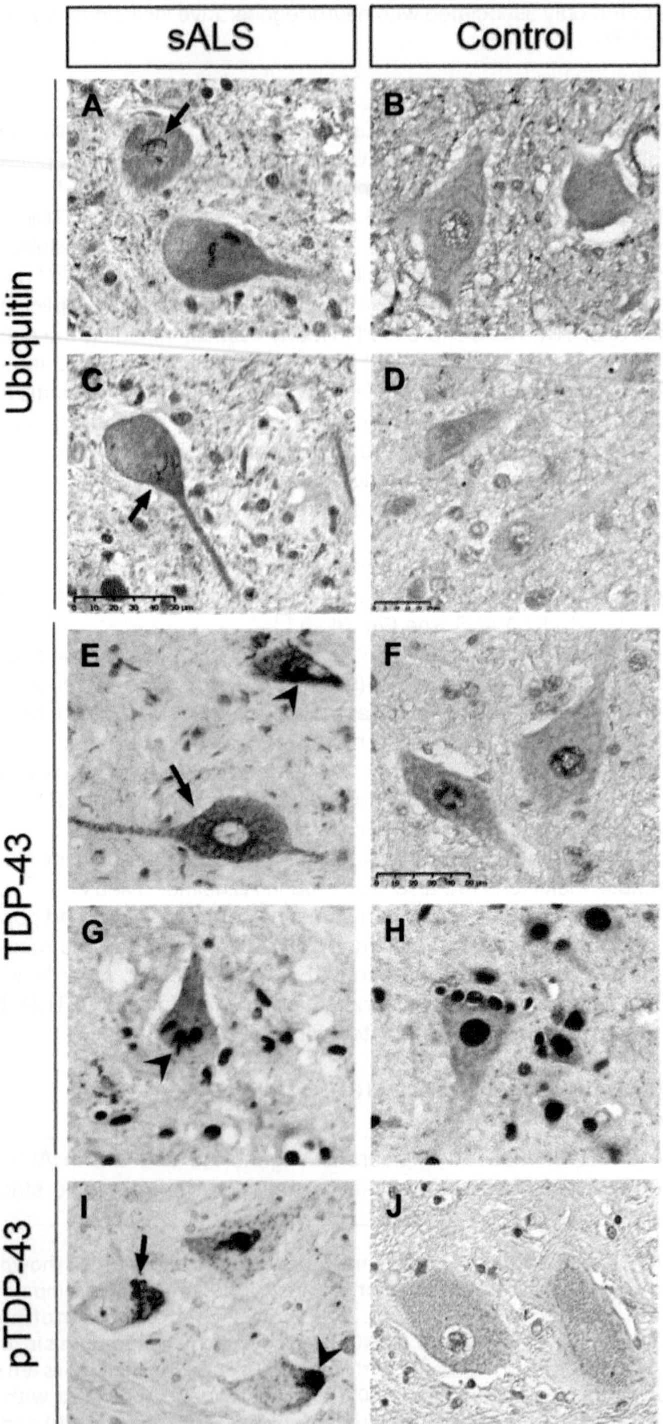
sALS
Control
Ubiquitin
TDP-43
pTDP-43
A
B
C
D
E
F
G
H
I
J

death are not clear. It is commonly believed that motor neuron death in ALS closely resembles apoptosis, although the evidence for this is incomplete.[85] Martin[86] postulated 3 stages of neuronal death in motor neurons of patients with ALS: chromatolysis (dissolution of the Nissl bodies in the cell body of a neuron), somatodendritic attrition, and apoptosis. This process of neuronal death is accompanied by morphologic findings such as cytoplasmic and nuclear condensation and darkness, DNA fragmentation in the presence of DNA fragmentation activation factor, as well as a lack of appreciable vacuolar and edematous cytoplasm in dying neurons. Based on these observations, Martin concluded that apoptosis plays a role in neuronal death in ALS cases. Increased levels of proapoptotic proteins Bax and Bak and decreased levels of antiapoptotic protein Bcl-2 in vulnerable central nervous systems (CNS) regions in patients with ALS compared with controls were also observed, further strengthening the link between motor neuron death and apoptosis.[86] A related question about ALS regards the spread of the disease and the cell-to-cell spread of disease. A neuropathologic correlate of this subject is that LMN loss is greatest at the region of onset and decreased outward.[87,88] Recently, necroptosis, a form of programmed necrosis involving receptor interacting protein 1 and the mixed lineage kinase domainlike protein, has been postulated to be an important driver of motor neuron death,[89] although the neuropathologic underpinnings remain to be established.

### *Anatomic Distribution of Pathologic Changes*

Staging of ALS neuropathology, similar to Alzheimer and Parkinson diseases, has been proposed by Braak and colleagues[90] and Brettschneider and colleagues.[91] In this staging, stage 1 disease is characterized by mild burden of pTDP-43 disease involving motor cortex, brainstem motor nuclei, and spinal motoneurons. Stage 2 disease involves mild-moderate burden of pTDP-43 with dissemination into the prefrontal neocortex (middle frontal gyrus), reticular formation, and precerebellar nuclei. Stage 3 disease involves moderate burden of pTDP-43 with dissemination into the basal ganglia and prefrontal and postcentral neocortex and striatum. Stage 4 disease involves severe burden of pTDP-43 including the hippocampal formation. In the spinal cord, severity of pTDP-43 disease in the lamina IX motor nuclei and neuronal loss correlated closely with gray and white matter oligodendroglial involvement and was linked to onset of disease.[87] pTDP-43 disease sometimes included the Onuf nucleus and neurons of the Clarke column but rarely in the intermediolateral nucleus. Gray matter oligodendroglial pTDP-43 inclusions were present in areas devoid of neuronal pTDP-43 aggregates and neuronal loss and suggested involvement is an early event. This staging classification is based on neuropathology, not clinical disease severity (all nervous systems were from patients who died of end-stage disease), and clinical-pathologic correlations remain to be established.

**Fig. 3.** Inclusions in ALS neuropathology. Ubiquitin skein-like inclusions (*arrows*) are shown in spinal motor neurons of the lumbar anterior horn (*A*) and Betz cells of the motor cortex (*C*) in ALS but not control (*B, D*). TDP-43 inclusions are shown to be diffuse (*arrow*) and skein-like (*arrowhead*) and there is nuclear clearing in the spinal motor neurons of ALS (*E*), features not seen in controls. Note the normal nuclear TDP-43 in control (*F*). TDP-43 dense round inclusions (*arrowhead*) are shown in the motor cortex of ALS (*G*) but not in controls, which show normal nuclear TDP-43 (*H*). Phospho-TDP-43 staining shows skein-like (*arrow*) and dense round (*arrowhead*) inclusions in ALS LMNs (*I*), which are not seen in controls. Note pTDP is not seen in normal nuclei (unlike TDP-43) (*J*). All images are 40X.

**Table 1**
**ALS proteinopathies: main molecular neuropathologic features**

| | | | Main Molecular Features | | | | |
|---|---|---|---|---|---|---|---|
| **Proteinopathy** | **Phenotype** | **Gene** | **Motor Cortex (UMN)** | **Spinal Anterior Horn or Brain Stem Motor Nuclei (LMN)** | **Frontotemporal Regions** | **Miscellaneous (Cerebellum, Hippocampus)** | **Descending Axonal Pathways (eg, Lateral Columns)** |
| FUS pathology<br>FUS proteinopathy | Juvenile ALS<br>Rare adult ALS (usually with atypical symptoms, eg, oculomotility, autonomic, cerebellar or cognitive dysfunction)<br>FTD | FUS-TLS | Basophilic inclusions especially juvenile cases<br>FUS+, TDP43−, NCIs especially juvenile cases<br>FUS+, TDP43−, GCIs especially adult cases | Basophilic inclusions especially juvenile cases<br>FUS+, TDP43−, NCIs all cases<br>FUS+, TDP43−, GCIs especially adult cases | Rare or none basophilic inclusions<br>Rare or none FUS+, TDP43−, NCIs<br>FUS+, TDP43−, GCIs in adult cases | Rare basophilic inclusions<br>FUS+, TDP43−, NCIs and GCIs in other regions including substantia nigra, nuclei raphe, inferior olives, and dentate nucleus in adult cases | Degeneration and sclerosis |
| SOD1 disease[a] | ALS, usually LMN predominant features<br>Very rare FTD | SOD1 | Infrequent abnormalities as seen in spinal anterior horns | Weakly, ubiquitin+, TDP43−, SOD1-neurofilament + intracytoplasmic hyaline conglomerates | Few reports, presumptively same as motor cortex | Changes also in Clarke nucleus, dorsal horn, nucleus ambiguous, and Onuf nucleus | Distal axonal degeneration<br>Also, degeneration in dorsal columns |

| | | | | | | | |
|---|---|---|---|---|---|---|---|
| TDP43 disease (non-C9ORF72 related)<br>TDP43 proteinopathies<br>Ubiquitinated disease | ALS<br>ALS-FTD<br>FTD | Most non-SOD1-associated FALS, including TARDBP<br>All SALS | Ubiquitin+, TDP43+, NCIs and GCIs | Ubiquitin+, TDP43+, NCIs and GCIs | Ubiquitin+, TDP43+, NCIs and GCIs | No significant p62+ or UBQLN+, NCIs or GCIs in cerebellum and hippocampus | Degeneration and sclerosis |
| TDP43 disease or TDP43 proteinopathies, C9ORF72 variant | ALS<br>ALS-FTD<br>FTD | C9ORF72 | Ubiquitin+, TDP43+, NCI and GCI | Ubiquitin+, TDP43+, NCI and GCI | Ubiquitin+, TDP43+, NCI and GCI | p62+, UBQLN+, TDP43−, NCIs and GCIs in cerebellum and hippocampus; TDP+ disease present but separable from p62 and UBQLN | Degeneration and sclerosis |
| Tau pathology (including FTLD-tau with Pick bodies)[b]<br>Tauopathies | FTD<br>Progressive supranuclear palsy<br>Corticobasal syndrome<br>Multiple system atrophy | MAPT | Signature tau+, ubiquitin−, TDP43−, NCIs and GCIs | Few reports, presumptively negative (see 3) | Signature tau+, ubiquitin−, TDP43−, NCIs and GCIs | Pick bodies = 3R tau+ globular or spherical NCIs in the granule cells of dentate gyrus | Presumptively negative |

*Abbreviations:* GCI, glial cytoplasmic inclusions; NCI, nuclear cytoplasmic inclusions.
[a] No primary FTD phenotypes have been defined by SOD1 disease.
[b] Included here for comparison: no primary ALS phenotypes have been defined by tau+ neuropathology.

## FAMILIAL AMYOTROPHIC LATERAL SCLEROSIS: GENETICS AND ASSOCIATED DISEASE

Approximately 90% of all ALS cases occur sporadically, with no associated family history. The remaining 10% of ALS cases are FALS, and are usually the result of dominantly inherited autosomal mutations. The most common mutations occur in SOD1, TDP-43, FUS, and C9orf72, although several other genes have been identified (reviewed in Ref.[92]). The reader is also referred to the article titled "Familial amyotrophic lateral sclerosis" elsewhere in this issue.[93] Each genetic cause correlates with a relatively distinctive neuropathologic signature (see **Table 1**).

### *SOD1*

Mutations in the superoxide dismutase 1 (*SOD1*) gene account for 20% of all FALS cases. Mutations throughout the gene have been linked to ALS. In general, updating of SOD1 neuropathology is critically needed,[94] but it is clear that patients with SOD1 ALS show more severe LMN degeneration than UMN degeneration. UMN degeneration is suggested to be a distal axonopathy.[95] Anterior horn motor neurons also show Lewy body–like inclusions (LBLIs), which consist of a hyalinized, poorly stainable

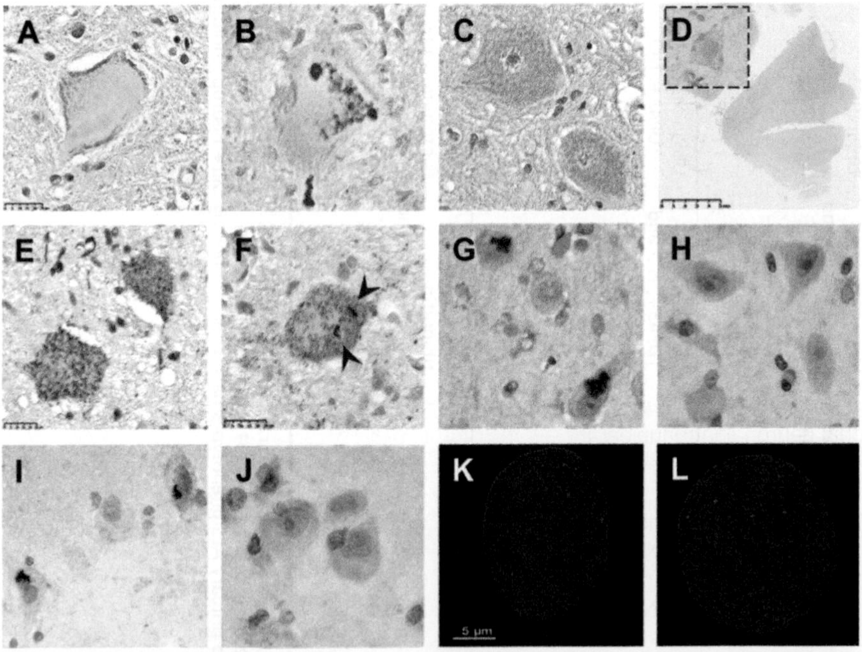


**Fig. 4.** Neuropathology of FALS. Inclusions in a spinal motor neuron from a nervous system of a patient with an SOD1 A4V mutation (*A*, 40X). A subsequent histologic section showing co-localization of misfolded SOD1 and the inclusion (*B*, 40X). Misfolded SOD1 is not seen in spinal motor neurons of controls (*C*, 40X) or in the motor cortex of SOD1 patients (*D*, insert 40X). Skein-like and diffuse inclusions in spinal motor neurons of lumbar spinal cord of a nervous system of a patient with repeat expanded C9orf72 using anti-TDP antibody (*E*, 40X). Diffuse and dense round inclusions (*arrowheads*) are seen in the same C9 patient using an anti-phosphoTDP-43 antibody (*F*, 40X). PolyGA dipeptide repeat proteins in the hippocampus of a nervous system from a patient with a repeat expansion in C9orf72 (*G*, 100X) that are not seen in SALS (*H*, 100X). PolyGP dipeptide repeat proteins in the hippocampus of a nervous system from a patient with repeat expansion in C9orf72 (*I*, 100X) are not seen in SALS (*J*, 100X). RNA foci from the sense (*K*) and antisense (*L*) directions from cultured fibroblasts of a patient with repeat expansion in C9orf72 using FISH.

substance (**Fig. 4**A), which by immunohistochemistry are positive for SOD1, ubiquitin, phosphorylated neurofilaments, and various chaperone proteins,[96,97] but negative for TDP-43, p-TDP-43, and FUS.[98] Isotype-specific antibodies can uniquely detect misfolded SOD1 in spinal cord motor neurons of patients with *SOD1* mutations (see **Fig. 4**B, C). This misfolded SOD1 is absent in the Betz cells in the motor cortex (see **Fig. 4**D). Based on the morphology of the motor neurons and the fact that they are TDP-43 negative,[99] neuropathology suggests that molecular mechanisms of SOD1 mutant FALS may be distinct from SALS. However, misfolded SOD1 aggregates have been reported in SALS as well as mutant SOD1 FALS,[100–102] thus suggesting that SOD1 protein misfolding may play a role in sporadic disease, although such findings remain controversial.[103–105]

### *TDP-43*

The discovery of TDP-43 proteinopathy in 2006 was quickly followed by the identification of mutations in the *TARDBP* gene that encodes it. Mutations are responsible for 2% to 5% of FALS cases. Approximately 30 mutations have been identified throughout *TARDBP*,[16,106] nearly all of them in the glycine-rich domain, which is responsible for regulating gene expression and protein-protein interactions.[107] The TDP-43 and pTDP-43 proteinopathy that is observed in SALS is also observed in FALS caused by *TARDBP* mutations. In a neuropathologic study of patients with the Gly298Ser TDP-43 mutation, inclusions were observed in various locations throughout the CNS, including the substantia nigra, dentate gyrus, cingulate gyrus, amygdala, and the frontal and temporal cortices. The quantity of TDP-43 preinclusions in patients with FALS with this mutation seems to be greater than in patients with SALS.[108]

### *Fused in Sarcoma/Translocated in Sarcoma*

In 2009, mutations in the RNA-binding protein fused in sarcoma (FUS)/translocated in sarcoma in a subset of patients with FALS were identified.[17,18] FUS mutations are responsible for 5% of FALS cases and are distinct from TDP-43 proteinopathies but follow a similar motif wherein a protein involved in RNA metabolism is mislocalized from the nucleus and aggregates in the cytoplasm of neurons. Mutant FUS forms large, ubiquitinated, TDP-43 negative neuronal cytoplasmic inclusions (NCI) and occasional neuronal intranuclear inclusions in the spinal cords and brains of affected patients.[109] These inclusions take the form of fine and coarse granules, as well as filaments, and can be seen in neurons and glia. They are believed to interfere with RNA processing[110] and cause the formation of cytoplasmic stress granules.[111] In contrast with TDP-43 NCIs, cytoplasmic FUS aggregates and nonpathogenic nuclear FUS are not exclusive and can be observed in the same cell. There is 1 report[112] that FUS immunoreactive NCIs may be present in SALS, but the specificity of the antibodies was not proved and there has been no further confirmation. Bunina bodies are absent after H&E staining; however, basophilic cytoplasmic inclusions are present. Specific FUS-ALS mutations may cause distinctive severity and neuropathology[113]: the p.P525L FUS mutation, with early onset, has basophilic inclusions and round FUS-positive NCI, whereas the p.R521C mutation has tanglelike NCI and numerous cytoplasmic inclusions in oligodendroglia. FUS proteinopathy is now understood to account for cases of FTLD-U that are TDP-43-negative[114] and thus cause an ALS-FTLD spectrum.[115]

### *C9orf72*

In 2011, abnormally expanded GGGGCC hexanucleotide repeats in C9orf72 were identified as the most common genetic cause of FALS and FTD.[19,20] This finding not only linked ALS and FTD at the genetic level but connected them to the repeat expansion diseases. C9orf72 neuropathology shows the signature ubiquitin-positive, TDP-43-positive immunoreactive aggregates in neuronal cytoplasm and thus is a TDP-43 proteinopathy (see **Fig. 4**E, F). However, it is unique among the TDP-43 proteinopathies in several respects. Most of the ubiquitinated inclusions in C9orf72-ALS are p62 positive but TDP-43 negative.[116,117] Nucleoporin 62 (p62) is a component of the nuclear envelope and believed to be involved in mRNA and protein trafficking into and out of the nucleus.[118] Another signature is the production of dipeptide repeats proteins (DPRs) resulting from repeat-associated non-ATG translation, which occurs bidirectionally. DPRs translated from the sense strand are poly Gly-Ala (see **Fig. 4**G, H), poly Gly-Pro (see **Fig. 4**I, J), and poly Gly-Arg. DPRs translated from the antisense strand are poly Gly-Pro (also coded by sense), poly Ala-Pro, and poly Pro-Arg. All have been observed in CNS material of C9orf72 cases, although DPRs originating from the sense strand seem to be more frequent than antisense-related dipeptides.[119,120] DPRs colocalize with p62 but not TDP-43.[121,122] DPR aggregates can be seen in different parts of the CNS, including, frontal, occipital, temporal, and motor cortex as well as subcortical areas, midbrain, cerebellum, and spinal cord, but TDP-43 disease may not correlate better with disease stage.[123] Another signature of C9-ALS neuropathology is foci of RNA of the expanded repeat (see **Fig. 4**K, L). These foci are detected by fluorescent in situ hybridization (FISH)[119] and are a feature of several of the repeat expansion diseases.[124] The RNA foci are bidirectionally transcribed and both sense-directed and antisense-directed expansions are seen.[125,126] The foci are in multiple cell types, including motor neurons, microglia, and astrocytes,[20] and in multiple regions of the nervous system, including frontal cortex, motor cortex, hippocampus, cerebellum, and spinal cord, as well as lymphoblasts, fibroblasts, and induced pluripotent stem cell–derived neurons.[123,127,128] RNA foci seem to accumulate in cells with TDP-43 protein abnormalities.[129]

## AMYOTROPHIC LATERAL SCLEROSIS VARIANTS

There are many clinical variants of ALS that seem to be distinctive, and a key debate is whether these are distinct disease entities with different biologies or ends of a continuum. The neuropathologic evidence is scarce but suggests the latter, that they share a similar neuropathology and differences are based on the anatomic distribution of the pathologic burden rather than biological differences. Separate from this debate about ALS are the important genetic syndromes that affect the motor system but are clearly different from ALS; because these may be confusing, they are reviewed here for clarification.

### *Primary Lateral Sclerosis*

Primary lateral sclerosis (PLS) is characterized by its UMN pattern with little or no apparent LMN involvement.[130–132] In this issue, a detailed description can be found in the article titled "Primary lateral sclerosis."[133] By some estimates, PLS is approximately 0.5% as prevalent as ALS. The most commonly reported differences in neuropathology between ALS and PLS lie in which regions have greater demyelination. PLS reportedly shows the greatest demyelination near the corpus callosum, whereas in ALS demyelination occurs most in the superior frontal gyrus.[134] However, PLS neuropathology does show changes in LMNs and these changes are of the same molecular pattern as is seen in typical ALS disease, including TDP-43 disease, at least in some cases.[131,135] Further study is needed to characterize the hallmarks of ALS, including TDP-43 and Bunina bodies, in PLS.

### *Progressive Muscular Atrophy*

Progressive muscular atrophy (PMA) is characterized by it LMN pattern with little or no UMN involvement.[136] The reader is also referred to the article elsewhere in this issue titled "Progressive muscular atrophy."[137] ALS and PMA also share similar genetic mutations in familial cases.[138] Despite the predominant involvement of LMNs clinically, neuropathologic studies have shown degeneration of the corticospinal tract even in the absence of symptoms or signs of UMNs.[139] PMA neuropathology may show abnormalities of the UMN by way of CD68 staining of the descending corticospinal tract, abnormalities identified in 50% of patients with clinically isolated LMN disease.[139] Distinct pathologic change is identified in the motor and extramotor areas of the brains as well as the spinal cords of patients whose disease was clinically limited to the LMN, and these changes seem independent of progression rate.[140] As is seen in ALS, inclusions positive for ubiquitin, TDP-43, and FUS are frequently present.[139,141] Thus, the strongest evidence points to PMA being part of a disease spectrum, not a different disease.

### *Overlap FTD*

The clinical overlap of ALS and FTD[142,143] is mirrored at the neuropathologic level. Nearly all SALS and most FALS (except SOD1 and FUS) show TDP-43 proteinopathy, whereas only about 50% of FTLD is a TDP-43 proteinopathy. Most of the remaining cases of FTLD are considered as tauopathies, and a small percentage are FUS proteinopathies. The discovery of repeat expanded C9orf72 showed a common genetic link between ALS and FTD and highlighted the fact that both ALS and FTD are phenotypes of disease, as well as diseases. C9-ALS and C9-FTD share many pathologic markers (as outlined earlier), and it remains to be shown whether or not C9-ALS, C9-ALS/FTD, and C9-FTD are different neuropathologically; the assumption is that they are not.[121]

### *Spinal Muscular Atrophy*

Spinal muscular atrophy (SMA), like PMA, is also characterized by degeneration of LMNs[144] and results from homozygous mutations in the *SMN1* gene.[145] SMA affects infants, juveniles, and young adults and is the leading genetic cause of infant death.[146] A detailed review of SMA is discussed in the article elsewhere in this issue. Affected individuals show muscle weakness and atrophy of muscle fibers.[144] There is also extensive motor neuron loss, gliosis, neuronophagia, and chromatolysis in the anterior horn.[144,147] Reduction in the number of Betz cells in the motor cortex has also been observed.[147] TDP-43 proteinopathy does not seem to contribute to SMA biology, at least in mouse models.[148]

### *Hereditary Spastic Paraparesis*

Hereditary spastic paraparesis (HSP) is a group of genetically heritable diseases that present with late-onset slowly progressive spasticity of the lower limbs. The neuropathologic findings are almost entirely limited to the pyramidal tracts of the spinal cord and most significantly affect the longest ascending and descending axons. This axonal degeneration is particularly noticeable in the lumbar region of the spinal cord. Some degeneration of the anterior corticospinal and spinocerebellar tracts is also observed, as well as occasional loss of the cells in the anterior horn.[149,150] Only 1 mutation of HSP has been studied neuropathologically, and it did show evidence of TDP-43 proteinopathy.[151]

## FUTURE DIRECTIONS AND FINAL REMARKS

The clinical syndrome called ALS is named by its neuropathology, amyotrophy and lateral sclerosis. With the rapid progress in our understanding of phenotypes, genetics, and molecular biology and with the availability of new microscopic technologies including immunohistochemistry, immunofluorescence, and in situ hybridization, we are beginning to appreciate the extraordinary microscopic and molecular complexity underlying ALS neuropathology and its importance in unraveling the mystery of disease biology.

## ACKNOWLEDGMENTS

Amish Rohatgi created **Fig. 1**. Work has been supported by grants from the National Institutes of Health (NS051738), ALS Association, Target ALS, Microsoft Research, Wyckoff family, Moyer Foundation, Mrs Lois Caprile, and Benaroya Foundation.

## REFERENCES

1. Tyler HR, Shefner J. Amyotrophic lateral sclerosis. Handb Clin Neurol 1991;15: 169–215.
2. Aran F. Recherches sur une maladie non encore décrite du système musculaire (atrophie musculaire progressive). Arch Gen Med 1850;24:172.
3. Cruveilhier J. Sur la paralysie musculaire progressive atrophique. Arch Gen Med 1853;91:561–603.
4. Duchenne de Boulogne G. Recherches électro-physiologiques et thérapeutiques. Comp Rend Seances Acad Sci 1851;32:506.
5. Charcot JM, Joffroy A. Deux cas d'atrophie musculaire progressive: avec lésions de la substance grise et des faisceaux antérolatéraux de la moelle épinière. Paris: Masson; 1869.
6. Charcot J. De la sclérose latérale amyotrophique. Prog Med 1874;2:341–453.
7. Brodmann K. Vergleichende Lokalisationslehre der Grosshirnrinde in ihren Prinzipien dargestellt auf Grund des Zellenbaues. Leipzig (Germany): Barth; 1909.
8. Bunina T. On intracellular inclusions in familial amyotrophic lateral sclerosis. Zh Nevropatol Psikhiatr Im S S Korsakova 1961;62:1293–9 [in Russian].
9. Leigh P, Anderton B, Dodson A, et al. Ubiquitin deposits in anterior horn cells in motor neurone disease. Neurosci Lett 1988;93:197–203.
10. Lowe J, Lennox G, Jefferson D, et al. A filamentous inclusion body within anterior horn neurones in motor neurone disease defined by immunocytochemical localisation of ubiquitin. Neurosci Lett 1988;94:203–10.
11. Arai T, Hasegawa M, Akiyama H, et al. TDP-43 is a component of ubiquitin-positive tau-negative inclusions in frontotemporal lobar degeneration and amyotrophic lateral sclerosis. Biochem Biophys Res Commun 2006;351:602–11.
12. Neumann M, Sampathu DM, Kwong LK, et al. Ubiquitinated TDP-43 in frontotemporal lobar degeneration and amyotrophic lateral sclerosis. Science 2006; 314:130–3.
13. Hudson AJ. Amyotrophic lateral sclerosis and its association with dementia, parkinsonism and other neurological disorders: a review. Brain 1981;104: 217–47.
14. Kiernan JA, Hudson AJ. Frontal lobe atrophy in motor neuron diseases. Brain 1994;117(Pt 4):747–57.
15. Rosen DR, Siddique T, Patterson D, et al. Mutations in Cu/Zn superoxide dismutase gene are associated with familial amyotrophic lateral sclerosis. Nature 1993; 362(6415):59–62.
16. Sreedharan J, Blair IP, Tripathi VB, et al. TDP-43 mutations in familial and sporadic amyotrophic lateral sclerosis. Science 2008;319:1668–72.

17. Vance C, Rogelj B, Hortobagyi T, et al. Mutations in FUS, an RNA processing protein, cause familial amyotrophic lateral sclerosis type 6. Science 2009;323:1208–11.
18. Kwiatkowski TJ Jr, Bosco DA, Leclerc AL, et al. Mutations in the FUS/TLS gene on chromosome 16 cause familial amyotrophic lateral sclerosis. Science 2009;323:1205–8.
19. Renton AE, Majounie E, Waite A, et al. A hexanucleotide repeat expansion in C9ORF72 is the cause of chromosome 9p21-linked ALS-FTD. Neuron 2011;72:257–68.
20. DeJesus-Hernandez M, Mackenzie IR, Boeve BF, et al. Expanded GGGGCC hexanucleotide repeat in noncoding region of C9ORF72 causes chromosome 9p-linked FTD and ALS. Neuron 2011;72:245–56.
21. Ellison D, Love S, Chimelli LMC, et al. Neuropathology: a reference text of CNS pathology. London: Elsevier Health Sciences; 2012.
22. Chang J, Lomen-Hoerth C, Murphy J, et al. A voxel-based morphometry study of patterns of brain atrophy in ALS and ALS/FTLD. Neurology 2005;65:75–80.
23. Abrahams S, Goldstein L, Suckling J, et al. Frontotemporal white matter changes in amyotrophic lateral sclerosis. J Neurol 2005;252:321–31.
24. Murphy JM, Henry RG, Langmore S, et al. Continuum of frontal lobe impairment in amyotrophic lateral sclerosis. Arch Neurol 2007;64:530–4.
25. Kassubek J, Unrath A, Huppertz HJ, et al. Global brain atrophy and corticospinal tract alterations in ALS, as investigated by voxel-based morphometry of 3-D MRI. Amyotroph Lateral Scler Other Motor Neuron Disord 2005;6:213–20.
26. Roccatagliata L, Bonzano L, Mancardi G, et al. Detection of motor cortex thinning and corticospinal tract involvement by quantitative MRI in amyotrophic lateral sclerosis. Amyotroph Lateral Scler 2009;10:47–52.
27. Hammer RP, Tomiyasu U, Scheibel AB. Degeneration of the human Betz cell due to amyotrophic lateral sclerosis. Exp Neurol 1979;63:336–46.
28. Nihei K, McKee AC, Kowall NW. Patterns of neuronal degeneration in the motor cortex of amyotrophic lateral sclerosis patients. Acta Neuropathol 1993;86:55–64.
29. Dickson D, Weller RO. Neurodegeneration: the molecular pathology of dementia and movement disorders. Singapore: John Wiley & Sons; 2011.
30. Stephens B, Guiloff RJ, Navarrete R, et al. Widespread loss of neuronal populations in the spinal ventral horn in sporadic motor neuron disease. A morphometric study. J Neurol Sci 2006;244:41–58.
31. Piao YS, Wakabayashi K, Kakita A, et al. Neuropathology with clinical correlations of sporadic amyotrophic lateral sclerosis: 102 autopsy cases examined between 1962 and 2000. Brain Pathol 2003;13:10–22.
32. Tomonaga M, Saito M, Yoshimura M, et al. Ultrastructure of the Bunina bodies in anterior horn cells of amyotrophic lateral sclerosis. Acta Neuropathol 1978;42:81–6.
33. Kuroda S, Ishizu H, Kawai K, et al. Bunina bodies in dendrites of patients with amyotrophic lateral sclerosis. Acta Med Okayama 1990;44:41–5.
34. Okamoto K, Mizuno Y, Fujita Y. Bunina bodies in amyotrophic lateral sclerosis. Neuropathology 2008;28:109–15.
35. Sasaki S, Maruyama S. Immunocytochemical and ultrastructural studies of the motor cortex in amyotrophic lateral sclerosis. Acta Neuropathol 1994;87:578–85.
36. Okamoto K, Hirai S, Ishiguro K, et al. Light and electron microscopic and immunohistochemical observations of the Onuf's nucleus of amyotrophic lateral sclerosis. Acta Neuropathol 1991;81:610–4.

37. Okamoto K, Hirai S, Amari M, et al. Bunina bodies in amyotrophic lateral sclerosis immunostained with rabbit anti-cystatin C serum. Neurosci Lett 1993; 162:125–8.
38. Mizuno Y, Fujita Y, Takatama M, et al. Peripherin partially localizes in Bunina bodies in amyotrophic lateral sclerosis. J Neurol Sci 2011;302:14–8.
39. Mizuno Y, Amari M, Takatama M, et al. Transferrin localizes in Bunina bodies in amyotrophic lateral sclerosis. Acta Neuropathol 2006;112:597–603.
40. Sasaki S, Komori T, Iwata M. Neuronal inclusions in sporadic motor neuron disease are negative for alpha-synuclein. Neurosci Lett 2006;397:15–9.
41. Mizuno Y, Amari M, Takatama M, et al. Immunoreactivities of p62, an ubiquitin-binding protein, in the spinal anterior horn cells of patients with amyotrophic lateral sclerosis. J Neurol Sci 2006;249:13–8.
42. Murayama S, Mori H, Ihara Y, et al. Immunocytochemical and ultrastructural studies of lower motor neurons in amyotrophic lateral sclerosis. Ann Neurol 1990;27:137–48.
43. Boillée S, Vande Velde C, Cleveland Don W. ALS: a disease of motor neurons and their nonneuronal neighbors. Neuron 2006;52:39–59.
44. McGeer PL, McGeer EG. Inflammatory processes in amyotrophic lateral sclerosis. Muscle Nerve 2002;26:459–70.
45. Boillée S, Yamanaka K, Lobsiger CS, et al. Onset and progression in inherited ALS determined by motor neurons and microglia. Science 2006;312: 1389–92.
46. Yamanaka K, Chun SJ, Boillee S, et al. Astrocytes as determinants of disease progression in inherited amyotrophic lateral sclerosis. Nat Neurosci 2008;11: 251–3.
47. Schiffer D, Fiano V. Astrogliosis in ALS: possible interpretations according to pathogenetic hypotheses. Amyotroph Lateral Scler 2004;5:22–5.
48. Barbeito LH, Pehar M, Cassina P, et al. A role for astrocytes in motor neuron loss in amyotrophic lateral sclerosis. Brain Res Brain Res Rev 2004;47:263–74.
49. Lasiene J, Yamanaka K. Glial cells in amyotrophic lateral sclerosis. Neurol Res Int 2011;2011:718987.
50. Henkel J, Beers D, Zhao W, et al. Microglia in ALS: the good, the bad, and the resting. J Neuroimmune Pharmacol 2009;4:389–98.
51. Leigh P, Whitwell H, Garofalo O, et al. Ubiquitin-immunoreactive intraneuronal inclusions in amyotrophic lateral sclerosis morphology, distribution, and specificity. Brain 1991;114:775–88.
52. Bergmann M, Kuchelmeister K, Schmid K, et al. Different variants of frontotemporal dementia: a neuropathological and immunohistochemical study. Acta Neuropathol 1996;92:170–9.
53. Ikeda K, Akiyama H, Arai T, et al. Morphometrical reappraisal of motor neuron system of Pick's disease and amyotrophic lateral sclerosis with dementia. Acta Neuropathol 2002;104:21–8.
54. Jackson M, Lennox G, Lowe J. Motor neurone disease-inclusion dementia. Neurodegeneration 1996;5:339–50.
55. Okamoto K, Murakami N, Kusaka H, et al. Ubiquitin-positive intraneuronal inclusions in the extramotor cortices of presenile dementia patients with motor neuron disease. J Neurol 1992;239:426–30.
56. Okamoto K, Hirai S, Yamazaki T, et al. New ubiquitin-positive intraneuronal inclusions in the extra-motor cortices in patients with amyotrophic lateral sclerosis. Neurosci Lett 1991;129:233–6.

57. Wightman G, Anderson V, Martin J, et al. Hippocampal and neocortical ubiquitin-immunoreactive inclusions in amyotrophic lateral sclerosis with dementia. Neurosci Lett 1992;139:269–74.
58. Kawashima T, Kikuchi H, Takita M, et al. Skeinlike inclusions in the neostriatum from a case of amyotrophic lateral sclerosis with dementia. Acta Neuropathol 1998;96:541–5.
59. Arai T, Nonaka T, Hasegawa M, et al. Neuronal and glial inclusions in frontotemporal dementia with or without motor neuron disease are immunopositive for p62. Neurosci Lett 2003;342:41–4.
60. Geser F, Lee VM, Trojanowski JQ. Amyotrophic lateral sclerosis and frontotemporal lobar degeneration: a spectrum of TDP-43 proteinopathies. Neuropathology 2010;30:103–12.
61. Ayala YM, De Conti L, Avendaño-Vázquez SE, et al. TDP-43 regulates its mRNA levels through a negative feedback loop. EMBO J 2011;30:277–88.
62. Volkening K, Leystra-Lantz C, Yang W, et al. Tar DNA binding protein of 43 kDa (TDP-43), 14-3-3 proteins and copper/zinc superoxide dismutase (SOD1) interact to modulate NFL mRNA stability. Implications for altered RNA processing in amyotrophic lateral sclerosis (ALS). Brain Res 2009;1305:168–82.
63. Buratti E, De Conti L, Stuani C, et al. Nuclear factor TDP-43 can affect selected microRNA levels. FEBS J 2010;277:2268–81.
64. Kawahara Y, Mieda-Sato A. TDP-43 promotes microRNA biogenesis as a component of the Drosha and Dicer complexes. Proc Natl Acad Sci U S A 2012;109:3347–52.
65. Godena VK, Romano G, Romano M, et al. TDP-43 regulates *Drosophila* neuromuscular junctions growth by modulating Futsch/MAP1B levels and synaptic microtubules organization. PLoS One 2011;6:e17808.
66. Wang I, Wu LS, Chang HY, et al. TDP-43, the signature protein of FTLD-U, is a neuronal activity-responsive factor. J Neurochem 2008;105:797–806.
67. Buratti E, Baralle FE. Characterization and functional implications of the RNA binding properties of nuclear factor TDP-43, a novel splicing regulator of CFTR Exon 9. J Biol Chem 2001;276:36337–43.
68. Giordana MT, Piccinini M, Grifoni S, et al. TDP-43 redistribution is an early event in sporadic amyotrophic lateral sclerosis. Brain Pathol 2010;20:351–60.
69. Thorpe JR, Tang H, Atherton J, et al. Fine structural analysis of the neuronal inclusions of frontotemporal lobar degeneration with TDP-43 proteinopathy. J Neural Transm 2008;115:1661–71.
70. Geser F, O'Dwyer L, Hardiman O, et al. On the development of markers for pathological TDP-43 in amyotrophic lateral sclerosis with and without dementia. Prog Neurobiol 2011;95:649–62.
71. Mackenzie IR, Neumann M, Baborie A, et al. A harmonized classification system for FTLD-TDP pathology. Acta Neuropathol 2011;122:111–3.
72. Davidson Y, Kelley T, Mackenzie IR, et al. Ubiquitinated pathological lesions in frontotemporal lobar degeneration contain the TAR DNA-binding protein, TDP-43. Acta Neuropathol 2007;113:521–33.
73. Hasegawa M, Arai T, Nonaka T, et al. Phosphorylated TDP-43 in frontotemporal lobar degeneration and amyotrophic lateral sclerosis. Ann Neurol 2008;64:60–70.
74. Braak H, Ludolph A, Thal DR, et al. Amyotrophic lateral sclerosis: dash-like accumulation of phosphorylated TDP-43 in somatodendritic and axonal compartments of somatomotor neurons of the lower brainstem and spinal cord. Acta Neuropathol 2010;120:67–74.

75. Mori F, Tanji K, Zhang H-X, et al. Maturation process of TDP-43-positive neuronal cytoplasmic inclusions in amyotrophic lateral sclerosis with and without dementia. Acta Neuropathol 2008;116:193–203.
76. Alves-Rodrigues A, Gregori L, Figueiredo-Pereira ME. Ubiquitin, cellular inclusions and their role in neurodegeneration. Trends Neurosci 1998;21:516–20.
77. Amador-Ortiz C, Lin WL, Ahmed Z, et al. TDP-43 immunoreactivity in hippocampal sclerosis and Alzheimer's disease. Ann Neurol 2007;61:435–45.
78. Higashi S, Iseki E, Yamamoto R, et al. Concurrence of TDP-43, tau and α-synuclein pathology in brains of Alzheimer's disease and dementia with Lewy bodies. Brain Res 2007;1184:284–94.
79. Uryu K, Nakashima-Yasuda H, Forman MS, et al. Concomitant TAR-DNA-binding protein 43 pathology is present in Alzheimer disease and corticobasal degeneration but not in other tauopathies. J Neuropathol Exp Neurol 2008;67:555.
80. Nakashima-Yasuda H, Uryu K, Robinson J, et al. Co-morbidity of TDP-43 proteinopathy in Lewy body related diseases. Acta Neuropathol 2007;114:221–9.
81. Yokota O, Davidson Y, Arai T, et al. Effect of topographical distribution of α-synuclein pathology on TDP-43 accumulation in Lewy body disease. Acta Neuropathol 2010;120:789–801.
82. Hasegawa M, Arai T, Akiyama H, et al. TDP-43 is deposited in the Guam parkinsonism–dementia complex brains. Brain 2007;130:1386–94.
83. McKee AC, Gavett BE, Stern RA, et al. TDP-43 proteinopathy and motor neuron disease in chronic traumatic encephalopathy. J Neuropathol Exp Neurol 2010; 69:918–29.
84. Geser F, Robinson JL, Malunda JA, et al. Pathological 43-kDa transactivation response DNA-binding protein in older adults with and without severe mental illness. Arch Neurol 2010;67:1238–50.
85. Sathasivam S, Ince P, Shaw P. Apoptosis in amyotrophic lateral sclerosis: a review of the evidence. Neuropathol Appl Neurobiol 2001;27:257–74.
86. Martin LJ. Neuronal death in amyotrophic lateral sclerosis is apoptosis: possible contribution of a programmed cell death mechanism. J Neuropathol Exp Neurol 1999;58:459–71.
87. Brettschneider J, Del Tredici K, Irwin DJ, et al. Sequential distribution of pTDP-43 pathology in behavioral variant frontotemporal dementia (bvFTD). Acta Neuropathol 2014;127:423–39.
88. Ravits J, Laurie P, Fan Y, et al. Implications of ALS focality rostral–caudal distribution of lower motor neuron loss postmortem. Neurology 2007;68:1576–82.
89. Re DB, Le Verche V, Yu C, et al. Necroptosis drives motor neuron death in models of both sporadic and familial ALS. Neuron 2014;81:1001–8.
90. Braak H, Brettschneider J, Ludolph AC, et al. Amyotrophic lateral sclerosis–a model of corticofugal axonal spread. Nat Rev Neurol 2013;9:708–14.
91. Brettschneider J, Del Tredici K, Toledo JB, et al. Stages of pTDP-43 pathology in amyotrophic lateral sclerosis. Ann Neurol 2013;74:20–38.
92. Renton AE, Chiò A, Traynor BJ. State of play in amyotrophic lateral sclerosis genetics. Nat Neurosci 2014;17:17–23.
93. Boylan K. Familial Amyotrophic Lateral Sclerosis. Neurol Clin 2015, in press.
94. Ince PG, Highley JR, Kirby J, et al. Molecular pathology and genetic advances in amyotrophic lateral sclerosis: an emerging molecular pathway and the significance of glial pathology. Acta Neuropathol 2011;122:657–71.
95. Ince PG, Tomkins J, Slade JY, et al. Amyotrophic lateral sclerosis associated with genetic abnormalities in the gene encoding Cu/Zn superoxide dismutase:

molecular pathology of five new cases, and comparison with previous reports and 73 sporadic cases of ALS. J Neuropathol Exp Neurol 1998;57:895–904.
96. Mizusawa H, Matsumoto S, Yen SH, et al. Focal accumulation of phosphorylated neurofilaments within anterior horn cell in familial amyotrophic lateral sclerosis. Acta Neuropathol 1989;79:37–43.
97. Okamoto Y, Shirakashi Y, Ihara M, et al. Colocalization of 14-3-3 proteins with SOD1 in Lewy body-like hyaline inclusions in familial amyotrophic lateral sclerosis cases and the animal model. PLoS One 2011;6:e20427.
98. Nakamura S, Wate R, Kaneko S, et al. An autopsy case of sporadic amyotrophic lateral sclerosis associated with the I113T SOD1 mutation. Neuropathology 2014;34:58–63.
99. Mackenzie IRA, Bigio EH, Ince PG, et al. Pathological TDP-43 distinguishes sporadic amyotrophic lateral sclerosis from amyotrophic lateral sclerosis with SOD1 mutations. Ann Neurol 2007;61:427–34.
100. Bosco DA, Morfini G, Karabacak NM, et al. Wild-type and mutant SOD1 share an aberrant conformation and a common pathogenic pathway in ALS. Nat Neurosci 2010;13:1396–403.
101. Forsberg K, Jonsson PA, Andersen PM, et al. Novel antibodies reveal inclusions containing non-native SOD1 in sporadic ALS patients. PLoS One 2010;5:e11552.
102. Forsberg K, Andersen PM, Marklund SL, et al. Glial nuclear aggregates of superoxide dismutase-1 are regularly present in patients with amyotrophic lateral sclerosis. Acta Neuropathol 2011;121:623–34.
103. Liu HN, Sanelli T, Horne P, et al. Lack of evidence of monomer/misfolded superoxide dismutase-1 in sporadic amyotrophic lateral sclerosis. Ann Neurol 2009;66:75–80.
104. Kerman A, Liu H-N, Croul S, et al. Amyotrophic lateral sclerosis is a non-amyloid disease in which extensive misfolding of SOD1 is unique to the familial form. Acta Neuropathol 2010;119:335–44.
105. Brotherton TE, Li Y, Cooper D, et al. Localization of a toxic form of superoxide dismutase 1 protein to pathologically affected tissues in familial ALS. Proc Natl Acad Sci U S A 2012;109:5505–10.
106. Yokoseki A, Shiga A, Tan CF, et al. TDP-43 mutation in familial amyotrophic lateral sclerosis. Ann Neurol 2008;63:538–42.
107. Pesiridis GS, Lee VM, Trojanowski JQ. Mutations in TDP-43 link glycine-rich domain functions to amyotrophic lateral sclerosis. Hum Mol Genet 2009;18:R156–62.
108. Van Deerlin VM, Leverenz JB, Bekris LM, et al. TARDBP mutations in amyotrophic lateral sclerosis with TDP-43 neuropathology: a genetic and histopathological analysis. Lancet Neurol 2008;7:409–16.
109. Verbeeck C, Deng Q, Dejesus-Hernandez M, et al. Expression of fused in sarcoma mutations in mice recapitulates the neuropathology of FUS proteinopathies and provides insight into disease pathogenesis. Mol Neurodegener 2012;7:53.
110. Takanashi K, Yamaguchi A. Aggregation of ALS-linked FUS mutant sequesters RNA binding proteins and impairs RNA granules formation. Biochem Biophys Res Commun 2014;452:600–7.
111. Vance C, Scotter EL, Nishimura AL, et al. ALS mutant FUS disrupts nuclear localization and sequesters wild-type FUS within cytoplasmic stress granules. Hum Mol Genet 2013;22:2676–88.

112. Deng HX, Zhai H, Bigio EH, et al. FUS-immunoreactive inclusions are a common feature in sporadic and non-SOD1 familial amyotrophic lateral sclerosis. Ann Neurol 2010;67:739–48.
113. Mackenzie IR, Ansorge O, Strong M, et al. Pathological heterogeneity in amyotrophic lateral sclerosis with FUS mutations: 2 distinct patterns correlating with disease severity and mutation. Acta Neuropathol 2011;122:87–98.
114. Mackenzie IR, Neumann M, Bigio EH, et al. Nomenclature and nosology for neuropathologic subtypes of frontotemporal lobar degeneration: an update. Acta Neuropathol 2010;119:1–4.
115. Snowden JS, Hu Q, Rollinson S, et al. The most common type of FTLD-FUS (aFTLD-U) is associated with a distinct clinical form of frontotemporal dementia but is not related to mutations in the FUS gene. Acta Neuropathol 2011;122: 99–110.
116. Pikkarainen M, Hartikainen P, Alafuzoff I. Neuropathologic features of frontotemporal lobar degeneration with ubiquitin-positive inclusions visualized with ubiquitin-binding protein p62 immunohistochemistry. J Neuropathol Exp Neurol 2008;67:280–98.
117. King A, Al-Sarraj S, Shaw C. Frontotemporal lobar degeneration with ubiquitinated tau-negative inclusions and additional α-synuclein pathology but also unusual cerebellar ubiquitinated p62-positive, TDP-43-negative inclusions. Neuropathology 2009;29:466–71.
118. Bullock TL, Clarkson WD, Kent HM, et al. The 1.6 angstroms resolution crystal structure of nuclear transport factor 2 (NTF2). J Mol Biol 1996;260:422–31.
119. Zu T, Liu Y, Bañez-Coronel M, et al. RAN proteins and RNA foci from antisense transcripts in C9ORF72 ALS and frontotemporal dementia. Proc Natl Acad Sci U S A 2013;110:E4968–77.
120. Mori K, Weng S-M, Arzberger T, et al. The C9orf72 GGGGCC repeat is translated into aggregating dipeptide-repeat proteins in FTLD/ALS. Science 2013; 339:1335–8.
121. Al-Sarraj S, King A, Troakes C, et al. p62 positive, TDP-43 negative, neuronal cytoplasmic and intranuclear inclusions in the cerebellum and hippocampus define the pathology of C9orf72-linked FTLD and MND/ALS. Acta Neuropathol 2011;122:691–702.
122. Boxer AL, Mackenzie IR, Boeve BF, et al. Clinical, neuroimaging and neuropathological features of a new chromosome 9p-linked FTD-ALS family. J Neurol Neurosurg Psychiatry 2011;82:196–203.
123. Mackenzie IR, Frick P, Neumann M. The neuropathology associated with repeat expansions in the C9ORF72 gene. Acta Neuropathol 2014;127:347–57.
124. Wojciechowska M, Krzyzosiak WJ. Cellular toxicity of expanded RNA repeats: focus on RNA foci. Hum Mol Genet 2011;20:3811–21.
125. Lagier-Tourenne C, Baughn M, Rigo F, et al. Targeted degradation of sense and antisense C9orf72 RNA foci as therapy for ALS and frontotemporal degeneration. Proc Natl Acad Sci U S A 2013;110:E4530–9.
126. Mizielinska S, Lashley T, Norona FE, et al. C9orf72 frontotemporal lobar degeneration is characterised by frequent neuronal sense and antisense RNA foci. Acta Neuropathol 2013;126:845–57.
127. Gendron TF, Bieniek KF, Zhang YJ, et al. Antisense transcripts of the expanded C9ORF72 hexanucleotide repeat form nuclear RNA foci and undergo repeat-associated non-ATG translation in c9FTD/ALS. Acta Neuropathol 2013;126: 829–44.

128. Mori K, Arzberger T, Grasser FA, et al. Bidirectional transcripts of the expanded C9orf72 hexanucleotide repeat are translated into aggregating dipeptide repeat proteins. Acta Neuropathol 2013;126:881–93.
129. Cooper-Knock J, Higginbottom A, Stopford MJ, et al. Antisense RNA foci in the motor neurons of C9ORF72-ALS patients are associated with TDP-43 proteinopathy. Acta Neuropathol 2015;130:1–13.
130. Ravits J. Focality, stochasticity and neuroanatomic propagation in ALS pathogenesis. Exp Neurol 2014;262(Pt B):121–6.
131. Kosaka T, Fu YJ, Shiga A, et al. Primary lateral sclerosis: upper-motor-predominant amyotrophic lateral sclerosis with frontotemporal lobar degeneration–immunohistochemical and biochemical analyses of TDP-43. Neuropathology 2012;32: 373–84.
132. Pringle CE, Hudson AJ, Munoz DG, et al. Primary lateral sclerosis: clinical features, neuropathology and diagnostic criteria. Brain 1992;115:495–520.
133. Statland JM, Barohn RJ, Dimachkie MM, et al. Primary Lateral Sclerosis. Neurol Clin 2015, in press.
134. Kolind S, Sharma R, Knight S, et al. Myelin imaging in amyotrophic and primary lateral sclerosis. Amyotroph Lateral Scler Frontotemporal Degener 2013;14: 562–73.
135. Dickson DW, Josephs KA, Amador-Ortiz C. TDP-43 in differential diagnosis of motor neuron disorders. Acta Neuropathol 2007;114:71–9.
136. Swank RL, Putnam TJ. Amyotrophic lateral sclerosis and related conditions: a clinical analysis. Arch Neurol Psychiatry 1943;49:151–77.
137. Liewluck T, Saperstein DS. Progressive Muscular Atrophy. Neurol Clin 2015, in press.
138. van Blitterswijk M, Vlam L, van Es MA, et al. Genetic overlap between apparently sporadic motor neuron diseases. PLoS One 2012;7:e48983.
139. Ince P, Evans J, Knopp M, et al. Corticospinal tract degeneration in the progressive muscular atrophy variant of ALS. Neurology 2003;60:1252–8.
140. Geser F, Stein B, Partain M, et al. Motor neuron disease clinically limited to the lower motor neuron is a diffuse TDP-43 proteinopathy. Acta Neuropathol 2011; 121:509–17.
141. Riku Y, Atsuta N, Yoshida M, et al. Differential motor neuron involvement in progressive muscular atrophy: a comparative study with amyotrophic lateral sclerosis. BMJ Open 2014;4:e005213.
142. Lomen-Hoerth C, Anderson T, Miller B. The overlap of amyotrophic lateral sclerosis and frontotemporal dementia. Neurology 2002;59:1077–9.
143. Lomen-Hoerth C, Murphy J, Langmore S, et al. Are amyotrophic lateral sclerosis patients cognitively normal? Neurology 2003;60:1094–7.
144. Lunn MR, Wang CH. Spinal muscular atrophy. Lancet 2008;371:2120–33.
145. Alías L, Bernal S, Fuentes-Prior P, et al. Mutation update of spinal muscular atrophy in Spain: molecular characterization of 745 unrelated patients and identification of 4 novel mutations in the SMN1 gene. Hum Genet 2009;125:29–39.
146. Zhang Z, Pinto AM, Wan L, et al. Dysregulation of synaptogenesis genes antecedes motor neuron pathology in spinal muscular atrophy. Proc Natl Acad Sci U S A 2013;110:19348–53.
147. Araki S, Hayashi M, Tamagawa K, et al. Neuropathological analysis in spinal muscular atrophy type II. Acta Neuropathol 2003;106:441–8.
148. Turner BJ, Bäumer D, Parkinson NJ, et al. TDP-43 expression in mouse models of amyotrophic lateral sclerosis and spinal muscular atrophy. Neurosci 2008;9:104.

149. Behan WM, Maia M. Strümpell's familial spastic paraplegia: genetics and neuropathology. J Neurol Neurosurg Psychiatry 1974;37:8–20.
150. Harding A. Hereditary spastic paraplegias. Semin Neurol 1993;13:333.
151. Martinez-Lage M, Molina-Porcel L, Falcone D, et al. TDP-43 pathology in a case of hereditary spastic paraplegia with a NIPA1/SPG6 mutation. Acta Neuropathol 2012;124(2):285–91.

# Potential Environmental Factors in Amyotrophic Lateral Sclerosis

Björn Oskarsson, MD[a,*], D. Kevin Horton, DrPH, MSPH, CPH[b], Hiroshi Mitsumoto, MD, DSc[c]

**KEYWORDS**

- ALS • Epidemiology • Environmental risk factors • Smoking • Gender
- Military service • Oxidative stress

**KEY POINTS**

- Proven risk factors for ALS are genetic variants, male gender, and advanced age.
- The only environmental factor that is generally accepted to be associated with ALS is smoking.
- Some evidence supports US military service, lead exposure, physical activity, β-N-methylamino-L-alanine (BMAA), head trauma, electromagnetic fields, agricultural chemicals, and heavy metals as possible factors.
- ALS/Parkinson-dementia complex of Guam and the western Pacific is a distinct clinicopathologic entity; its cause may be different from ALS.
- Oxidative stress is a plausible mechanism through which many environmental risk factors may affect ALS.

## INTRODUCTION

The causes of amyotrophic lateral sclerosis (ALS) are unknown for most patients. ALS is a clinically defined syndrome where upper and lower motor neurons degenerate, but

---

The authors have nothing to disclose.
Disclaimer: The conclusions of this article are those of the authors and do not necessarily represent the views of the federal Agency for Toxic Substances and Disease Registry, the Centers for Disease Control and Prevention, or the US Department of Health and Human Services.
This work was supported in part by grant funds from the National Institutes of Health (UL1 TR000002, R01 ES 016848-01A2 and KL2 TR000134).
[a] UC Davis Multidisciplinary ALS Clinic, An ALS Association Certified Center of Excellence, University of California Davis Medical Center, 4860 Y Street, Suite 3700, Sacramento, CA 95817, USA; [b] Division of Toxicology and Human Health Sciences, ATSDR/CDC, 4770 Buford Highway Northeast, Atlanta, GA 30341, USA; [c] The Eleanor and Lou Gehrig MDA/ALS Research Center, The Neurological Institute, Columbia University Medical Center, 710 West 168th Street, Floor 9, New York, NY 10032, USA
* Corresponding author.
*E-mail address:* boskarsson@ucdavis.edu

Neurol Clin 33 (2015) 877–888
http://dx.doi.org/10.1016/j.ncl.2015.07.009 neurologic.theclinics.com
0733-8619/15/$ – see front matter 

it is not clear that the pathogenesis is identical across individual cases. It has been suggested that, for all cases, multiple events need to occur or multiple factors need to be present for the disease to manifest. Presumably these would include genetic susceptibility factors and the environmental or random factors that influence them. As of yet there are not any specific environmental factors that are proven to cause ALS, apart from smoking, but this article discusses several factors that have been examined, and their possible mechanisms. We summarize these in the table (**Table 1**) and rate of the strength of the association using the grading system proposed by Armon. Many proposed factors are not covered because there are more than 1000 epidemiologic ALS studies published. Controversy exists in regards to each of these factors ranging from limited data to conflicting evidence.

## GENE-ENVIRONMENT INTERACTION

No gene conferring susceptibility to a certain environmental exposure has been established in ALS, but the search continues.[1] Several candidate ALS risk genes have emerged from association studies, but these results have not been replicable in other populations outside of where they were identified. Theoretically this could

**Table 1**
**Proposed Risk factors for ALS**

| Proposed Risk Factor | Level of Increased Risk | Strength[62] and Type of Evidence | Proposed Mechanisms | References |
|---|---|---|---|---|
| Male gender | OR, 1.5 | Level A | Early testosterone exposure | 4 |
| Smoking | OR, 1.1 | Level A | Oxidative stress<br>Lead<br>Other toxins | 63 |
| US military service | OR, 0.22 to SMR, 1.92 | Level B | Multiple | 29 |
| Lead | OR, 1.81 | Level B | Neurotoxicity | 42 |
| Pesticides | OR<br>Men, 1.88<br>Women, 1.31 | Level B | Neurotoxic | 51 |
| Physical activity (or predilection thereof) | Unknown | Level U | Physical fitness, early testosterone exposure | 43,44 |
| Head trauma | Unknown | Level U | Direct neuronal injury | 64 |
| Electromagnetic radiation | Unknown | Level U | Electromagnetic field | 37 |
| Low body mass index | Unknown | Level U | Higher metabolism | 45 |
| Statin treatment | Unknown | Level U | Altered lipid metabolism | 47 |
| BMAA | Unknown | Level U | Neurotoxicity | 17,18 |

*Abbreviations:* BMAA, β-*N*-methylamino-L-alanine; OR, odds ratio; SMR, standardized morbidity/mortality ratio.

Level A rating: This is an established risk factor, Level B rating: This is a probable risk factor ('more likely than not'), Level C rating: This is a possible risk factor (does not attain a 'more likely than not' status). Better-designed studies may be warranted with regard to this risk factor, Level U rating: It is unknown whether this is a risk factor.

be caused by differing environmental exposures. For a condition to be influenced by an environmental factor there must be susceptibility, and there is evidence that susceptibility can vary among individuals in conditions related to exposure to a toxic risk factor. Examples from the neuromuscular field include where certain gene variations confer increased susceptibility: statins (SLCO1B1), azathioprine (TPMT), and vincristine (PMP 22). Varied susceptibility makes the relationship between exposure and disease more complex. A long delay between exposure and clinical disease also complicates ascertainment of risk factors. The onset of clinical ALS has generally been thought of as the disease onset, but a long preclinical phase of neuronal dysfunction may precede frank cell death. Other more common neurodegenerative diseases, such as Alzheimer's and Parkinson's disease, have a preclinical disease phase and this is certainly also possible in ALS. Epigenetic modifications caused by environmental factors may be the mediators of such delayed mechanisms.[2]

Most of the monogenetic types of familial ALS (fALS) do not lead to ALS in utero or in childhood years, but rather these diseases manifest later in adult life. Yet, on average fALS presents at an earlier age than sporadic ALS (sALS). Mathematical modeling using multistep disease occurrence borrowed from the cancer field suggests that, to develop ALS, six events need to occur in an individual.[3] The presence of a fALS gene is one such event. This type of modeling data implies that environmental factors also play a role in the cause of ALS, not just sALS. As the understanding of genetics and environmental medicine improves, gene-environment interactions will become clearer.

Age is a known strong risk factor for ALS. The incidence of ALS increases markedly with older age. There does, however, seem to be a slight reduction of incidence after the eighth or ninth decade, a finding that contrasts with many other neurodegenerative diseases. This could support the idea that only a portion of the human population is susceptible to ALS. By the time the ninth decade is reached, most people at risk of developing ALS have developed the disease, and this could explain the diminishing incidence. Otherwise the accrual of risk factors for ALS to manifest would be expected to increase, resulting in an ever increasing incidence for fALS and sALS.

## PROPOSED ENVIRONMENTAL FACTORS

### *Gender*

The strongest risk factor for ALS outside of fALS is male gender. Male gender is consistently detected as a factor associated with a 1.5 times increased risk of developing ALS compared with female gender.[4] Human males and females differ genetically, physiologically socially, and in their activities and environmental exposures. It is likely that multiple factors contribute to the observed gender difference in ALS incidence. A direct genetic connection seems likely, but the only X-linked fALS identified to date is a very rare defect in Ubiquilin 2; otherwise there is no proven direct gender-genetic connection. After menopause the incidence of ALS becomes nearly equal between the genders in many series.

The increased male risk could be mediated by the sex hormone testosterone, one of the major determinants of male sex characteristics. Testosterone begins to affect an individual in utero and fetal testosterone has been suggested as a risk factor for ALS, with anthropomorphic measures supporting this connection. The relative length of the second and fourth finger is influenced by the level of fetal testosterone,[5] and patients with ALS have relative finger length difference that are statistically greater than the mean population.[6] Later in life men are also more likely to be exposed to many environmental risk factors, including physical activity, head trauma, military service, heavy metal exposure, high field electromagnetic exposure, and other professions that have been suggested as risk factors.

### *Geographic Region*

Environmental exposures and disparate genetic heritage can be expected to vary by region in the world and a varying incidence of ALS across different regions would therefore seem likely. The best current nationwide epidemiologic data are from different industrial nations, mostly from Western Europe or countries with majority European emigrant populations. At the large national scale these first-world countries show no large differences. In European studies the estimated incidence is around 1.47 per 100,000, with most studies ranging from 1.0 to 3.0 per 100,000.[7] Prevalence in Western Europe was estimated at 4.06 per 100,000.[7] North American studies have estimated incidences around 1.75.[7] The US National ALS Registry has provided US prevalence estimates of 3.9 per 100,000 for 2010 to 2011.[4] Thus the differences between Western Europe and the United States are small. Japanese estimates have consistently been slightly higher with the latest incidence and prevalence being 2.2 and 9.9, respectively.[8] Japanese prevalence numbers could be higher because of a relatively higher use of mechanical ventilation as treatment, thereby prolonging survival of patients.

In less developed countries the estimated prevalence of ALS is generally lower and this is most likely because of less complete case ascertainment and diagnoses. Alternatively there are important environmental risk factors that are increased with highly developed countries, but in general exposures to known environmental toxins are higher in developing nations.[9] Lower and higher rates have been suggested for sub-Saharan Africa, but no good quality data exist.[10]

### *Clusters*

Regional geographic variability in ALS incidence has been shown many times. Generally these variations are small (relative risk, 0.5–2) but statistically significant. Different analysis strategies of the same data may also provide different conclusions, as demonstrated in the rigorous national Irish 1995 to 2013 cohort.[11] In this well-regarded study two types of analysis were done. Bayesian risk mapping identified several clusters of increased incidence, but with even more sophisticated formal cluster analysis (conducted by the same group of investigators) the clusters disappeared, but similar areas of relatively low incidence were identified again. It is worth keeping in mind that an uneven distribution could be the result of random variation, particularly when small numbers of cases are considered.

Most published studies looking to identify clusters have done so. Examples include Italian,[12] English,[13] French,[14] and Japanese[15] cluster studies. Differing explanations have been proposed, such as two Finnish clusters attributed to genetics or perinatal factors,[16] and both northeastern United States[17] and French[18] clusters proposed to be caused by proximity to water where cyanobacterial blooms occur, possibly mediated by β-*N*-methylamino-L-alanine (BMAA). Such connections are at this time speculative and require further study for verification.[19]

### *Amyotrophic Lateral Sclerosis/Parkinson-Dementia Complex*

The most well established geographic cluster of an ALS-like disease has been on the island of Guam. This cluster, with an incidence of 140 per 100,000 population, is not only limited geographically, but also temporally. On Guam there was a marked increase in incidence of ALS among the Chamorro people that decreased from the early

1950s to the 1980s, with much fewer cases reported since that time.[20] This Guamanian ALS is distinct from sALS and fALS. It clinically associates with Parkinson disease and dementia and is labeled ALS/Parkinson-dementia complex (ALS/PDC).

Neuropathologically ALS/PDC is a tauopathy and this may suggest a quite different pathologic process from ALS; however, both share ubiquitin and TDP43 pathology.[21] Some Chamorros without ALS/PDC also demonstrate tau pathology. This could suggest either a premanifestation state or that the tauopathy is not purely a consequence of the ALS/PDC. Clinically the presentation can be typical for ALS, Parkinson, or a dementia, but often overlapping features exist. The mechanism behind ALS/PDC remains unproved and the disappearance of the disease from Guam makes it harder to study. Some Filipino immigrants to Guam who adopted the native lifestyle also developed the disease, suggesting an acquired nature. Natives who emigrated at an early age later developed the disease, possibly indicating that early life exposure could affect later manifestation. Extensive genetic studies have also failed to yield any genetic associations.

The current leading hypothesis behind ALS/PDC is neurotoxicity from BMAA. This amino acid is produced by blue-green algae and it is a neurotoxin that can cause motor neuron disease in animal models.[22] BMAA is present in high levels in the cycad plants native to Guam and further bioaccumulated by fruit bats, which were a popular food for the decades preceding the ALS/PDC outbreak. BMAA has been proposed to be an environmental risk factor not just for ALS/PDC, but for ALS, Parkinson disease, Alzheimer disease, and other neurodegenerative diseases. This remains controversial and only limited evidence supports this idea. Blue-green algae and BMAA are nearly ubiquitous so if this connection could be established it might have wide ranging implications. On Japan's Kii peninsula ALS/PDC also occurred,[23] and a third focus for ALS/PDC exists in western Papua.[24] Both clusters seem to be disappearing, but still have higher than expected rates for ALS. Cycads grow and are used as medicines and food in both regions.

### *Smoking*

Tobacco smoking has been posited to increase the risk for ALS in several studies.[25] Pooled analysis[26] and meta-analysis supports this notion, at least in women.[27] A minority of studies suggest a reduced risk.[28] It is not known whether the association between ALS and smoking is caused by nicotine, oxidative stress, or one of the many other known toxic substances in tobacco smoke.

### *Occupational Risks*

Many occupations share common exposures and arguably many of the occupations proposed to predispose to ALS are physically active ones with high risk for trauma. No causal factors have been identified.

US military service has been suggested as being a risk factor for ALS in several studies examining the topic.[29] The risk has been estimated with an odds ratio of 0.22,[30] to a standardized morbidity/mortality ratio of 1.92.[31] No singular factor has been discernable; no link to combat, service branch, or place of deployment has been consistently identified. Other exposures that are common in military service are strenuous physical exertion, poor sleep, trauma, psychological stress, and lead exposure (some of which are discussed later).

Furthermore, there does not seem to be a general association between ALS and military service. French,[32] Italian,[33] and British[34] data do not suggest a positive association between ALS and their respective militaries. The Institute of Medicine determined that the evidence is limited but suggestive, and recommends further studies.[35] US medical providers should be aware that there are special veteran's benefits for all US veterans with ALS.

High linesmen and electricians and other professions with exposure to high-strength electromagnetic fields have been suggested as having an increased risk of ALS. Odds ratios as high as 6.7 have been proposed,[36] but the association is not consistent. Residential exposure to electromagnetic fields does not seem to infer a risk of developing ALS.[37]

Other occupations that have been proposed to have an increased risk of ALS include welders,[36] agricultural workers,[38] and soccer players.[39] The methodology used for the many studies trying to discern occupational risk for developing ALS are varied, which complicates attempts to conduct systematic reviews. However, in one systematic review military service was considered to be a likely factor, and health care workers (including veterinarians), hairdressers, and power plant and electrical workers were candidate professions with a possibility for increased risk.[40] The US National ALS Registry is currently collecting data related to occupation and it is hoped this will lead to a better understanding of occupational risk within the United States.

### *Lead*

Many metals, including lead, are neurotoxic and can cause neuropathies with strong motor nerve involvement. Several studies have found a connection between lead and ALS, whereas others have found no relationship.[41] A recent meta-analysis does support the connection,[42] but flaws in the original retrospective case control studies, particularly in regard to ascertainment of exposure, makes the conclusion arguable. The connection between lead and ALS is unproven and unclear. Many of the lead studies have also seen prolonged survival in patients with ALS who have higher lead levels. This could mean that lead is a risk factor for developing ALS and a protective factor that slows ALS disease progression. Selenium, mercury, and other metals are less well studied and no firm connections with ALS are established.

### *Physical Exercise*

Physical exercise and activity has been positively correlated with ALS incidence in many studies, but not all.[43] The American moniker for ALS - "Lou Gehrig's disease" – after the baseball player who succumbed to the disease - exemplifies and/or contributes to this idea. A dose relationship between physical exercise and ALS has not been shown and it has been suggested that the increased risk is not due to actual physical activity itself, but instead it is due to unknown congenital factors predisposing individuals to physical activity and fitness.[44] It has been proposed that it is this "athletic phenotype" that conveys the increased risk of ALS.[45] There are several plausible explanations for how exercise directly could cause ALS including increased oxidative stress and potentiation of environmental toxins.[45,46]

### *Trauma*

A relationship between head trauma and ALS has not been definitively proved, but several studies have examined head trauma as a risk factor for ALS.[47,48] Head trauma can cause a neurodegenerative disease called chronic traumatic encephalopathy (CTE). A misclassification of some patients with CTE as having ALS has been proposed as a possible explanation for the apparent increase of ALS cases in patients with prior head trauma. CTE shares tau and TDP43 pathologic features with ALS/PDC, and is more clearly differentiated from sALS.

Limb or other injury is frequently described preceding the first manifestation of disease by patients with ALS. A positive linear relationship between ALS severity and number of trauma events has been observed,[49] but other studies were unable to find a relationship between trauma and ALS. Weakness from ALS commonly result in traumatic falls, when they occur prior to the ALS diagnosis patients may interpret the trauma as the cause of the ALS.

### *Agricultural Chemicals*

Many pesticides are known to be neurotoxic and such substances as organophosphates have a direct effect on the lower motor neuron synapse.[50] Farm workers[51,52] and athletes working on grass covered playing fields[52] may have increase incidences of ALS. Several studies have found an association between ALS and chemicals including pesticides and herbicides, but a meta-analysis does not confirm this relationship.[51]

### *Other*

An association between cancers and ALS has been considered,[53] but such a connection has not been found in methodologically rigorous studies.[47,54]

Statin medications have been suggested both to increase the risk[55] of ALS and decrease it.[47] At this time the evidence favors a protective or null effect.[56] Other protective environmental factors that have been suggested include vitamins E[57] and D, but strong evidence is lacking.[58]

## COMBINED OXIDATIVE STRESS THEORY

Any factor that favors a pro-oxidative state could contribute to oxidative stress, and there are many indicators that oxidative stress is one of the central pathways in motor neuron disease.[59,60] Oxidative stress could potentially be the common aspect of many studied environmental risk factors in ALS, including lead (and other heavy metals), organophosphate pesticides, trauma, physical activity, and smoking. Studies evaluating a potential factor individually, along with biomarkers measuring a summation of oxidative factors, could help better define their contribution to ALS risk.[61]

**CASE VIGNETTE**

*A 45-year-old US Navy veteran presents to the ALS clinic after a referral from his Veterans Affairs neurologist for suspected ALS. He started developing slurring of his speech 9 months earlier and this has gradually progressed. He also noted choking on liquids in the last 2 months. He is no longer working as an electrician and he is less interested in pursuing his action shooting hobby and is no longer recharging his casings. He notes no cognitive change but his wife thinks that he is a bit more withdrawn and more easily frustrated. Despite this he is generally quite positive and considers himself blessed with a very good life up until this point. His past medical history includes two concussions and hyperlipidemia. He has been taking a statin medication for the last 4 years. The only neurologic disease that he knows of in his family is dementia. His mother is 75 years old and has dementia; she lives in a nursing home. She had been "acting strangely" even before her "memory got bad" and she still easily recognizes her family members. Her father also had dementia with onset in his 70s.*

*His general examination reveals a well-nourished man in no distress; he communicates using a writing board. His mental status examination is grossly intact with a normal Folstein mini-mental status examination, but a bedside frontal lobe instrument reveals mild impairment. His cranial nerves are notable for mild facial weakness and a tongue with atrophy and fasciculation. On motor examination he has increased tone and mild atrophy of his cervical paraspinal muscles. He has moderate weakness for neck extension and mild weakness in his shoulders. His tendon reflexes are brisk and his sensory examination normal.*

*Records of his electromyogram at the Veterans Affairs show acute and chronic denervation changes in the tongue, cervical and thoracic paraspinal muscles, and muscles of both arms. He had a brain MRI that has been read as normal, but on review you appreciate a slight hyperintensity of the corticospinal tracts. His blood work has been unremarkable except for a mildly elevated serum lead level.*

*You conclude that he has clinically probable ALS and one issue that you discuss is genetic testing. After education the patient is interested in getting C9ORF72 gene sequencing, which shows an abnormal repeat expansion of 800 times. Thus it is likely that his ALS relates to the C9ORF72 repeat expansion, and he has a family history consistent with this dominantly inherited gene. Additional environmental factors could also be playing a role, which is suggested by his phenotype being different than the dementia that affected his other relatives, and by his relatively younger age of ALS onset. In his case ALS risk factors could include male gender/testosterone exposure, US military service, head trauma, and low-level lead exposure.*

## SUMMARY

The current state of research in environmental risk factors of ALS has provided many intriguing possible associations. Yet only one-smoking is at this time firmly established. The methodologic difficulties with studying a rare disease that occurs late in life, which could be related to exposures many decades ago, make relationships dauntingly difficult to prove. Despite continued improvement in methodology, significant challenges remain. The diagnostic criteria for ALS are complicated and there are continued efforts to improve them. As they are, the criteria do not yet capture all people with ALS, which further complicates epidemiologic studies. It is hoped that larger datasets with better characterization of different clinical features and laboratory markers will provide more robust estimates of risk factors in ALS in the years to come. A better understanding of environmental risk factors could help reduce exposures and it is hoped markedly reduce ALS incidence over time. Epidemiologic research is critical to advance this field, but the relative rarity of ALS and the current notion that exposures may affect the risk of ALS only decades later make such projects complex with many challenges. One US project of great potential is the National ALS Registry. It is a congressionally-mandated prospective population-based registry encompassing the entire US population. In addition to quantifying the incidence, prevalence, and demographics of ALS in the US, another main goal of the Registry is to examine the risk factors for the disease through online risk factor modules. There are currently 17 different risk factor modules that persons with ALS can complete including, but not limited to, cigarette smoking, alcohol consumption, military service history, occupational history, and a family history of ALS. Since the Registry's launch in October 2010, over 45,000 online risk factor modules have been completed. To our knowledge, this is the largest and most geographically diverse collection of risk factor data available about adults with ALS. Findings from these surveys may provide important insights into the pathology of ALS.

## REFERENCES

1. Al-Chalabi A, Hardiman O. The epidemiology of ALS: a conspiracy of genes, environment and time. Nat Rev Neurol 2013;9:617–28.
2. Eisen A, Kiernan M, Mitsumoto H, et al. Amyotrophic lateral sclerosis: a long preclinical period? J Neurol Neurosurg Psychiatry 2014;85:1232–8.
3. Al-Chalabi A, Calvo A, Chio A, et al. Analysis of amyotrophic lateral sclerosis as a multistep process: a population-based modelling study. Lancet Neurol 2014;13: 1108–13.

4. Mehta P, Antao V, Kaye W, et al. Prevalence of amyotrophic lateral sclerosis—United States, 2010-2011. MMWR Surveill Summ 2014;63(Suppl 7):1–14.
5. Manning JT, Bundred PE. The ratio of 2nd to 4th digit length: a new predictor of disease predisposition? Med Hypotheses 2000;54:855–7.
6. Vivekananda U, Manjalay ZR, Ganesalingam J, et al. Low index-to-ring finger length ratio in sporadic ALS supports prenatally defined motor neuronal vulnerability. J Neurol Neurosurg Psychiatry 2011;82:635–7.
7. Chio A, Logroscino G, Traynor BJ, et al. Global epidemiology of amyotrophic lateral sclerosis: a systematic review of the published literature. Neuroepidemiology 2013;41:118–30.
8. Doi Y, Atsuta N, Sobue G, et al. Prevalence and incidence of amyotrophic lateral sclerosis in Japan. J Epidemiol 2014;24:494–9.
9. Smith KR, Corvalan CF, Kjellstrom T. How much global ill health is attributable to environmental factors? Epidemiology 1999;10:573–84.
10. Lekoubou A, Echouffo-Tcheugui JB, Kengne AP. Epidemiology of neurodegenerative diseases in sub-Saharan Africa: a systematic review. BMC Public Health 2014;14:653.
11. Rooney J, Vajda A, Heverin M, et al. Spatial cluster analysis of population amyotrophic lateral sclerosis risk in Ireland. Neurology 2015;84(15):1537–44.
12. Uccelli R, Binazzi A, Altavista P, et al. Geographic distribution of amyotrophic lateral sclerosis through motor neuron disease mortality data. Eur J Epidemiol 2007;22:781–90.
13. Scott KM, Abhinav K, Stanton BR, et al. Geographical clustering of amyotrophic lateral sclerosis in South-East England: a population study. Neuroepidemiology 2009;32:81–8.
14. Boumediene F, Druet-Cabanac M, Marin B, et al. Contribution of geolocalisation to neuroepidemiological studies: incidence of ALS and environmental factors in Limousin, France. J Neurol Sci 2011;309:115–22.
15. Doi Y, Yokoyama T, Tango T, et al. Temporal trends and geographic clusters of mortality from amyotrophic lateral sclerosis in Japan, 1995-2004. J Neurol Sci 2010;298:78–84.
16. Sabel CE, Boyle PJ, Loytonen M, et al. Spatial clustering of amyotrophic lateral sclerosis in Finland at place of birth and place of death. Am J Epidemiol 2003; 157:898–905.
17. Caller TA, Chipman JW, Field NC, et al. Spatial analysis of amyotrophic lateral sclerosis in Northern New England, USA, 1997-2009. Muscle Nerve 2013;48: 235–41.
18. Masseret E, Banack S, Boumediene F, et al. Dietary BMAA exposure in an amyotrophic lateral sclerosis cluster from southern France. PLoS One 2013;8: e83406.
19. Delzor A, Couratier P, Boumediene F, et al. Searching for a link between the L-BMAA neurotoxin and amyotrophic lateral sclerosis: a study protocol of the French BMAALS programme. BMJ Open 2014;4:e005528.
20. Galasko D, Salmon DP, Craig UK, et al. Clinical features and changing patterns of neurodegenerative disorders on Guam, 1997-2000. Neurology 2002;58:90–7.
21. Geser F, Winton MJ, Kwong LK, et al. Pathological TDP-43 in parkinsonism-dementia complex and amyotrophic lateral sclerosis of Guam. Acta Neuropathol 2008;115:133–45.
22. Yin HZ, Yu S, Hsu CI, et al. Intrathecal infusion of BMAA induces selective motor neuron damage and astrogliosis in the ventral horn of the spinal cord. Exp Neurol 2014;261:1–9.

23. Mimuro M, Kokubo Y, Kuzuhara S. Similar topographical distribution of neurofibrillary tangles in amyotrophic lateral sclerosis and parkinsonism-dementia complex in people living in the Kii peninsula of Japan suggests a single tauopathy. Acta Neuropathol 2007;113:653–8.
24. Okumiya K, Wada T, Fujisawa M, et al. Amyotrophic lateral sclerosis and parkinsonism in Papua, Indonesia: 2001-2012 survey results. BMJ Open 2014;4:e004353.
25. de Jong SW, Huisman MH, Sutedja NA, et al. Smoking, alcohol consumption, and the risk of amyotrophic lateral sclerosis: a population-based study. Am J Epidemiol 2012;176:233–9.
26. Wang H, O'Reilly EJ, Weisskopf MG, et al. Smoking and risk of amyotrophic lateral sclerosis: a pooled analysis of 5 prospective cohorts. Arch Neurol 2011;68:207–13.
27. Alonso A, Logroscino G, Hernan MA. Smoking and the risk of amyotrophic lateral sclerosis: a systematic review and meta-analysis. J Neurol Neurosurg Psychiatry 2010;81:1249–52.
28. Fang F, Bellocco R, Hernan MA, et al. Smoking, snuff dipping and the risk of amyotrophic lateral sclerosis: a prospective cohort study. Neuroepidemiology 2006;27:217–21.
29. Beard JD, Kamel F. Military service, deployments, and exposures in relation to amyotrophic lateral sclerosis etiology and survival. Epidemiol Rev 2015;37:55–70.
30. Qureshi MM, Hayden D, Urbinelli L, et al. Analysis of factors that modify susceptibility and rate of progression in amyotrophic lateral sclerosis (ALS). Amyotroph Lateral Scler 2006;7:173–82.
31. Horner RD, Kamins KG, Feussner JR, et al. Occurrence of amyotrophic lateral sclerosis among Gulf War veterans. Neurology 2003;61:742–9.
32. Drouet A, Desjeux G, Balaire C, et al. Retrospective study of ALS in French military personnel. Rev Neurol (Paris) 2010;166:621–9 [in French].
33. Binazzi A, Belli S, Uccelli R, et al. An exploratory case-control study on spinal and bulbar forms of amyotrophic lateral sclerosis in the province of Rome. Amyotroph Lateral Scler 2009;10:361–9.
34. Gale CR, Braidwood EA, Winter PD, et al. Mortality from Parkinson's disease and other causes in men who were prisoners of war in the Far East. Lancet 1999;354:2116–8.
35. Medicine Io. Amyotrophic Lateral Sclerosis in Veterans: Review of the Scientific Literature. Washington, DC: The National Academies Press; 2006.
36. Gunnarsson LG, Bodin L, Söderfeldt B, et al. A case-control study of motor neurone disease: its relation to heritability, and occupational exposures, particularly to solvents. Br J Ind Med 1992;49:791–8.
37. Seelen M, Vermeulen RC, van Dillen LS, et al. Residential exposure to extremely low frequency electromagnetic fields and the risk of ALS. Neurology 2014;83:1767–9.
38. Rosati G, Pinna L, Granieri E, et al. Studies on epidemiological, clinical, and etiological aspects of ALS disease in Sardinia, Southern Italy. Acta Neurol Scand 1977;55:231–44.
39. Belli S, Vanacore N. Proportionate mortality of Italian soccer players: is amyotrophic lateral sclerosis an occupational disease? Eur J Epidemiol 2005;20:237–42.
40. Sutedja NA, Fischer K, Veldink JH, et al. What we truly know about occupation as a risk factor for ALS: a critical and systematic review. Amyotroph Lateral Scler 2009;10:295–301.

41. Callaghan B, Feldman D, Gruis K, et al. The association of exposure to lead, mercury, and selenium and the development of amyotrophic lateral sclerosis and the epigenetic implications. Neurodegener Dis 2011;8:1–8.
42. Wang MD, Gomes J, Cashman NR, et al. A meta-analysis of observational studies of the association between chronic occupational exposure to lead and amyotrophic lateral sclerosis. J Occup Environ Med 2014;56:1235–42.
43. Hamidou B, Couratier P, Besancon C, et al. Epidemiological evidence that physical activity is not a risk factor for ALS. Eur J Epidemiol 2014;29:459–75.
44. Huisman MH, Seelen M, de Jong SW, et al. Lifetime physical activity and the risk of amyotrophic lateral sclerosis. J Neurol Neurosurg Psychiatry 2013;84:976–81.
45. Mattsson P, Lonnstedt I, Nygren I, et al. Physical fitness, but not muscle strength, is a risk factor for death in amyotrophic lateral sclerosis at an early age. J Neurol Neurosurg Psychiatry 2012;83:390–4.
46. Longstreth WT, Nelson LM, Koepsell TD, et al. Hypotheses to explain the association between vigorous physical activity and amyotrophic lateral sclerosis. Med Hypotheses 1991;34:144–8.
47. Seelen M, van Doormaal PT, Visser AE, et al. Prior medical conditions and the risk of amyotrophic lateral sclerosis. J Neurol 2014;261:1949–56.
48. McKee AC, Gavett BE, Stern RA, et al. TDP-43 proteinopathy and motor neuron disease in chronic traumatic encephalopathy. J Neuropathol Exp Neurol 2010;69:918–29.
49. Pupillo E, Messina P, Logroscino G, et al. Trauma and amyotrophic lateral sclerosis: a case-control study from a population-based registry. Eur J Neurol 2012;19:1509–17.
50. Singh G, Khurana D. Neurology of acute organophosphate poisoning. Neurol India 2009;57:119–25.
51. Malek AM, Barchowsky A, Bowser R, et al. Pesticide exposure as a risk factor for amyotrophic lateral sclerosis: a meta-analysis of epidemiological studies: pesticide exposure as a risk factor for ALS. Environ Res 2012;117:112–9.
52. Chio A, Calvo A, Dossena M, et al. ALS in Italian professional soccer players: the risk is still present and could be soccer-specific. Amyotrophic lateral sclerosis : official publication of the World Federation of Neurology Research Group on Motor Neuron Diseases 2009;10:205–9.
53. Corcia P, Gordon PH, Camdessanche JP. Is there a paraneoplastic ALS? Amyotrophic lateral sclerosis & frontotemporal degeneration 2015;16:252–7.
54. Fang F, Al-Chalabi A, Ronnevi LO, et al. Amyotrophic lateral sclerosis and cancer: a register-based study in Sweden. Amyotroph Lateral Scler Frontotemporal Degener 2013;14:362–8.
55. Edwards IR, Star K, Kiuru A. Statins, neuromuscular degenerative disease and an amyotrophic lateral sclerosis-like syndrome: an analysis of individual case safety reports from vigibase. Drug Saf 2007;30:515–25.
56. Zheng Z, Sheng L, Shang H. Statins and amyotrophic lateral sclerosis: a systematic review and meta-analysis. Amyotroph Lateral Scler Frontotemporal Degener 2013;14:241–5.
57. Ascherio A, Weisskopf MG, O'Reilly EJ, et al. Vitamin E intake and risk of amyotrophic lateral sclerosis. Ann Neurol 2005;57:104–10.
58. Camu W, Tremblier B, Plassot C, et al. Vitamin D confers protection to motoneurons and is a prognostic factor of amyotrophic lateral sclerosis. Neurobiol Aging 2014;35:1198–205.
59. Simpson EP, Yen AA, Appel SH. Oxidative stress: a common denominator in the pathogenesis of amyotrophic lateral sclerosis. Curr Opin Rheumatol 2003;15:730–6.

60. D'Amico E, Factor-Litvak P, Santella RM, et al. Clinical perspective on oxidative stress in sporadic amyotrophic lateral sclerosis. Free Radic Biol Med 2013;65: 509–27.
61. Mitsumoto H, Factor-Litvak P, Andrews H, et al. ALS Multicenter Cohort Study of Oxidative Stress (ALS COSMOS): study methodology, recruitment, and baseline demographic and disease characteristics. Amyotroph Lateral Scler Frontotemporal Degener 2014;15:192–203.
62. Armon C. An evidence-based medicine approach to the evaluation of the role of exogenous risk factors in sporadic amyotrophic lateral sclerosis. Neuroepidemiology 2003;22:217–28.
63. Armon C. Smoking may be considered an established risk factor for sporadic ALS. Neurology 2009;73:1693–8.
64. Armon C, Nelson LM. Is head trauma a risk factor for amyotrophic lateral sclerosis? An evidence based review. Amyotroph Lateral Scler 2012;13:351–6.

# Symptom Management and End-of-Life Care in Amyotrophic Lateral Sclerosis

Carlayne E. Jackson, MD[a], April L. McVey, MD[b], Stacy Rudnicki, MD[c], Mazen M. Dimachkie, MD[b,*], Richard J. Barohn, MD[b]

**KEYWORDS**

- Sialorrhea • Pseudobulbar affect • Noninvasive ventilation • Secretion management
- Laryngospasm • Edema • Urinary urgency • Constipation

**KEY POINTS**

- Sialorrhea should initially be treated with anticholinergic medications. For patients who remain medically refractory, treatment with botulinum toxin type B (level B; recommendation by the American Academy of Neurology Practice Parameters Committee) or low-dose radiation therapy to the salivary glands (level C) should be considered.
- Pseudobulbar affect can be successfully treated with selective serotonin reuptake inhibitors, tricyclic antidepressants, and serotonin-norepinephrine reuptake inhibitors. A combination of dextromethorphan/quinidine should also be considered (level B).
- Noninvasive ventilation (NIV) should be considered to treat respiratory insufficiency, both to lengthen survival and to slow the rate of forced vital capacity decline (level B). NIV has demonstrated a positive impact on quality of life (level C). Mechanical insufflation/exsufflation may be considered to clear secretions, particularly during an acute chest infection (level C). NIV may be considered at the earliest sign of nocturnal hypoventilation in order to improve compliance (level C).
- Although enteral nutrition may help with weight stabilization, studies that have investigated possible survival benefits have provided mixed results. There are no conclusive data regarding specific diets and possible benefits in amyotrophic lateral sclerosis (ALS). Multiple studies have found that weight loss is associated with a worse prognosis.
- End-of-life discussions are difficult for patients, families, and physicians but must not be avoided. Advance directives should be addressed soon after the diagnosis. Hospice services are essential in the management of end-of-life issues in patients with ALS and optimize the likelihood of a peaceful and dignified death. Despite its advantages, it is generally underused or initiated too late in the disease course.

Disclosure: See last page of article.

[a] Department of Neurology, University of Texas Health Science Center, 8300 Floyd Curl Drive, Mail Code 7883, San Antonio, TX 78229-3900, USA; [b] Department of Neurology, University of Kansas Medical Center, 3901 Rainbow Boulevard, Mailstop 2012, Kansas City, KS 66160, USA; [c] Department of Neurology, University of Arkansas for Medical Sciences, 501 Jackson Stephens Drive, Room 769, Little Rock, AR 72205-7199, USA
* Corresponding author.
*E-mail address:* mdmachkie@kumc.edu

Neurol Clin 33 (2015) 889–908
http://dx.doi.org/10.1016/j.ncl.2015.07.010 neurologic.theclinics.com

## SIALORRHEA

Sialorrhea is a socially embarrassing symptom related to pharyngeal muscle weakness, which can lead to aspiration pneumonia, the most common cause of death in ALS other than respiratory failure.[1] The prevalence of the sialorrhea among patients with ALS is estimated at 50%.[2] Patients frequently have to wipe their mouth with a tissue or, in extreme cases, may need to insert a paper towel or washcloth into their mouths to absorb the saliva.

The American Academy of Neurology's (AAN) practice parameter for the care of patients with ALS published in 1999 recommended both pharmacologic interventions and nonpharmacologic approaches, such as suctioning.[3] Treatment with anticholinergic medication (**Table 1**)[4] is considered first-line pharmacologic therapy; however, the benefits of this class of medication can be insufficient to completely address the symptom. In addition, common side effects associated with anticholinergic therapy include constipation, fatigue, impotence, urinary retention, blurred vision, tachycardia, orthostatic hypotension, and dizziness. These side effects occur most commonly in elderly patients. In addition, anticholinergic medications are relatively contraindicated in patients with a history of glaucoma, benign prostatic hypertrophy, or cardiac conduction disorders (especially bifascicular block, left bundle branch block, and a prolonged QT interval).

Selection of a particular medication often depends on the severity and frequency of the drooling. Sialorrhea associated with mealtimes or a particular time of day may be treated with as-needed administration of atropine, hyoscyamine, or glycopyrrolate. Transdermal scopolamine, botulinum toxin, or antidepressant medications provide a more continuous effect. Patients who have difficulty swallowing medications may prefer an agent that can be given sublingually or transdermally or is available in a liquid form that can be administered directly through a percutaneous endoscopic gastrostomy (PEG) tube.

Data from the national ALS Patient CARE database indicate that more than 70% of patients with ALS treated with atropine, glycopyrrolate, or amitriptyline reported these modalities were helpful.[2,4,5] By inference, approximately 30% of patients were not helped by these therapies. There remains, to date, no randomized trial comparing the efficacy of these different agents in the ALS population. In general, all of these medications may cause or aggravate existing problems with constipation; therefore, it is recommended that a stool softener be initiated at the same time the anticholinergic agent is prescribed.

**Table 1**
**Medications commonly used for sialorrhea**

| Medication | Dosage |
|---|---|
| Amitriptyline | 25–75 mg qhs |
| Nortriptyline | 20–100 mg qhs |
| Atropine | 0.4 mg q 4–6 h<br>1–2 ophthalmic drops SL q 4–6 h |
| Glycopyrrolate | 1–2 mg tid |
| Scopolamine patch | Apply behind ear q3d |
| Hyoscyamine sulfate | 0.125 mg–0.25 mg q 4–6 h (available as oral tablets, elixir, or sublingual tablets) |
| Botulinum toxin type A<br>Botulinum toxin type B | — |

Botulinum toxin is the newest mode of sialorrhea therapy and has, thus far, shown to have great promise in patients resistant to conventional medical therapy.[6–10] In a double-blind controlled trial of botulinum toxin type B (BTxB) in 20 patients with ALS with refractory sialorrhea,[10] patients were randomized to 2500 U of BTxB or placebo into bilateral parotid and submandibular glands. Treated patients reported a global improvement of 82% at 2 and 4 weeks compared with 38% in the placebo group ($P$ <.05). At 12 weeks, 50% of patients receiving BTxB were improved compared with 14% receiving placebo. There were no significant adverse events.

Radiation therapy for medically refractory sialorrhea reduced salivary production; but side effects included erythema, sore throat, and nausea.[11] A satisfactory response was observed, and the saliva secretion rate diminished with a single dose of 7.0 to 7.5 Gy bilaterally.[12]

Based on the AAN's practice guidelines published in 2009,[13] in patients with ALS who have medically refractory sialorrhea, BTxB should be considered (level B) and low-dose radiation therapy to the salivary glands may be considered (level C).

Sticky secretions can also be problematic for patients with ALS. These secretions may originate not only from the salivary glands but also mucous from the nose and mouth.[14] Sticky secretions can be a symptom of dehydration, and encouraging patients to increase fluid intake may be helpful. Using a room humidifier for those not using noninvasive ventilation (NIV) and bleeding humidified air into the machine for those who do may reduce their tenacity. An open-label trial of 16 patients with thick secretions who had failed anticholinergic therapy and were treated with either propanolol 10 mg twice a day or metoprolol 25 mg twice a day found that 75% of patients reported decreased secretions, with sustained short-term efficacy in most.[15] Drinking papaya or pineapple juice and reducing caffeine, milk, or alcohol have been anecdotally suggested.[16]

## PSEUDOBULBAR AFFECT

Pseudobulbar affect (PBA) affects 20% to 50% of patients with ALS, especially in patients with bulbar onset.[17] The characteristics of PBA include uncontrolled laughter or crying, often with minimal or no provocation. Episodes are often sudden involuntary outbursts of emotion inappropriate to the context of the situation. Patients experiencing uncontrolled crying are more common than those with uncontrolled laughter; however, the symptoms can result in significant disability, limiting social interactions and impairing quality of life (QoL).

Although it is not a mood disorder, selective serotonin reuptake inhibitors, tricyclic antidepressants, and some serotonin-norepinephrine reuptake inhibitors have been used for treatment of PBA (**Table 2**).[4]

A novel combination of dextromethorphan (20 mg) and quinidine sulfate (10 mg) (Nuedexta) has been shown to be effective in a large phase 3 multicenter randomized trial.[18] Nuedexta patients reported significantly less emotional lability, improved QoL, and improved quality of relationship scores. Side effects included dizziness, nausea, and somnolence. These side effects can be minimized by initiating the dosage at 1 tablet at bedtime for 7 days followed by twice-a-day dosing. The AAN's practice guidelines[13] recommend that if side effects are acceptable, dextromethorphan/quinidine should be considered for symptoms of PBA in patients with ALS (level B).

## SLEEP DISRUPTION

Sleep disruption in patients with ALS is frequently multifactorial in cause and may be caused by respiratory muscle weakness, difficulty repositioning in bed, anxiety,

**Table 2**
**Medications for treatment of PBA**

| Drug | Dosage | Common Side Effects |
|---|---|---|
| SSRI antidepressants | | |
| Paroxetine<br>Fluoxetine<br>Fluvoxamine<br>Sertraline<br>Citalopram | 10–50 mg qd<br>10–30 mg qd<br>50 mg qd–bid<br>50–100 qd–bid<br>20–60 mg qd | Sexual dysfunction, akathisia, sleep disturbance, anxiety |
| Tricyclic antidepressants | | |
| Amitriptyline<br>Nortriptyline<br>Desipramine | 25–75 mg qhs | Dry mouth, fatigue, dizziness, urinary retention, constipation |
| Mirtazapine | 15 mg qhs | Abnormal dreams, mild cognitive change, constipation |
| Venlafaxine | 37.5–75.0 mg bid–tid | Anorexia, constipation, weight loss, impotence, anxiety, dizziness |
| Dextromethorphan/ quinidine | 20 mg/10 mg 1 tablet bid | Nausea, dizziness, somnolence, loose stools |

depression, and pain. Nocturnal hypoventilation results in frequent arousals and decreased total sleep time resulting in daytime fatigue and poor concentration. Overall, impaired sleep can markedly affect QoL and likely impact prognosis.

Available solutions to address impaired sleep are as varied as the diverse issues causing it. Simple physical adaptations, such as an electric hospital bed, can be ideal to enhance mobility and positioning. An alternating-pressure air mattress or gel overlay mattress can lessen the discomfort from limited mobility. Noninvasive positive pressure ventilation can significantly affect respiratory hygiene and improve sleep quality. Antidepressant medications are also effective at reducing anxiety and depression and promoting sleep. In that regard, mirtazapine (15 mg at bedtime) can be especially helpful. At higher doses (≥30 mg) mirtazapine may have a confounding effect caused by the enhancement of its noradrenergic effect. The anticholinergic action of the tricyclic antidepressant group can also be especially helpful, particularly in patients with sialorrhea.

Anxiolytic medications, such as benzodiazepines, used specifically to induce sleep can be helpful when used selectively. Zolpidem tartrate (10 mg qhs) is often effective and preferred because of the low risk of respiratory depression. Pharmacologic tolerance and withdrawal symptoms can become evident, however, with chronic use. Addressing the underlying cause of such anxiety (depression, fear, pain, and so forth) is a preferred method of treatment.

Alternative pharmacologic agents, such as melatonin, passionflower, lavender, and hops, have been effective for individual patients; however, their benefits are quite variable and untested.

## RESPIRATORY INSUFFICIENCY

Patients with ALS commonly develop respiratory failure as a result of decreased diaphragmatic and intercostal muscle strength and impaired glottis function resulting in an ineffective cough.[19] Dyspnea is an uncommon presenting symptom of chronic respiratory failure. Rather, patients usually present insidiously with symptoms related to nocturnal oxygen desaturations, such as frequent nighttime arousals, morning headache, excessive daytime sleepiness, orthopnea, and fatigue.

Patients with ALS should have an assessment of pulmonary function every 3 to 6 months. Forced vital capacity (FVC) is the most commonly used respiratory measurement in ALS and is a significant predictor of survival.[20] In most cases, however, the earliest detectable abnormality is a reduction in maximum inspiratory pressure (MIP), sniff nasal pressure (SNP), sniff transdiaphragmatic pressure or nocturnal oximetry (desaturations <90% for 1 cumulative minute).[21] Supine FVC, although more difficult to perform, may be a better predictor of diaphragm weakness than erect FVC.[22,23]

When FVC decreases to less than 50% of normal or the MIP is less than 60 cm, noninvasive ventilation (NIV) should be initiated. Discussions about respiratory interventions should always take place in concert with a pulmonologist or respiratory therapist expert in managing neuromuscular patients, and the opinions and wishes of patients and family should be the prime consideration. If the topics of a living will and durable power of attorney for health care have not yet been addressed, they should be discussed.[24,25]

NIV should be considered to treat respiratory insufficiency in ALS, both to lengthen survival and to slow the rate of FVC decline (level B).[26] In a randomized controlled study, patients using NIV experienced a median survival benefit of 205 days.[27] NIV was initiated based on orthopnea with an MIP less than −60 cm or symptomatic hypercapnia. FVC declined more slowly after introducing NIV (-2.2%/month before compared to −1.1%/month after), and the decline was slower in those who used NIV greater than >4 hours per /day.

NIV has demonstrated a positive impact on QoL in several studies (level C).[21,26,28,29] There were improvements noted in energy, vitality,[28,30] shortness of breath, daytime somnolence, depression, concentration, sleep quality, and physical fatigue for 10 months or more.[29]

NIV may be considered at the earliest sign of nocturnal hypoventilation or respiratory insufficiency in order to improve compliance (level C).[26,31,32] Orthopnea has been shown to be a strong predictor of benefit and also has better compliance with NIV.[27] NIV use correlated with symptoms of orthopnea and dyspnea as well as with the use of PEG, speech devices, and riluzole.[33] Young age and preserved upper limb function have also predicted better compliance.

Noncompliance with NIV was seen in 75% of patients with ALS and frontotemporal dysfunction versus 38% in patients with classic ALS (relative risk 2.0).[34] Low compliance has also been reported in bulbar patients,[27,35] but cognitive/executive function was not described. Compliance can be improved by prescribing a variety of different interfaces, including nasal mask, nasal pillows, full-face masks, or mouthpieces in order to maximize patient comfort and minimize pressure sores. NIV should be started at low pressures to maximize patients' tolerance to the device. Generally the inspiratory pressure (IPAP) is set at 6 to 8 cm $H_2O$ and the expiratory pressure at 3 to 5 cm $H_2O$. The IPAP can then be titrated in 1–2 cm increments based on patient tolerance and clinical status. The device should be placed on a spontaneous timed mode with a backup rate set at the patients' nocturnal respiratory rate (generally 8–10). Frequent follow-up by a trained respiratory therapist is crucial to deal with any problems affecting patient tolerance. A heated humidifier should be prescribed if patients develop symptoms of nasal dryness or congestion.

Expiratory respiratory muscle weakness can lead to ineffective cough, retained upper airway secretions, and pulmonary infections. Peak cough expiratory flows (PCEFs) greater than 160 L/min are needed to clear secretions[36] when the PCEF decreases to less than 270 L/min[37]; mechanical insufflation/exsufflation (MIE) may be considered to clear secretions, particularly during an acute chest infection (level C).[26] These devices allow delivery of pressurized air (30–50 cm $H_2O$) followed by an immediate forced exsufflation of negative pressure (30–50 cm $H_2O$) for several seconds via a mouthpiece or naso-oral mask. The use of MIE safely allows patients with respiratory tract infections and profuse mucus production to clear their secretions and permit the ongoing use of NIV. MIE pressures should be set to the maximum comfortable level tolerated by each patient in order to eliminate airway secretions. In general inspiratory pressures are set at 20 to 40 cm $H_2O$, and expiratory pressures are set at 5 to 20 cm $H_2O$. Another device useful for helping patients clear secretions is a high frequency chest wall oscillation device (HFCWO) that rapidly inflates and deflates resulting in a vibratory-like manner up to 25 chest wall compressions per second. This device helps dislodge mucus from the bronchial walls for removal via cough or a insufflation-exsufflation device. There are currently insufficient data to support or refute HFCWO for clearing airway secretions in patients with ALS (level U).[26]

Medications with mucolytics like guaifenesin or N-acetylcysteine, a β-receptor antagonist (such as metoprolol or propanolol), nebulized saline, or an anticholinergic bronchodilator (such as ipratropium) are widely used; however, no controlled studies exist in ALS.

The Centers for Disease Control and Prevention recommends that essentially all patients with significant neuromuscular illness should receive one or more doses of the pneumococcal vaccine and annual vaccines for the pertinent influenza virus. Adequate hydration must also be maintained to assure easy mobilization of secretions.

Acute respiratory failure in patients with ALS is usually precipitated by an acute infection or pulmonary embolism and is seldom caused by muscle weakness alone. For dyspneic or obtunded patients, emergency evaluation for endotracheal intubation may be necessary. If hypoxia alone is present and patients are alert, oxygen at low-flow rates (<1 L/min) may correct hypoxia, although such therapy must be administered with caution because patients with neuromuscular disease are often hypercapneic, and oxygen often depresses ventilatory drive and exacerbates hypoventilation.[38] NIV is usually tried initially if control of secretions and cough assistance is successful.[39] Whether intubation or NIV is utilized, patients sometimes can be weaned following the precipitating respiratory crisis; others may require ventilation assistance indefinitely. Pulmonary consultation is always indicated in these patients.

NIV is contraindicated in patients with copious secretions, cognitive impairment, or lack of caregiver support.[40,41] In these instances, ventilation may be more easily managed with tracheostomy and positive-pressure ventilation (**Fig. 1**). Initiation of chronic respiratory support poses major practical, financial, medical, and ethical responsibilities for patients and families; it is often helpful for patients to discuss the procedure with others receiving such support. The input of experienced pulmonary consultants and palliative medicine services can be invaluable in these instances.

## FATIGUE

Fatigue is reported in 44% to 83% of patients with ALS and likely is multifactorial with sleep disruption, nocturnal complaints (such as nocturia and cramps), nutritional status, weakness, vital capacity, functional status, depression, and medications, including riluzole, all potentially playing a role.[42–45] In a given patient, it may be challenging to tease out the biggest contributors; but treating those that are readily identified to see if fatigue improves is a practical approach. Overall and physical fatigue but not mental fatigue was found more often in patients with ALS compared

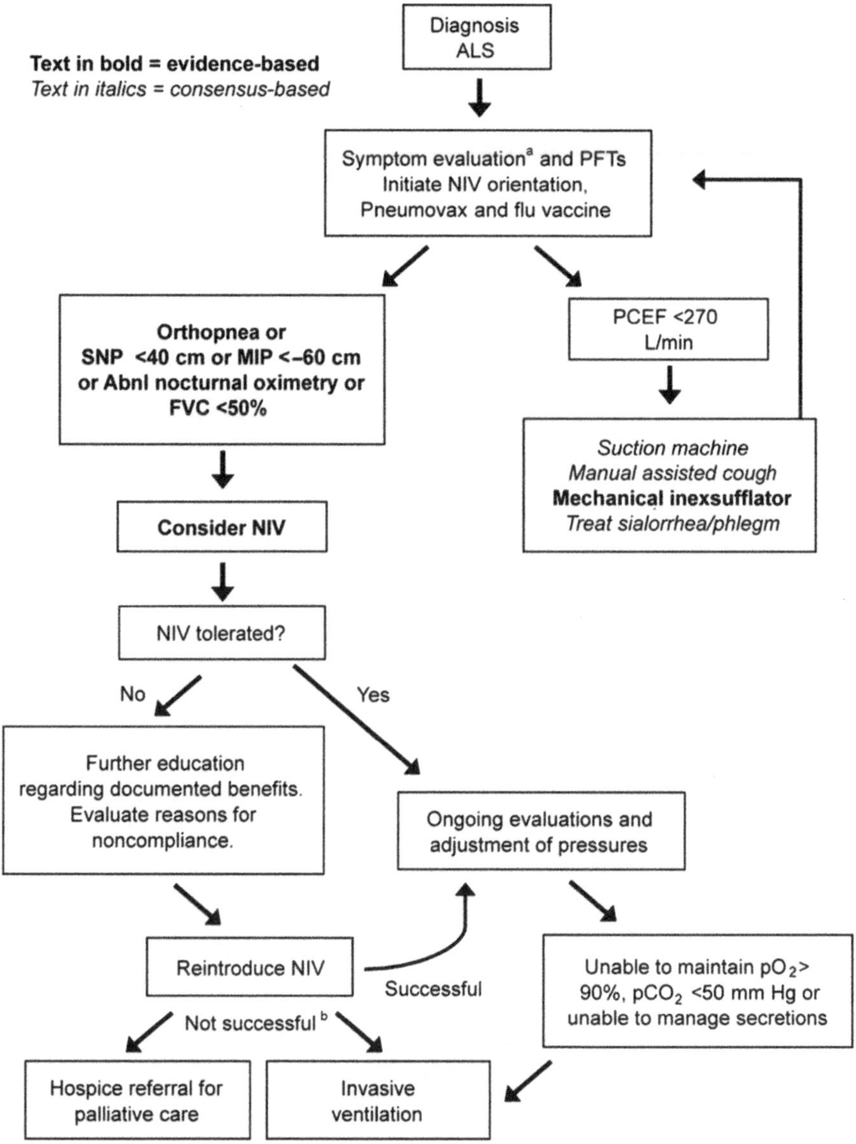


**Fig. 1.** Respiratory management algorithm. Abnl.nocturnal oximetry, pO2 <4% from baseline; FVC, forced vital capacity (supine or erect); MIP, maximal inspiratory pressure; NIV, noninvasive ventilation; PCEF, peak cough expiratory flow; PFT, pulmonary function tests; SNP, sniff nasal pressure. [a] Symptoms suggestive of nocturnal hypoventilation: frequent arousals, morning headaches, excessive daytime sleepiness, vivid dreams. [b] If NIV is not tolerated or accepted in the setting of advancing respiratory compromise, consider invasive ventilation or referral to hospice. (*From* Miller RG, Jackson CE, Kasarskis EJ, et al. Practice parameter update: the care of the patient with amyotrophic lateral sclerosis: drug, nutritional, and respiratory therapies (an evidence-based review) report of the Quality Standards Subcommittee of the American Academy of Neurology. Neurology 2009;73:1222; with permission.)

with controls.[46] Modafinil in dosages ranging from 100 to 300 mg daily in a placebo-controlled trial for 4 weeks resulted in a statistically significant improvement in the Clinical Global Impression score (the study's primary end point) in 19 out of 25 on active drug and in 1 out of 7 on placebo ($P = .003$) as well as improvement on the visual analog scale (VAS) for energy ($P = .039$) and the VAS for stamina ($P = .009$) but not in the Fatigue Severity Scale ($P = .066$).[47]

## NUTRITION

Weight loss in patients with ALS may occur because of dysphagia, muscle atrophy, poor appetite related to depression, and hypermetabolic state.[48–50] In addition, caloric needs in patients with ALS may be underestimated using traditional equations in part because of the increased work of using weak muscles as well as energy expenditure associated with cramps, spasticity, fasciculations, and pseudobulbar manifestations. A potentially more accurate way to measure the total daily caloric needs of a patient with ALS uses the Harris-Benedict equation but also incorporates scores of 6 items from the ALS functional rating scale relating to speech, handwriting, dressing and hygiene, turning in bed, walking, and dyspnea.[51]

Weight loss of greater than 10%,[52] rapid changes in body mass index (BMI) from the time of symptom onset to diagnosis[53] as well as greater BMI changes in the first 2 years of being diagnosed with ALS[54] are all associated with a worse prognosis. Patients with a BMI classification of mild obesity at the time of study entry had a better prognosis.[55] In a prospective nutritional and cancer study of more than a half a million subjects followed for 14 to 28 years, higher body fat was associated with a lower risk of dying from ALS.[56]

Despite these data, there is mixed evidence regarding survival benefits of providing enteral nutrition through gastrostomy tubes in patients with ALS. In the absence of randomized controlled trials, physicians are left with case-controlled studies and prospective and retrospective cohort studies.[57] Survival benefits for those undergoing a gastrostomy include studies authored by Chiò and colleagues[58] and Czaplinski and colleagues,[59] whereas examples of those finding no benefit have been reported by Forbes and colleagues[60] and Mitchell and colleagies.[61] Possible reasons for failure to always demonstrate a benefit may be patients' reluctance to do the procedure until they have lost a substantial amount of weight and so are already malnourished when the procedure is performed. Another challenge with enteral nutrition is that noncompliance with the nutritionist's recommendations is not uncommon.[62]

Enteral nutrition has resulted in stabilization and/or improvement in the BMI following gastrostomy placement.[63,64] It also allows patients to stay hydrated and provides a safe manner to administer medications. Radiographically inserted gastrostomy tubes may confer both a survival benefit[65] as well as be associated with fewer insertional failures and postprocedure episodes of aspiration[66] compared with endoscopically placed tubes.

Only small relatively short-duration studies have investigated different types of diets in patients with ALS to determine if there is a preferred diet that could influence disease progression, with variable findings as described in **Table 3**.

Early swallowing problems are addressed with changes made while eating, including smaller bites, slowing down, and avoiding talking while eating. Consistency changes may be suggested, including blending solid foods or adding thickener to liquids. Speech therapists may provide instructions in chin tuck or head turning to improve the ease and safety of a swallow. As the disease progresses, these are frequently not sufficient, and a feeding tube is considered. Reasons to recommend

**Table 3**
**Diets studied in ALS**

| Author | Diet | N | Duration | Results |
|---|---|---|---|---|
| Stanich et al,[67] 2002 | High protein | 20 | 6 mo | No change in muscle mass or disease progression |
| Silva et al,[68] 2010 | High protein | 16 | 4 mo | Stabilization of ALS-FRS-R |
| Dorst et al,[69] 2013 | High fat, high calorie<br>High carbohydrate, high calorie | 22<br>16 | 3 mo | Weight stabilized<br>ALS-FRS progressed<br>High dropout rate with high carbohydrate/high calorie |
| Willis et al,[70] 2014 | High fat, high calorie<br>High carbohydrate, high calorie<br>Control | 8<br>9<br>7 | 3 mo | High carbohydrate, high calorie group had fewer adverse events, dropouts, and deaths |

*Abbreviation:* ALS-FRS, ALS-functional rating score.

a gastrostomy tube include malnutrition/weight loss, long meal times, evidence for aspiration, and dehydration.[3] Although the AAN's practice guidelines support placement when the vital capacity is greater than 50% because of concerns of increased risk as this value decreases,[26] recent data provide evidence that a gastrostomy tube can be safely placed with vital capacities less than this value, particularly when NIV can be used during the procedure.[71]

## PAIN

Pain is reported in 57% to 72% of patients with ALS and may involve the extremities, neck, back, or trunk.[72,73] Pain can occur at any time during the course of the disease and does not necessarily correlate with depression but is associated with more impaired functional status and worse QoL.[72,74,75] Although nonsteroidal antiinflammatory drugs are frequently used, several therapies are prescribed, including nonopioid analgesics, opioids, muscle relaxants, quinine sulfate, gabapentin, steroids, botulinum toxin, and physical therapy.[73] It is thought that the more common causes of pain are related to limited range of motion in joints, general immobility, spasticity, and/or cramps. Descriptions of pain include burning, aching, cramping, and shock-like pain.[76]

A Cochrane review on this subject in 2013 found no controlled or quasi-controlled studies of treating pain in patients with ALS.[77] Therefore, one cannot endorse specific ways to treat pain in ALS, though sorting out the type of pain may help the physician develop a rational approach to developing a treatment plan. In addition, if pain is related to immobility, trying to improve the comfort of what patients sit or sleep on, such as changing the cushion on their wheelchair or suggesting an alternating pressure mattress, may be practical interventions to consider.

## SPASTICITY

Spasticity, in addition to being a source of pain in patients with ALS, can also limit mobility and function. Studies specifically investigating the treatment of spasticity in patients with ALS are limited. Common medications used to treat spasticity in patients with ALS include baclofen, tizanidine, benzodiazepines, and dantrolene. None of these have been specifically studied in ALS but rather in other disorders, such as multiple sclerosis and cerebral palsy associated with spasticity.[16,26] One concern in using these medications in patients with ALS is that they can potentially worsen weakness, which could adversely impact function.

Eight patients with pain attributed to spasticity who had failed oral medication management received an intrathecal baclofen pump. There was a significant reduction in the mean pain score, and 6 out of 8 patients had a reduction in their pain score, including 3 who became pain free. The mean preoperative Ashworth spasticity score was 2.93; a year following pump placement, the mean score was 1.72.[78] In an unblinded trial, 14 patients were randomized to a moderate exercise program and 11 to their usual activities. At 3 months but not at 6 months, patients performing moderate exercise showed less deterioration on the Ashworth spasticity scale; at 9 and 12 months, patient dropouts made it impossible to compare the groups.[79] An open-label trial of levetiracetam in 20 patients found it improved cramps as well as the phasic but not tonic spasticity.[80] Marked spasticity of masseter muscles preventing jaw opening has been effectively treated in open-label studies with botulinum toxin.[81,82] Hydrotherapy, cryotherapy, heat, and ultrasound have also been used despite the lack of controlled trials.[83]

#### *Laryngospasm*

Laryngospasm is the sudden sensation that air cannot be moved in and out, usually lasting seconds accompanied by inspiratory stridor or audible respirations caused by a rapid and forceful contraction of laryngeal adductors. It is extremely frightening because patients cannot take a breath or call for help. In a study on laryngospasm, 2% of a control group of 122 patients in the early stages of ALS reported laryngospasm,[84] though up to 19% of patients have reported it in later stages.[1] Common causes of laryngospasm in ALS are liquid or saliva in contact with the larynx, acid reflux, smoke, strong smells, emotion, alcohol, cold bursts of air, and even spicy foods. Nonpharmacologic measures help in many patients. A rapid change to the upright position of the upper body, fixation of the arms to stabilize the body, breathing through the nose, swallowing repetitively, and breathing with slow exhalation through the lips have been reported to shorten episodes. If frequent enough and nonpharmacologic measures are ineffective, benzodiazepines twice a day or 3 times a day can be used.[4,85–87] In the case of gastroesophageal reflux disease, treat with antireflux therapy and prokinetic drugs like metoclopramide before meals and at bedtime.

#### *Jaw Quivering/Cheek Biting*

Patients with ALS may report jaw quivering or clenching caused by spasticity precipitated by pain, anxiety, or cold. Jaw clenching can be severe enough to interfere with oral hygiene. Treatment includes benzodiazepines as listed in **Table 4**. Botulinum toxin injected at 2 sites within the masseters on each side has been reported anecdotally to be effective.[4] Dental guards can alleviate cheek biting at night.

**Table 4**
**Medications used for jaw clenching**

| Medication | Dosage |
|---|---|
| Clonazepam | 0.5–1.0 mg tid |
| Diazepam | 2.5–5.0 mg tid |
| Lorazepam | 0.5–1.0 mg tid |
| Alprazolam | 0.25–0.5 mg tid |

### *Edema*

Dependent edema of the hands and feet occurs in weak limbs because of immobility and reduced muscle pump activity. If severe, it can be associated with painful burning sensations and fragile, easily damaged skin. Limb elevation is the primary intervention. A reclining wheelchair with leg elevation above the heart and a hospital bed are probably the most comfortable and efficient, especially because patients can reposition frequently. Moving the legs as much as possible, passive range of motion, and stretching exercises performed by a caregiver several times a day, though labor intensive, are also helpful. Some patients can benefit from compression stockings, but they require proper fitting and are very difficult to put on and take off. Diuretics are avoided unless edema is severe because fluid overload is not the issue, patients with ALS already have trouble with maintaining good hydration, and diuretics worsen muscle cramps.[88] If the edema is worse in one limb or is not improved by elevating the limbs or asymmetrical, consider evaluating patients for deep venous thrombosis because, if chronic, patients may not complain of calf pain or have erythema.

### *Constipation and Urinary Urgency*

Autonomic symptoms have been reported in up to 29% of patients with ALS.[89,90] Common symptoms involve urinary and gastrointestinal dysfunction.[91] Changes in the intermediolateral columns and the Onuf nucleus provide an anatomic explanation. Causes of constipation are multifactorial and include reduced mobility, reduced fluid and food intake, and medications, such as anticholinergics, tricyclic antidepressants, narcotics, muscle relaxants, and sedatives. Long delays in getting to the bathroom contribute to the problem. Abdominal muscles weaken and make it difficult to expel stool, even if soft. Treatment can start with increased dietary fiber and water as well as prune juice. Fiber laxatives (methylcellulose, bran, psyllium) are bulk forming agents and require 8 ounces of fluid (preferably water) taken immediately with each dose and maintaining good hydration to prevent intestinal blockage. In patients with dysphagia, failure to drink enough water to swallow the fiber laxative might allow swelling in the esophagus. They can also cause abdominal distension. Stool softeners should be recommended on a daily basis and reduce the amount of straining needed for a bowel movement. Stimulant or irritant laxatives like senna, cascara, and bisacodyl tablets and suppositories should be used at the lowest effective dose and not in slowly progressive disease as they can cause an atonic colon if used for years. They can cause abdominal cramps after each dose and, if overused, fluid and electrolyte disturbances. Lactulose and polyethylene glycol are effective osmotic agents. They can cause abdominal distension, diarrhea, flatulence, and nausea. More intensive treatments, such as enemas, magnesium citrate, and manual disimpaction, are last resorts. Another option is to adjust the tube feeding formula to one with higher fiber content. Patients who are bedridden or receiving narcotics should be given mild laxatives prophylactically.

Urinary frequency and urgency are common in patients with ALS. Some patients feel the need to urinate every 1 to 2 hours. For weak patients, transferring to and from a toilet every few hours can be difficult and time consuming. Some patients will not leave their home because they cannot get to a bathroom fast enough and do not want to wear a diaper. Nonpharmacologic interventions include avoiding caffeine and alcohol, timed voiding and the use of a urinal and condom catheter for men. Although physicians are reluctant to use Foley catheters or refer a patient to the urologist for a suprapubic catheter, many patients are willing to accept the risk of infection and nursing care, as they are no longer confined to home. Anticholinergic medications are used after urinary tract infections or an enlarged prostate is ruled out. Medications may improve urinary urgency and frequency in some patients but not all. It is uncommon for symptoms to resolve completely. Oxybutynin is commonly tried first at 5 mg twice a day or 3 times a day. It is inexpensive and can be crushed and used with a PEG tube. Extended-release oxybutynin at doses of 5, 10, and 15 mg are used once a day but cannot be crushed for PEG tube use. An oxybutynin chloride (Oxytrol) skin patch delivers a continuous amount of medication. Tolterodine tartrate (Detrol), darifenacin (Enablex), solifenacin (Vesicare), Trospium (Sanctura), and Fesoterodine (Toviaz) are other options. Although beneficial, anticholinergics may produce dry mouth, constipation, blurred vision, drowsiness, and confusion in elderly patients with dementia (**Table 5**).

**Table 5**
**Medications used for urinary urgency and frequency (lower doses with comorbidities)**

| | | |
|---|---|---|
| Amitriptyline | 12.5–75.0 mg qhs | — |
| Oxybutynin (Ditropan) | 2.5–5.0 mg bid | Dry mouth can be significant |
| Oxybutynin chloride (Oxytrol) | 3.9-mg patch qd<br>Gel | Skin irritation, minimal dry mouth<br>Gel without skin irritation |
| Tolterodine (Detrol LA) | 1–2 mg bid | — |
| Darifenacin hydrobromide (Enablex ER) | 7.5–15.0 mg qd | Less impact on cognitive function |
| Solifenacin (Vesicare) | 5–10 mg qd | — |
| Trospium (Sanctura) | 20 mg bid | Less interaction with CYP-450 drugs |
| Trospium (Sanctura XR) | 60 mg qd | — |
| Fesoterodine (Toviaz) | 4–8 mg qd | Superior to tolterodine |
| Mirabegron (Myrbetriq) | 25–50 mg qd | Cannot use in renal, hepatic, or uncontrolled hypertension |

### *Depression and Anxiety*

The reported prevalence of depression in patients with ALS varies widely and depends on which assessment measure is used.[92,93] The ALS Depression Inventory (ADI-12) is a self-reported questionnaire developed specifically to screen for depression in ALS and does not refer to motor-related symptoms in ALS. Using the ADI-12, Atassi and colleagues,[92] in 2011, reported that the prevalence of mild and severe depression was 29% and 6%, respectively, compared with 10% of the general population with major depression. The lower rate of severe depression was attributed to patients receiving antidepressants to treat sialorrhea, PBA, and insomnia. The ALS Cosmos study reported that 88% of 329 patients had no depressive disorder based on structured telephone interviews. Minor depression was found in 7%, and 5% had a current major depressive disorder by the *Diagnostic and Statistical Manual of Disorders* (Fourth Edition) criteria. Demographic, financial, and employment factors were unrelated to depression, as were the duration of ALS symptoms and respiratory status. Also, of the 19% of the sample who expressed a wish to die, only 37% were clinically depressed.[93] Several classes of medications are used for the treatment of depression in ALS and are used depending on their side-effect profile. There have been no controlled clinical studies of these medications in patients with ALS. Tricyclic antidepressants like amitriptyline can be prescribed if anticholinergic effects are desired simultaneously for treating sialorrhea, PBA, or insomnia.

Prevalence rates for anxiety in patients with ALS range from 0% to 30%.[94–96] The early disease phase, especially during the diagnostic period, has been reported to be associated with a higher level of stress and anxiety.[97,98] Anxiety is usually treated with anxiolytics like benzodiazepines, but again there have been no systematic studies of these drugs in patients with ALS. Treatment of depression and anxiety can involve both cognitive behavioral therapy and pharmacologic intervention. There are no clinical trials that allow a recommendation of pharmacotherapy over psychotherapy. A positive patient-physician relationship and easy access in communicating with their physician reduces levels of anxiety in patients. Patients may benefit from a range of approaches, including relaxation strategies, such as meditation and biofeedback. Cognitive behavioral therapy equips patients with the skills to overcome maladaptive thought patterns and encourages emotional readjustment (**Table 6**).

**Table 6**
**Medications used for depression and anxiety (also see side effects in Table 2)**

| | Dosage |
|---|---|
| Depression | |
| Selective serotonin reuptake inhibitor antidepressants | |
| Sertraline (Zoloft) | 50–200 mg/d |
| Fluoxetine (Prozac) | 10–60 mg/d |
| Paroxetine (Paxil) | 10–50 mg/d |
| Paroxetine CR | 12.5–62.5 mg/d |
| Citalopram (Celexa) | 20–40 mg/d |
| Escitalopram (Lexapro) | 10–20 mg/d |
| Tricyclic antidepressants | |
| Amitriptyline (Elavil) | 50–200 mg qhs |
| Nortriptyline (Pamelor) | 50–150 mg qhs |
| Serotonin norepinephrine reuptake inhibitors | |
| Venlafaxine (Effexor) | 37.5–225.0 mg qd |
| Duloxetine (Cymbalta) | 30–60 mg qd |
| Norepinephrine dopamine reuptake inhibitor | |
| Bupropion hydrochloride (Wellbutrin) | 300–450 mg qd |
| Norepinephrine serotonin modulator | |
| Mirtazapine (Remeron) | 15–45 mg qhs |
| Anxiety | |
| Benzodiazepines | |
| Alprazolam (Xanax) | 0.25–1.0 mg tid |
| Lorazepam (Ativan) | 0.5–2.0 mg tid |
| Diazepam (Valium) | 2–10 mg tid |
| Clonazepam (Klonopin) | 0.5–2.0 mg qhs |
| 5HT1A agonists | |
| Buspirone | 10 mg tid |

## *End of Life*

End-of-life conversations can be a source of great anxiety and discomfort for patients, their families, and health care professionals; as a result, such discussions may be avoided. The issue of advance directives should be raised soon after the diagnosis.

Palliative care can start any time after the diagnosis of ALS and permits the use of high-tech assistive communication devices, power wheelchairs, hospitalization, NIV and PEG tubes. The referring physician is responsible initially for managing all medical treatment until patients are admitted to hospice for continued palliative care. Dyspnea, despite liberal use of NIV, can be treated with morphine starting at 2.5 to 5.0 mg every 4 hours and increased in dose and frequency as needed. Anxiety and restlessness can be treated with lorazepam 0.5 to 2.0 mg every 4 hours as needed.[91] Opiates and anxiolytics doses should be increased if they are not providing satisfactory control.

Palliative care is most often done in the hospital setting, though more community-based outpatient services have become available in large metropolitan areas. Hospice care provides interdisciplinary case management, medications, durable medical equipment, and supplies. The hospice medical director manages medical treatment. Some hospices offer hospice residential care. Hospice care is appropriate for patients with an FVC less than 30% of predicted and an estimated 6 months of life. In a study of the last month of life in patients with ALS, the most common symptoms were difficulty communicating, dyspnea, choking episodes, insomnia, and pain. Many of these symptoms were often inadequately controlled.[99] A significant number of caregivers reported depressed mood (40%), anxiety (30%), and confusion (10%) in patients.[99] Hospice services are essential in the management of end of life in patients with ALS and optimize the likelihood of a peaceful and dignified death. Despite its advantages, it is generally underused or initiated too late in the disease course.[100]

Failure to address advance directives can result in a difficult situation in which a patient who did not want tracheostomy mechanical ventilation (TMV) is intubated. Less than 10% of patients with ALS in the United States use invasive ventilation.[101] Factors influencing patients against selecting invasive ventilation include high cost for home care on a ventilator, increased caregiver burden, and continued progression of the disease. Patients with TMV may end up in an extended care facility if round-the-clock care is not available in their home. Many caregivers report TMV at home a major burden, which impacts their own health. The locked-in state occurs in 18% of patients with ALS surviving more than 5 years on TMV.[102] Withdrawal of invasive ventilation is usually carried out with the use of high-dose opiates and benzodiazepines. A Danish palliative care study on withdrawal of invasive mechanical ventilation at home in patients with advanced ALS reported median time from discontinuation to apnea was 15 minutes (range 0–18 hours).[103] Doses of morphine were in the range of 60 to 400 mg (median 100 mg) and doses of diazepam in the range of 20 to 120 mg (median of 100 mg) before the ventilator was disconnected.

## SUMMARY

Patients with ALS should be provided opportunities for multidisciplinary care because the spectrum of available treatments can markedly impact both QoL and survival. ALS should no longer be considered untreatable based on the broad range of interventions that can be prescribed for symptom management.

## DISCLOSURE

S. Rudnicki has received research grants for Cytokinetics. A.L. McVey has received research grants from Cytokinetics. C.E. Jackson is a consultant and has received research support from OneWorld Meds regarding use of Myobloc for sialorrhea. She also serves on the speaker's bureau for Nuedexta for PBA. M.M. Dimachkie is on the speaker's bureau or is a consultant for Baxter, Biomarin, Catalyst, CSL-Behring, Depomed, Genzyme, Merck, NuFactor, and Pfizer. He has also received grants from Catalyst, CSL-Behring, FDA/OPD, GSK, MDA, NIH, and TMA. R.J. Barohn has served as a consultant and received consulting fees from Baxter, CSL Behring, Genzyme, Grifols, Novartis, and NuFactor. He has received research grants from Biomarin, Cytokinetics, Eli Lilly, FDA/OPD, GSK, MDA, MGFA, Neals, NIH, NINDS, Novartis, PTC, Sanofi/Genzyme, and Teva. This publication was also supported by an Institutional Clinical and Translational Science Award, NIH/NCATS grant numbers UL1TR000001. Its contents are solely the responsibility of the authors and do not necessarily represent the official views of the NIH.

## REFERENCES

1. Forshew DA, Bromberg MB. A survey of clinicians' practice in the symptomatic treatment of ALS. Amyotroph Lateral Scler Other Motor Neuron Disord 2003;4: 258–63.
2. Sufit R, Miller R, Mitsumoto H, et al. Prevalence and treatment outcomes of sialorrhea in amyotrophic lateral sclerosis patients as assessed by the ALS patient care database. Ann Neurol 1999;46:506.
3. Miller RG, Rosenberg JA, Gelinas DF, et al. Practice parameter: the care of the patient with amyotrophic lateral sclerosis (an evidence-based review): report of the Quality Standards Subcommittee of the American Academy of Neurology: ALS Practice Parameters Task Force. Neurology 1999;52:1311–23.
4. Jackson CE, Rosenfeld J. Symptomatic pharmacotherapy: bulbar and constitutional symptoms. In: Mitsumoto, Przedborski, Gordon, et al, editors. Amyotrophic lateral sclerosis. New York: Taylor & Francis Group; 2006. p. 649–64.
5. Bradley WG, Anderson F, Bromberg M, et al. Current management of ALS: comparison of the ALS CARE Database and the AAN Practice Parameter. The American Academy of Neurology. Neurology 2001;57:500–4.
6. Portis M, Gamba M, Bertaccji G, et al. Treatment of sialorrhea with ultrasound guided botulinum toxin type A injection in patients with neurological disorders. J Neurol Neurosurg Psychiatry 2001;70:538–40.
7. Giess R, Naumann M, Werner E, et al. Injections of botulinum toxin A into the salivary glands improve sialorrhoea in amyotrophic lateral sclerosis [see comment]. J Neurol Neurosurg Psychiatry 2000;69:121–3.
8. Rowe D, Erjavec S. An open-label pilot study of intra-parotid botulinum toxin A injections in the treatment of sialorrhea in motor neuron disease. Amyotroph Lateral Scler Other Motor Neuron Disord 2003;4:53–4.
9. Bhatia KP, Munchau A, Brown P. Botulinum toxin is a useful treatment in excessive drooling in saliva. J Neurol Neurosurg Psychiatry 1999;67:697.
10. Jackson CE, Gronseth G, Rosenfeld J, et al. Randomized double-blind study of botulinum toxin type B in ALS patients. Muscle Nerve 2009;39:137–43.
11. Harriman M, Morrison M, Hay J, et al. Use of radiotherapy for control of sialorrhea in patients with amyotrophic lateral sclerosis. J Otolaryngol 2001;30: 242–9.
12. Andersen PM, Gronberg H, Franze L, et al. External radiation of the parotid glands significantly reduces drooling in patients with motor neuron disease with bulbar paresis. J Neurol Sci 2001;191:111–4.
13. Miller RG, Jackson CE, Kasarskis EJ, et al. Practice parameter update: the care of the patient with amyotrophic lateral sclerosis: multidisciplinary care, symptom management, and cognitive/behavioral impairment (an evidence-based review) report of the quality standards Subcommittee of the American Academy of Neurology. Neurology 2009;73:1227–33.

14. Marin MG. Pharmacology of airway secretion. Pharmaocl Rev 1986;38:273–89.
15. Newall AR, Orser R, Hunt M. The control of oral secretions in bulbar ALS/MND. J Neurol Sci 1996;139:43–4.
16. Radunovic A, Mitsumotor H, Leigh PN. Clinical care of patients with amyotrophic lateral sclerosis. Lancet Neurol 2007;6(10):913–25.
17. McCullagh S, Moore M, Gawel M, et al. Pathological laughing and crying in amyotrophic lateral sclerosis: an association with prefrontal cognitive dysfunction. J Neurol Sci 1999;169:43–8.
18. Brooks BR, Thisted RA, Appel SH, et al. Treatment of pseudobulbar affect in ALS with dextromethorphan/quinidine: a randomized trial. Neurology 2004;63: 1364–70.
19. Arnulf I, Similowski T, Salachas F, et al. Sleep disorders and diaphragmatic function in patients with amyotrophic lateral sclerosis. Am J Respir Crit Care Med 2000;161:849–56.
20. Czaplinski A, Yen AA, Appel SH. Forced vital capacity (FVC) as an indicator of survival and disease progression in an ALS clinic population. J Neurol Neurosurg Psychiatry 2006;77:390–2.
21. Jackson CE, Rosenfeld J, Moore DH, et al. A preliminary evaluation of a prospective study of pulmonary function studies and symptoms of hypoventilation in ALS/MND patients. J Neurol Sci 2001;191:75–8.
22. Lechtzin N, Wiener CM, Shade DM, et al. Spirometry in the supine position improves the detection of diaphragmatic weakness in patients with amyotrophic lateral sclerosis. Chest 2002;121:436–42.
23. Varrato J, Siderowf A, Damiano P, et al. Postural change of forced vital capacity predicts some respiratory symptoms in ALS. Neurology 2001;57:357–9.
24. Vaszar LT, Weinacker AB, Henig NR, et al. Ethical issues in the long-term management of progressive degenerative neuromuscular diseases. Semin Respir Crit Care Med 2002;23:307–14.
25. Hull J, Aniapravan R, Chan E, et al. British Thoracic Society guideline for respiratory management of children with neuromuscular weakness. Thorax 2012; 67(Suppl 1):i1–40.
26. Miller RG, Jackson CE, Kasarskis EJ, et al. Practice parameter update: the care of the patient with amyotrophic lateral sclerosis: drug, nutritional, and respiratory therapies (an evidence-based review) report of the quality standards subcommittee of the American Academy of Neurology. Neurology 2009;73:1218–26.
27. Bourke SC, Tomlinson M, Williams TL, et al. Effects of non-invasive ventilation on survival and quality of life in patients with amyotrophic lateral sclerosis: a randomised controlled trial. Lancet Neurol 2006;5:140–7.
28. Bourke SC, Bullock RE, Williams TL, et al. Noninvasive ventilation in ALS: indications and effect on quality of life. Neurology 2003;61:171–7.
29. Butz M, Wollinsky KH, Wiedemuth-Catrinescu U, et al. Longitudinal effects of noninvasive positive-pressure ventilation in patients with amyotrophic lateral sclerosis. Am J Phys Med Rehabil 2003;82:597–604.
30. Lyall RA, Donaldson N, Fleming T, et al. A prospective study of quality of life in ALS patients treated with noninvasive ventilation. Neurology 2001;57:153–6.
31. Pinto A, de Carvalho M, Evangelista T, et al. Nocturnal pulse oximetry: a new approach to establish the appropriate time for non-invasive ventilation in ALS patients. Amyotroph Lateral Scler Other Motor Neuron Disord 2003;4:31–5.
32. Aboussouan LS, Khan SU, Meeker DP, et al. Effect of noninvasive positive-pressure ventilation on survival in amyotrophic lateral sclerosis. Ann Intern Med 1997;127:450–3.

33. Jackson CE, Lovitt S, Gowda N, et al. Factors correlated with NPPV use in ALS. Amyotroph Lateral Scler 2006;7:80–5.
34. Olney RK, Murphy J, Forshew D, et al. The effects of executive and behavioral dysfunction on the course of ALS. Neurology 2005;65:1774–7.
35. Gruis KL, Brown DL, Schoennemann A, et al. Predictors of noninvasive ventilation tolerance in patients with amyotrophic lateral sclerosis. Muscle Nerve 2005; 32:808–11.
36. Bach JR. Amyotrophic lateral sclerosis: predictors for prolongation of life by noninvasive respiratory aids. Arch Phys Med Rehabil 1995;76:828–32.
37. Tzeng AC, Bach JR. Prevention of pulmonary morbidity for patients with neuromuscular disease. Chest 2000;118:1390–6.
38. Mangera Z, Panesar G, Makker H. Practical approach to management of respiratory complications in neurological disorders. Int J Gen Med 2012;5:255–63.
39. Garpestad E, Hill N. Noninvasive ventilation for patients with neuromuscular disease and acute respiratory failure. Chest 2008;133:315 [author reply: 315].
40. Perrin C, Unterborn JN, Ambrosio CD, et al. Pulmonary complications of chronic neuromuscular diseases and their management. Muscle Nerve 2004;29:5–27.
41. Park JH, Kang SW, Lee SC, et al. How respiratory muscle strength correlates with cough capacity in patients with respiratory muscle weakness. Yonsei Med J 2010;51:392–7.
42. McElhiney MC, Rabkin JG, Gordon PH, et al. Prevalence of fatigue and depression in ALS patients and change over time. J Neurol Neurosurg Psychiatry 2009; 80:1146–9.
43. Lo Coco D, La Bella V. Fatigue, sleep, and nocturnal complaints in patients with amyotrophic lateral sclerosis. Eur J Neurol 2012;19:760–3.
44. Ramirez C, Piemonte ME, Callegaro D, et al. Fatigue in amyotrophic lateral sclerosis: frequency and associated factors. Amyotroph Lateral Scler 2008;9:75–80.
45. Bensimon G, Lacomblez L, Meininger VA. A controlled trial of riluzole in amyotrophic lateral sclerosis. ALS/Riluzole Study Group. N Engl J Med 1994;330: 585–91.
46. Lou J-S, Reeves A, Benice T, et al. Fatigue and depression are associated with poor quality of life in ALS. Neurology 2003;60:122–3.
47. Rabkin JG, Gordon PH, McElhiney M, et al. Modafinil treatment of fatigue in patients with ALS: a placebo controlled study. Muscle Nerve 2009;39:297–303.
48. Mascaritioli M, Kushta I, Molfino A, et al. Nutritional and metabolic support in patients with amyotrophic lateral sclerosis. Nutrition 2012;28:959–66.
49. Desport JC, Preux PM, Magy L, et al. Factors associated with hypermetabolism in patients with amyotrophic lateral sclerosis. Am J Clin Nutr 2001;74:328–34.
50. Dupuis L, Pradat P-F, Ludolph AC, et al. Energy metabolism in amyotrophic lateral sclerosis. Lancet Neurol 2011;10:75–82.
51. Kasarskis EF, Mendiondo MS, Matthews DE, et al. Estimating daily energy expenditure in individuals with amyotrophic lateral sclerosis. Am J Clin Nutr 2014;99:792–803.
52. Limousin N, Blasco H, Corcia P, et al. Malnutrition at the time of diagnosis is associated with a shorter disease duration in ALS. J Neurol Sci 2010;297:36–9.
53. Shimuzu T, Nagaoka U, Nakayama Y, et al. Reduction rate of body mass index predicts prognosis for survival in amyotrophic lateral sclerosis: a multicenter study in Japan. Amyotroph Lateral Scler 2012;13:363–6.
54. Jawaid A, Murphy SB, Wilson AM, et al. A decrease in body mass index is associated with faster progression of motor symptoms and shorter survival in ALS. Amyotroph Lateral Scler 2010;11:542–8.

55. Paganoni S, Deng J, Jaffa M, et al. Body mass index, not dyslipidemia, is an independent predictor of survival in amyotrophic lateral sclerosis. Muscle Nerve 2011;44:20–4.
56. Gallo V, Wark P, Jenab M, et al. Prediagnostic body fat and risk of death from amyotrophic lateral sclerosis. Neurology 2013;80:829–38.
57. Katzberg HD, Benatar M. Enteral tube feeding for amyotrophic lateral sclerosis/motor. Neuron disease. Cochrane Database Syst Rev 2011;(1):CD004030.
58. Chiò A, Bottacchi E, Buffa C, et al, PARALS. Positive effects of tertiary centres for amyotrophic lateral sclerosis on outcomes and use of hospital facilities. J Neurol Neurosurg Psychiatry 2006;77:948–50.
59. Czaplinski A, Yen AA, Simpson ER, et al. Slower disease progression and prolonged survival in contemporary patients with amyotrophic lateral sclerosis: is the natural history of amyotrophic lateral sclerosis changing? Arch Neurol 2006;63:1139–43.
60. Forbes RB, Colvisse S, Swingler RJ, Scottish Motor Neurone Disease Research Group. Frequency, timing and outcome of gastrostomy tubes for amyotrophic lateral sclerosis/motor neurone disease - a record linkage study from the Scottish Motor Neuron Disease Registry. J Neurol 2004;251(7):813–7.
61. Mitchell JD, O'Brien MR, Joshi M. Audit of outcomes in motor neuron disease (MND) patients treated with riluzole. Amyotroph Lateral Scler 2006;7(2):67–71.
62. Zhang M, Hubbard J, Rudnicki SA, et al. Survey of current enteral nutrition practices in treatment of amyotrophic lateral sclerosis. ESPEN J 2013;8:e25–8. Available at: http://www.sciencedirect.com/science/article/pii/S2212826312000619.
63. Desport JC, Preux PM, Truong CT, et al. Nutritional assessment and survival in ALS patients. Amyotroph Lateral Scler Other Motor Neuron Disord 2000;1(2):91–6.
64. Mazzini L, Corra T, Zaccala M, et al. Percutaneous endoscopic gastrostomy and enteral nutrition in amyotrophic lateral sclerosis. J Neurolog y 1995;242(10):695–8.
65. Chiò A, Galetti R, Finocchiaro C, et al. Percutaneous radiological gastrostomy: a safe and effective method of nutritional tube placement in advanced ALS. J Neurol Neurosurg Psychiatry 2004;75:645–6.
66. Allen JA, Chen R, Ajroud-Driss S, et al. Gastrostomy tube placement by endoscopy vs radiologic methods in patients with ALS: a retrospective study of complications and outcomes. Amyotroph Lateral Scler Frontotemporal Degener 2013;14(4):308–14.
67. Stanich P, Chiapetta A, Oliviera A, et al. Nutritional supplementation in patients with amyotrophic lateral sclerosis. Amyotroph Lateral Scler Other Motor Neuron Disord 2002;3:119.
68. Silva LB, Mourao LF, Silva AA, et al. Effect of nutritional supplementation with milk whey proteins in amyotrophic lateral sclerosis patients. Arq Neuropsiquiatr 2010;68(2):263–8.
69. Dorst J, Cypionka J, Ludolph AC. High-caloric food supplements in the treatment of amyotrophic lateral sclerosis: a prospective interventional study. Amyotroph Lateral Scler Frontotemporal Degener 2013;14(7–8):533–6.
70. Wills AM, Hubbard J, Macklin EA, et al. Hypercaloric enteral nutrition in patients with amyotrophic lateral sclerosis: a randomised, double-blind, placebo-controlled phase 2 trial. Lancet 2014;383(14):6065–72.
71. Czell D, Bauer M, Binek J, et al. Outcomes of percutaneous endoscopic gastrostomy tube insertion in respiratory impaired amyotrophic lateral sclerosis patients under noninvasive ventilation. Respir Care 2013;58(5):838–44.

72. Pizziementia A, Aragona M, Onesti E, et al. Depression, pain, and quality of life in patients with amyotrophic lateral sclerosis: a cross sectional study. Funct Neurol 2013;28(2):115–9.
73. Chio A, Canosa A, Gallo S, et al. Pain in amyotrophic lateral sclerosis: a population-based controlled study. Eur J Neurol 2012;19(4):551–5.
74. Ajroud-Driss S, Casey P, Heller S, et al. Prevalence and characteristics of pain in early and late stages of ALS. Amyotroph Lateral Scler Frontotemporal Degener 2013;14(5–6):369–72.
75. Pagnini F, Lunetta C, Banfi P, et al. Pain in amyotrophic lateral sclerosis: a psychological perspective. Neurol Sci 2012;33(5):1193–6.
76. Newrick PG, Langton-Hewer R. Pain in motor neuron disease. J Neurol Neurosurg Psychiatry 1985;48:838–40.
77. Brettschneider J, Kurent J, Ludolph A. Drug therapy for pain in amyotrophic lateral sclerosis or motor neuron disease [review]. Cochrane Database Syst Rev 2013;(6):CD005226.
78. McClelland S, Bethoux FA, Boulis NM, et al. Intrathecal baclofen for spasticity-related pain in amyotrophic lateral sclerosis: efficacy and factors associated with pain relief. Muscle Nerve 2008;37(3):396–8.
79. Drory VE, Goltsman E, Reznik JG, et al. The value of muscle exercise in patients with amyotrophic lateral sclerosis. J Neurol Sci 2001;191:133–7.
80. Bedlack RS, Pastula DM, Hawes J, et al. Open-label pilot trial of levetiracetam for cramps and spasticity in patients with motor neuron disease. Amyotroph Lateral Scler 2009;10(4):210–5.
81. Winterholler MG, Heckman JG, Hecht M, et al. Recurrent trismus and stridor in an ALS patient: successful treatment with botulinum toxin. Neurology 2002;58:502–3.
82. Restivo DA, Lanza S, Marchese-Raguna R, et al. Improvement of masseter spasticity by botulinum toxin facilitates PEG placement in amyotrophic lateral sclerosis. Gastroenterology 2002;123(5):1749–50.
83. Anderson PM, Abrahams S, Borasio G, et al. EFNS guidelines on the clinical management of amyotrophic lateral sclerosis (MALS) - revised report of an EFNS task force. Eur J Neurol 2012;19:360–75.
84. Sperfeld AD, Hanemann OC, Ludolph AC, et al. Laryngospasm: an underdiagnosed symptom of X-linked spinobulbar muscular atrophy. Neurology 2005; 64(4):753–4.
85. Kuhnlein P, Gdynia HJ, Sperfeld AD, et al. Diagnosis and treatment of bulbar symptoms in amyotrophic lateral sclerosis. Nat Clin Pract Neurol 2008;4(7): 366–74.
86. Jenkins TM, Hollinger H, McDermott CJ. The evidence for symptomatic treatments in amyotrophic lateral sclerosis. Curr Opin Neurol 2014;27:524–31.
87. Simmons Z. Management strategies for patients with amyotrophic lateral sclerosis from diagnosis through death. Neurologist 2005;11(5):257–70.
88. Borasio GD, Oliver D. The control of other symptoms. In: Oliver D, Borasio GD, Walsh D, editors. Amyotrophic lateral sclerosis. Oxford (United Kingdom): Oxford University Press; 2000. p. 72–9.
89. Piccione EA, Sletten DM, Staff NP, et al. Autonomic system and ALS. Muscle Nerve 2015;51(5):676–9.
90. Nubling GS, Bauer M, Bauer RM, et al. Increased prevalence of bladder and intestinal dysfunction in amyotrophic lateral sclerosis. Amyotroph Lateral Scler Frontotemporal Degener 2014;15(3–4):174–9.
91. Rocha JA, Reis C, Simoes F, et al. Diagnostic investigation and multidisciplinary management in motor neuron disease. J Neurol 2005;252:1435–47.

92. Atassi N, Cook A, Pineda CM, et al. Depression in amyotrophic lateral sclerosis. Amyotroph Lateral Scler 2011;12(2):109–12.
93. Rabkin JG, Goetz R, Factor-Litvak P, et al, The ALS Cosmos Study Group. Depression and wish to die in a multicenter cohort of ALS patients. Amyotroph Lateral Scler Frontotemporal Degener 2015;16(3–4):265–73.
94. Kurt A, Nijboer F, Maatuz T, et al. Depression and anxiety in individuals with amyotrophic lateral sclerosis: epidemiology and management. CNS Drugs 2007;21(4):279–91.
95. Chen D, Xiaoyan G, Sheng Z, et al. Depression and anxiety in amyotrophic lateral sclerosis: correlations between the distress of patients and caregivers. Muscle Nerve 2015;51:353–7.
96. Taylor L, Wicks P, Leigh PN, et al. Prevalence of depression in amyotrophic lateral sclerosis and other motor disorders. Eur J Neurol 2010;17:1047–53.
97. Vignola A, Guzzo A, Calvo A, et al. Anxiety undermines quality of life in ALS patients and caregivers. Eur J Neurol 2008;15(11):1231–6.
98. Tagami M, Kimura F, Nakajima H, et al. Tracheostomy and invasive ventilation in Japanese ALS patients: decision making and survival analysis: 1990–2010. J Neurol Sci 2014;344(1–2):158–64.
99. Ganzini L, Johnston WS, Silveira MJ. The final month of life in patients with ALS. Neurology 2002;59:428–31.
100. Blackhall LJ. Amyotrophic lateral sclerosis and palliative care: where we are, and the road ahead. Muscle Nerve 2012;45:311–8.
101. Rabkin J, Ogino M, Goetz R, et al. Tracheostomy with invasive ventilation for ALS patients: neurologist's roles in the US and Japan. Amyotroph Lateral Scler Frontotemporal Degener 2013;14(2):116–23.
102. Hayashi H, Oppenheier EA. ALS patients on TPPV: totally locked-in state, neurologic findings and ethical implications. Neurology 2003;61:135–7.
103. Dreyer PS, Felding M, Klitnaes CS, et al. Withdrawal of invasive home mechanical ventilation in patients with advanced amyotrophic lateral sclerosis: ten years of Danish experience. J Palliat Med 2012;15(2):205–9.

# Complementary and Alternative Therapies in Amyotrophic Lateral Sclerosis

Richard S. Bedlack, MD, PhD[a,*], Nanette Joyce, DO, MAS[b], Gregory T. Carter, MD, MS[c], Sabrina Paganoni, MD, PhD[d], Chafic Karam, MD[e]

**KEYWORDS**

- Complementary and alternative medicine • Paternalism • Autonomy

**KEY POINTS**

- Patients with amyotrophic lateral sclerosis (ALS) often consider complementary and alternative therapies they read about on the Internet.
- Common types of alternative therapies considered for ALS include special diets, nutritional supplements, cannabis, acupuncture, chelation, and energy healing.
- Physicians may handle discussions about alternative therapies via paternalism, autonomy, or shared decision making.
- ALSUntangled reviews alternative therapies via a shared decision making model.

## INTRODUCTION

Complementary and alternative medicine (CAM) is defined as nonmainstream treatment used in addition to (complementary) or instead of (alternative) standard evidence-based care.[1] At some point in their illness, most patients with amyotrophic

Disclosure statement: Dr R.S. Bedlack has received research support from the ALS Association and Motor Neurone Disease Association for ALSUntangled, and is a consultant for Neuraltus Pharmaceuticals. Dr S. Paganoni is funded by an NIH Career Development Award (2K12HD001097-16).
[a] Department of Neurology, Duke University Medical Center, Durham, NC 27702, USA; [b] Department of Physical Medicine and Rehabilitation, University of California, Davis School of Medicine, 4860 Y Street Suite 3850, Sacramento, CA 95817, USA; [c] Department of Physical Medicine and Rehabilitation, St. Luke's Rehabilitation Institute, 711 South Cowley, Spokane, WA 99202, USA; [d] Spaulding Rehabilitation Hospital, Boston VA Health Care System, Harvard Medical School, Massachussets General Hospital, Boston, MA 02114, USA; [e] Department of Neurology, University of North Carolina School of Medicine, 170 Manning Drive, Campus Box 7025, Chapel Hill, NC 27599-7025, USA
* Corresponding author.
*E-mail address:* Bedla001@mc.duke.edu

Neurol Clin 33 (2015) 909–936
http://dx.doi.org/10.1016/j.ncl.2015.07.008 neurologic.theclinics.com

lateral sclerosis (PALS) will try at least one type of CAM.[2,3] It is easy to see why. ALS rapidly disables and shortens the life span. Although symptom management has improved in recent years,[4–6] there remains no evidence-based clinically meaningful disease-modifying therapy to improve this dreaded condition. Surveys shed light on patient motivations and expectations for ALS CAMs: 10% think they will find a cure; 30% think they will improve; 50% think they will slow progression.[2,3] Other drivers the authors have encountered include peer pressure from family members and friends who have these expectations and the belief that nothing worse than the present disease could possibly be encountered.

The Internet has made it easier than ever for PALS to find CAMs. A Google search of *ALS treatment*, for example, yields more than 100 million hits.[7] Although this breadth is impressive, there is often little depth within Web sites offering CAMs. Claims such as *clinically proven* and *perfectly safe* are too often supported by data that range from absent, to flawed, to completely inaccurate. Real harms have come to PALS pursuing CAMs, including physical, financial, and psychological harms.[8,9] There is also the potential for scientific harms, as pursuit of CAM is sometimes undertaken in place of enrollment in a trial; meaning trials may take longer, cost more, and have to be stopped prematurely because of poor enrollment.[10]

In this article, the authors describe the types of ALS CAMs that they have been asked about most often over the years. The authors then discuss options for reviewing CAMs with PALS, including one called ALSUntangled.

## TYPES OF COMPLEMENTARY AND ALTERNATIVE MEDICINE THAT PEOPLE WITH AMYOTROPHIC LATERAL SCLEROSIS COMMONLY ASK ABOUT

### *Diets and Nutritional Supplements*

The importance of energy balance is well established in ALS, with both preclinical and human studies offering evidence to support a disease-influencing effect of premorbid weight, weight maintenance, and caloric intake.[11–13] Although studies in the healthy population suggest that reduced caloric intake provides survival benefits by reducing the risk for chronic disease, the opposite is true in ALS. ALS SOD1-mutant mice placed on a calorie-restricted diet showed reduced paw-grip strength and significantly reduced survival compared with animals receiving adequate nutrition.[14] In contrast, several studies examining the effects of high-calorie diets enriched in carbohydrates or fat have shown prolonged survival in SOD1 animals.[15–18]

Evidence supporting a survival benefit related to energy balance in PALS has been collected primarily from population studies that include assessment of body mass index (BMI) and malnutrition. Malnutrition in ALS has been defined as the loss of greater than 10% baseline body weight or a BMI lower than 18.5 kg/m$^2$; both are considered negative predictors of survival in ALS. Although the prevalence varies between studies, some report more than half of all PALS meet the criteria for malnutrition.[19] The literature consistently shows that a higher BMI, between 30 and 35 kg/m$^2$, is associated with decreased risk of disease, later disease onset, and prolonged survival.[20] Low BMI or rapid weight loss negatively affects disease progression, with reports suggesting a 7.7-fold relative risk of mortality in malnourished PALS.[12] In addition, Lindauer and colleagues,[21] in their prospective study assessing adiposity by MRI imaging, reported that increased subcutaneous fat mass was a statistically significant predictor of survival in men.

Weight loss is nearly ubiquitous in ALS and presents significant challenges for patients. In a cohort of 121 patients, queried by Körner and colleagues,[22] weight loss had a negative impact on quality of life (QOL) with perception of reduced physical functioning and vitality. Patients who had lost weight and were subsequently placed on high-calorie supplements or had undergone percutaneous endoscopic gastrostomy (PEG) (n = 23) reported weight stabilization or gain. Of those who chose PEG, 84.6% reported an improvement in QOL with no patients reporting worsened QOL. The cause of weight loss and subsequent malnutrition in ALS is multifactorial and includes dysphagia from bulbar dysfunction, upper extremity weakness, and hypermetabolism. Dysphagia is present in 45% of patients with bulbar-onset disease at diagnosis, and approximately 81% of all PALS will experience dysphagia as a symptom of ALS.[22] Because of the involvement of cranial nerves IX, X, and XII, patients with bulbar disease develop disruption in tongue, pharyngeal, and esophageal function resulting in difficulty chewing and swallowing. The weakened oral activities ultimately result in reduced calorie and fluid intake as patients often become fearful of choking and avoid eating and drinking or are unable to spend the increased time it takes to consume a meal safely. Upper extremity weakness also interferes with weight maintenance as it impairs self-feeding and prolongs mealtime, which often results in early satiety and reduced caloric intake. Dietary modification, with changes in food texture and liquid viscosity, as well as behavioral modification, including safe swallowing techniques and caregiver-assisted feeding, may help mitigate these problems, at least temporarily. For further discussion of nutrition, the reader is referred to the article in Ref.[23]

Hypermetabolism, defined as an increased resting metabolic rate, has been observed in PALS and SOD1 mice. The cause of the hypermetabolism in ALS is poorly described but has been attributed to increased energy utilization by weakened skeletal muscles; nonfunctional muscular activity, such as spasticity, cramps, fasciculations, and/or pseudobulbar motor activities (uncontrolled laughing or crying); and the metabolic cost of increased protein catabolism.[24,25] Calculating the total daily energy expenditure for PALS using standard methods, such as the Harris-Benedict equation, does not provide adequate estimation of total daily energy expenditure. It has been suggested that PALS require anywhere from 10% to 20% more calories than what these predication strategies indicate. Kasarskis and colleagues[26] followed 80 individuals with ALS, and their data provided evidence supporting the presence of hypermetabolism early in the disease and the potential for broad fluctuation of energy imbalance within a single patient with ALS (−2989 to +1395 kcal/d), illustrating the complexity of metabolic changes in ALS. This finding presents a challenge to the practitioner for providing accurate estimates and recommendations to meet each patient's nutritional needs over the course of the disease. From their data, the investigators developed a more accurate caloric estimation tool using the ALSFRS-R (Amyotrophic Lateral Sclerosis Functional Rating Scale-Revised Version) and the Harris-Benedict equation; both patients and practitioners can access this tool online and use it to guide nutrition-related interventions, including the need for gastrostomy.[27]

There have been conflicting opinions regarding the best diet to recommend for nutritional support in ALS. Some propose a diet high in carbohydrates, whereas others recommend a diet high in fat. Still others hypothesize that a ketogenic diet may have therapeutic potential in ALS based on preclinical data in SOD1 mice showing strength gains mid-disease when compared with mice fed a traditional diet.[28] Although high-calorie diets have shown survival benefit in SOD1 mice, the ketogenic diet did not. In a recent clinical trial, comparing the potential of high calorie diets enriched with either fat or carbohydrates to restore weight in 24 individuals with ALS, both strategies were reported as safe and effective after 12 weeks of treatment.[29] However, there was a trend toward greater weight gain that did not reach statistical significance for those who consumed the high-fat diet. This study was limited by a small sample size; no conclusion could be drawn about survival, as this was not an end point. In contrast, a second small but randomized, double-blind placebo-controlled phase II clinical study (n = 24) compared the safety and tolerability of 3 diets: a regular diet (Jevity 1.00; 29% fat calories), a hypercarbohydrate hypercaloric diet (Jevity 1.5; 29% fat calories), and a hyperfat hypercaloric diet (Oxepa; 55% fat calories with eicosapentaenoic acid and gamma-linolenic acid) with differing results.[30] Although this study was also limited by sample size, the data favored those who were treated with the hypercarbohydrate hypercaloric diet, who had fewer serious adverse events, including death, during the 5-month follow-up period (control deaths 3 of 7; hyperfat hypercaloric deaths 1 of 8; hypercarbohydrate hypercaloric deaths 0 of 9). Interestingly, the hyperfat hypercaloric cohort lost weight during the trial, calling into question the accuracy of their methods for assessing calorie requirements. In addition, preclinical data assessing the benefits of omega-3 fatty acids, and more specifically eicosapentaenoic acid, in ALS SOD1 mice showed reduced survival in the animals receiving the omega-3 fatty acids.[31] The investigators cautioned against its use in ALS. Further testing with a larger sample and perhaps using a different hyperfat hypercaloric supplement is needed. However, there seems to be sufficient data to conclude that a diet high in calories provides a benefit in ALS.

When PALS are unable to overcome negative energy balance and lose more than 10% of baseline body weight, a gastrostomy tube is often indicated. Argued advantages of gastrostomy include alleviation of patient and family stress, improvement in QOL, and increased survival. Although this has remained somewhat controversial, there is a growing body of evidence to support these benefits. Numerous studies have measured the mortality rate after the procedure, with respiratory insufficiency being the most common cause of periprocedural death. The American Academy of Neurology (AAN) recommends that gastrostomy be placed when the force vital capacity (FVC) is equal to or greater than 50% predicted to reduce the associated risks.[4] A study of 35 PALS with an FVC greater than 50%, observed in 3-month intervals after PEG tube placement for up to 2 years, did not differ significantly in mortality from patients without PEG at 6 months but did after 6 months, having lower mortality and significant improvement in BMI.[32] Intraprocedural mortality of PEG has been shown to be 1.8%, with a 24-hour in-hospital mortality rate of 3.6% and a 30-day mortality rate of 11.5%.[33] More recently, Dorst and colleagues[34] followed 89 patients in a multicenter prospective study observing the safety of PEG. They reported general safety of PEG placement with only 1.1% mortality in the periprocedural period. In addition, they had improved outcomes in patients receiving a single prophylactic injection of antibiotics during tube placement, slow initiation of nutritional supplementation (<200 kcal/d), and high-calorie nutritional supplementation once at goal. There were no reports of refeeding syndrome, and the patients who received high-calorie supplementation showed a survival benefit at 18 months after gastrostomy placement. In addition, the investigators concluded that the use of noninvasive ventilation in the periprocedural period decreased the risk associated with PEG, allowing safe placement later in the disease. However, some suggest that radiologically placed gastrostomy is safer than PEG.[35]

If nutrition has such a strong influence on disease onset and progression, are there disease-modifying effects of vitamin and mineral enriched diets? Supplements or nutraceuticals are "products intended to supplement the diet that contain one or more of the following dietary ingredients: a vitamin; a mineral; an herb or other botanic; or an amino acid used as a dietary substance for man to supplement the diet by increasing the total dietary intake to promote wellness."[36] Since the passing of the Dietary Supplement Health and Education Act of 1994, supplements have not been regulated by the Food and Drug Administration (FDA) and are widely available and easily obtained without physician oversight. In fact, there are few requirements, other than registering the manufacturing plant and following rules for labeling, that manufacturers have to meet to produce supplements or ensure product quality and safety. It is estimated that more than 50% of US citizens take supplements regularly for health. The prevalence of supplement users is even greater in the ALS community, with more than 75% of patients taking supplements as part of their health regimen.[4,37] In the setting of a terminal disease without ample choices for disease-modifying therapies, these patients assert their autonomy and report that they self-medicate with dietary supplements to improve general well-being and slow disease progression.[3] Importantly, as described in a study of 121 PALS, those who took supplements (52%) reported greater vitality, physical and social functioning, and an overall improved QOL in the early and midstages of the disease.[22] Whether this benefit was afforded or not by the physiologic effects of the supplements can be debated; however, the health benefit, as measured by QOL, of a self-determined choice should not be considered trivial and may be tightly bound to a patient's hope for improved health and prolonged life. Although most of the supplements have little or no supporting scientific evidence to back their use, patients will take them. Rosenthal and Ellis,[38] in their review of nutrition and dietary supplements for motor neuron disease, suggest that it is the responsibility of the practitioner to remain aware of known adverse effects and "offer advice or caution as our patients explore their own therapeutic combinations."[38]

The Deanna Protocol is a supplement regimen that many PALS currently ask about. It was developed by an orthopedic physician who became frustrated by the lack of effective disease-modifying treatments when his daughter was first diagnosed with ALS.[39] The regimen combines multiple supplements targeted to improve mitochondrial function and cellular energy production and to provide neuroprotection. The exact regimen itself changes; the most recent version can be found on the Winning the Fight Web site.[40] This Web site reports "Scientific studies have proven that the Deanna Protocol significantly slows the progression of ALS and extends life span."[40] The authors are aware of only 1 published study on the Deanna Protocol, and this was done in animals. Ari and colleagues[41] compared standard and ketogenic diets, both with and without added key supplements from the Deanna Protocol in SOD1 mutant mice. Their data demonstrated significant improvements in function mid-disease and prolonged longevity in animals fed both the supplemented diets compared with the nonsupplemented diets. Furthermore, the supplement-enriched standard diet provided the longest and most statistically significant survival benefit (7.5% increase; $P = .001$), whereas the mice fed the supplement-enriched ketogenic diet showed the earliest functional benefit with a shorter but still significant increase in survival (4.2% increase; $P = .006$). This animal study has multiple methodological flaws identified by published guidelines[42] and has not been independently replicated. There are anecdotal reports of patients having improved energy and slowed progression on the Deanna Protocol, but neither the ALS diagnosis nor the reported improvements could be independently validated.[39] The cost to obtain the entire supplement list from one version of the protocol has been estimated to be greater than $400.00 per month and is not reimbursable by insurance.[39] Further investigations are warranted to evaluate its efficacy.

Although limited, both preclinical and clinical studies have been completed for various nutritional supplements in ALS. Next is a select list of supplements, most with antioxidant properties, that have been proposed as potentially beneficial for PALS.

### *Catechins*

Catechins are polyphenolic flavonoids that possess strong antioxidant properties and include epigallocatechin, epicatechin, and epicatichin-3-gallate. Catechins are considered free radical scavengers found in high concentrations in some plants, fruits, and vegetables. They are considered the health-promoting constituent of green tea, blue berries, cocoa, prune juice, red wine, and *Ginkgo biloba*, to name a few. Studies have shown that catechins cross the blood-brain barrier and are incorporated into brain tissue where they exert potent neuroprotective actions by modulating the mitochondrial responses to oxidative insults. Clinical studies in Parkinson disease have had promising results; however, no clinical studies have been completed in ALS. Supporting biological plausibility for catechins in the treatment of ALS, in vitro studies revealed that epicatichin-3-gallate reduced hyperexcitability in SOD1 motor neurons by interfering with glutamate hyperexcitability and had a rescue effect in motor neurons exposed to hydrogen peroxide ($H_2O_2$).[43] Preclinical investigation in the G93A SOD1 mouse showed that presymptomatic oral administration of epicatichin-3-gallate significantly delayed the onset of disease and extended the life span. In addition, the treated mice had an increased number of motor neurons, diminished microglial activation, reduced immunohistochemical reaction of nuclear factor (NF)–kappaB, and cleaved caspase-3 as well as reduced protein levels of inducible nitric oxide synthase and NF-kappaB in the spinal cords.

### *Coenzyme Q10*

Coenzyme Q10 (CoQ10) is a fat-soluble vitaminlike substance found in mitochondria that is part of the electron transport chain, participating in aerobic cellular respiration and the generation of ATP. Both preclinical and clinic studies have been completed assessing CoQ10 in ALS. SOD1 transgenic mice, fed daily CoQ10, demonstrated an increase in survival by 6 days compared with controls, which met modest statistical significance.[44] Although high doses of up to 3000 mg/d were well tolerated in patients,[45] a phase II clinical trial did not confirm superiority of CoQ10 when compared with patients taking placebo.[46] Advancement to a phase III clinical trial was not recommended.

### *Creatine*

Creatine is a nitrogenous organic acid that participates in cellular energy production. In addition, creatine seems to have neuroprotective properties related to its role in stabilizing the mitochondrial membrane by suppressing the opening of the mitochondrial permeability transition pore and release of cellular proapoptotic factors.[47] In ALS, supplementation with creatine was found to improve motor performance, improve weight maintenance, and extend survival in G93A transgenic mice.[48] However, a second group showed no effect of creatine on muscle bulk and strength in SOD1 mice.[49] A randomized double-blind placebo-controlled trial in humans did not show significant benefits.[50,51] A recent Cochrane review, including 3 trials and 386 participants with ALS taking creatine, by Pastula and colleagues,[52] concluded that "in patients already diagnosed with clinically probable or definite ALS, creatine at doses ranging from 5 to 10 g per day did not have a statistically significant effect on survival, ALSFRS-R progression or percent predicted FVC progression."[52] However, it is unknown if, at higher doses, creatine may be beneficial to PALS.[53] A recent phase II study showed that high-dose creatine supplementation is safe, tolerable, and may have some positive effects in Huntington disease. The authors await further studies with high-dose creatine in PALS to determine whether it is beneficial.

### *Ibedenone*

Idebenone is a quinone analogue of CoQ10 that was developed in Japan in the 1980s for the treatment of neurodegenerative disorders. Idebenone is an antioxidant that has been shown to inhibit lipid peroxidation in brain mitochondria. In one series, idebenone was the most potent antioxidant of the 70 related quinones evaluated.[54] Idebenone has been most extensively evaluated in patients with Friedreich ataxia, a trinucleotide repeat disorder with impaired iron metabolism and redox homeostasis.[55] The results of multiple clinical trials in this patient population have been mixed, ranging from documented improvement in function to lack of efficacy.[55,56] Although there are concerns that idebenone has the potential to form superoxide radicals causing increased cellular damage, it was well tolerated in all clinical studies and was subsequently marketed in Canada. However, in 2013, Santhera Pharmaceuticals voluntarily pulled it from the market, citing lack of efficacy.[56] Idebenone continues to be available online through nutraceutical providers and is included as one of the key supplements in the Deanna Protocol. Although clinical trials are ongoing in multiple sclerosis (MS) and other neuromuscular diseases, no preclinical or clinical studies have been published in ALS.

### *L-carnitine*

An essential cofactor for the beta-oxidation of long-chain fatty acids, L-carnitine is a quaternary ammonium compound required for the transport of fatty acids into the mitochondrial matrix for use in energy metabolism. Its antioxidant properties include superoxide anion radical and hydrogen scavenging that reduces mitochondrial injury and apoptosis both in vitro and in vivo.[57] In transgenic mice carrying a human SOD1 gene, oral L-carnitine significantly delayed the onset of signs of disease, delayed deterioration of motor activity, and extended life span.[58] Furthermore, subcutaneous injection prolonged survival even when treatment was initiated after the onset of symptoms.[58] A small (n = 42 treated, 40 placebo) randomized double-blind placebo-controlled pilot study of acetyl-L-carnitine showed an increase in median survival and slower ALSFRS-R and FVC decline in the patients taking L-carnitine 3 g/d. No significant side effects were reported, and the investigators concluded that a phase III trial is needed to confirm these preliminary findings.[59]

### *Omega-3*

Omega-3 polyunsaturated fatty acids have been associated with significant health benefits.[60] Omega-3 is thought to reduce neuroexcitotoxicity and neuroinflammation and activate antiapoptotic pathways.[61] In a study combing the data from 5 large prospective cohorts, there was an associated reduced risk for developing ALS in those consuming a diet high in omega-3 polyunsaturated fatty acids.[62] A single preclinical study has been completed in transgenic SOD1 mice to evaluate disease-modifying effects of omega-3.[31] They fed the mice a diet high in eicosapentaenoic acid, a murine-derived omega-3 fatty acid. Omega-3 did not affect the course of motor deficit or the length of survival, whether administered at disease onset or if given during the symptomatic stage of the disease, and accelerated disease progression in those fed omega-3 during the presymptomatic stage of ALS. Those animals fed omega-3 fatty acids showed an increase in vacuolization of anterior horn cells and associated glial cell abnormalities. In their conclusion, the investigators advised against the use of omega-3 supplementation in PALS.[31] Although there have been no clinical trials directly assessing the efficacy of a diet high in omega-3 fatty acids, a small clinical trial discussed earlier in this article did compare a standard diet, high-carbohydrate diet, and a high-fat diet with 55% of its calories provided by omega-3 fatty acids. The high-fat diet had increased adverse events, including deaths, as compared with the high-carbohydrate diet.[29,30]

***Resveratrol***

Resveratrol is a polyphenol found in the skin of grapes, blueberries, raspberries, and mulberries. It is reported to have neuroprotective effects through cellular pathways affecting mitochondrial biogenesis and autophagy, with implicated pathways activating Sirtuins, AMPK, and PGC-1$\alpha$. A few preclinical studies have been completed studying the effects of resveratrol.[63–65] All studies reported a delay in disease onset and statistically significant increases in survival. In addition, resveratrol improved survival with post–disease-onset treatment in the SOD1 ALS mouse model.[63–65] More than 30 clinical trials have been conducted examining the effects of resveratrol in cancer, diabetes, and heart disease, to name a few.[66] The supplement has had varying affects but has been well tolerated in all the studies. There have been no clinical trials in PALS.

***Vitamin A***

Vitamin A is a fat-soluble vitamin with multiple functions, including growth and development, vision, and maintenance of the immune system. Although some investigators have suggested that retinoid signaling is altered in ALS, serum vitamin A levels have been evaluated and have not differed from controls.[67] A preclinical investigation using transgenic ALS mice demonstrated shortened life span in mice receiving daily retinoic acid supplementation. The investigators cautioned against its use in ALS.[68] Although there have been no human clinical trials assessing the efficacy of retinoic acid, it is not uncommon for PALS to take vitamin A 25,000 units daily as part of an antioxidant cocktail that also includes vitamins C and E (see later discussion).

***Homocysteine***

Homocysteine is involved in the formation of free radicals and cytosolic calcium accumulation, mitochondrial dysfunction, apoptotic pathway activation, and excitotoxic amino acid–mediated damage.[69] These pathologic pathways have been implicated in ALS. A small clinical study found that plasma homocysteine levels are increased in PALS compared with healthy controls. PALS with shorter time to diagnosis were found to have higher homocysteine levels. The investigators concluded that a higher plasma homocysteine may be linked to faster progression of the disease.[70] Another small study showed that the homocysteine level in the cerebrospinal fluid is also increased in PALS compared with healthy controls. The investigators hypothesized that homocysteine may be a biomarker of ALS and may be involved in the pathophysiology.[71] Folate and vitamin B12 are thought to reduce the level of homocysteine via remethylation. Studies using SOD1 mouse models have shown a beneficial effect of folate on reducing the levels of homocysteine, delaying the onset of disease, and prolonging the life span.[72] However, in one study, B12 alone did not show any effect on homocysteine levels, onset of the disease, or survival. However, a more recent in vitro study had opposite results, showing better survival against homocysteine toxicity in vitro, in cells pretreated with B12 but not in those treated with folate.[73] Furthermore, in one small preclinical study, ALS mice were supplemented with galactooligosaccharides (GOS), a prebiotic that is thought to improve the absorption and synthesis of B vitamins. GOS and prebiotics yogurt administration were shown to significantly delay the disease onset and prolong the life span in SOD1G93A mice. Also, these products increased the concentration of folate and vitamin B12 and reduced the level of homocysteine.[74] However, there have been no clinical trials examining the role of B12, folate, or GOS supplementation in ALS.

### *Thiamine*

The thiamin/thiamin monophosphate ratio has been shown to be reduced in the cerebrospinal fluid of PALS in 2 small studies. There have been no studies evaluating supplementation with thiamin (vitamin B1) in PALS.[75,76]

### *Riboflavin*

Riboflavin or vitamin B2 supplementation was evaluated in one preclinical study using the SOD1 transgenic mouse model. There was no significant effect of riboflavin on either survival or motor performance.[77]

### *Vitamin C*

Vitamin C is considered an antioxidant, but several studies have failed to show an association between vitamin C intake and ALS progression.[78] There have been no ALS clinical trials addressing vitamin C supplementation. Despite that, many PALS will take vitamin C 1 g, 3 times a day along with vitamins A and E.

### *Vitamin D*

Vitamin D is a fat-soluble secosteroid. Sources of vitamin D include direct skin exposure to sunlight, few foods, and dietary supplements. Skin exposure to ultraviolet B radiation from the sun provides the predominant source of vitamin D. After hydroxylation in the liver and kidney to 25-hydroxyvitamin D and 1,25-dihydroxyvitamin D, respectively, the active metabolite binds to the vitamin D receptor in a cell and induces transcription of a responsive gene. The vitamin D receptor has been found in many tissues, including motor neurons, bone, and muscle cells, suggesting wide physiologic influence. Vitamin D participates in several distinct pathways that are potentially important in ALS physiopathology, including calcium regulation and potentiation of protective neurotrophic factors.[79] In a retrospective study of 74 PALS, the risk of death was significantly increased in those with severe vitamin D deficiency (<25 nmol/L) compared with patients with normal vitamin D.[80] The investigators concluded that serum vitamin D may be a reliable prognostic indicator.[80] Supplementation with vitamin D in ALS mouse models has yielded mixed results.[81–83] A small clinical study showed that PALS tended to have low vitamin D levels and that oral vitamin D supplementation with 2000 IU/d was safe and may be of benefit.[84] Screening for 25-hydroxyvitamin D deficiency and providing vitamin D3 supplementation for those who are deficient are reasonable.[85]

### *Vitamin E*

Vitamin E is a fat-soluble antioxidant composed of tocopherols and tocotrienols. Studies in transgenic mice have shown that vitamin E can delay the onset of ALS but does not affect survival.[86] Randomized trials of vitamin E supplementation did not prove efficacy.[87,88] Interestingly, vitamin E intake may reduce the risk of developing ALS.[89] Patients who choose to augment their vitamin E by supplementation should be cautioned that hypervitaminosis E can increase the risk of bleeding. Many PALS safely take vitamin E 400 IU daily as part of an antioxidant cocktail.

## *Cannabis*

There is a growing body of evidence that that cannabinoids (the active ingredient in cannabis) may hold a significant therapeutic benefit for PALS. Moreover, through manipulation of the endocannabinoid system, cannabis may hold disease-modifying potential in ALS.[90–103] There are several animal studies that suggest that the endocannabinoid system is implicated in the pathophysiology of ALS.[91–97] This may be through a direct action or disease mechanism. Conversely this may be as part of a failure of homeostatic functioning of the neuromuscular system that may be governed by this system. There is now good animal-based evidence that cannabinoids are capable of slowing disease progression of ALS in mice.[91–94] The mechanisms are not entirely clear, but it is likely that this occurs partially by cannabinoids acting as antioxidants and neuromodulators, although other mechanisms are also likely.

Cannabis has also been reported to be useful in managing the symptoms in ALS.[102] There are many symptoms of the disease, including pain, spasticity, loss of appetite, depression, and management of saliva that could be helped by cannabis use. In a survey of 131 PALS, those who were able to obtain cannabis found it preferable to prescription medication in managing their symptoms.[102] However, this study also noted that the biggest reason PALS were not using cannabis was their inability to obtain it, either because of legal or financial reasons or lack of safe access.[102]

Thus, there could be a potential dual role of cannabis for both clinical symptom management and a positive disease-modifying effect. There are both physiologic and pharmacologic mechanisms identified to support these roles. The basic mechanism of action for cannabis is the endocannabinoid system. Our understanding of the receptors and ligands composing the endogenous cannabinoid system has increased tremendously over the past few decades.[104–109] There are now identified 2 major cannabinoid receptor subtypes.[109,110] The type 1 (CB1) cannabinoid receptor is predominantly expressed in the central nervous system (CNS), whereas the type 2 (CB2) receptor is primarily found in the peripheral nervous system, immune system, cardiovascular and gastrointestinal systems, among others.

***Biochemistry of the cannabis plant***

The cannabis plant is complex, with several types of subtypes of cannabis, each containing more than 400 chemical moieties.[111,112] Approximately 60 are chemically classified as cannabinoids.[112] The cannabinoids are 21 carbon terpenes, biosynthesized predominantly via a recently discovered deoxyxylulose phosphate pathway.[113] The molecular mechanism of action of the cannabinoids became much clearer with the characterization and cloning of the CB1 and CB2 receptors. Although these receptors seem to mediate most of the pharmacologic actions of cannabis, there may be other orphan receptors for plant-based cannabinoids (phytocannabinoids).[17,113] There are other natural plant-based compounds, including flavonoids, which are structurally similar to phytocannabinoids. Over the last decade, several potential alternative receptors for phytocannabinoids have been suggested, based on ligand-binding studies. This finding may also extend to the endocannabinoids and possibly even synthetic cannabinergic drugs.[114] The most recent data on these emerging non-CB1, non-CB2 receptors cannabinoid receptors suggest that there are still many uncharacterized or orphan endocannabinoid-mediated G-protein–coupled receptors that have yet to be fully delineated. Moreover, there are likely a whole host of cannabis plant–based terpenoids that may hold therapeutic promise, including compounds, such as limonene and myrcene.[115] Terpenoids share a precursor with phytocannabinoids but display unique therapeutic effects that may contribute meaningfully to the entourage effects of cannabis-based medicinal extracts. There continues to be growing evidence that these noncannabinoid components from the cannabis plant may have tremendous therapeutic potential for diseases, such as ALS, without any intoxicating effects.[115]

The cannabinoids themselves are all lipophilic and not soluble in water. Among the most psychoactive of the cannabinoids is delta-9-tetrahydrocannabinol (THC), the active ingredient in dronabinol.[116] This cannabinoid is the primary intoxicant in cannabis. Other major cannabinoids include cannabidiol (CBD) and cannabinol, both of which may modify the pharmacology of THC or have distinct effects of their own.[117] CBD is not psychoactive but has significant anticonvulsant, sedative, and other pharmacologic activity likely to interact with THC.[111,118–121]

***Clinical uses cannabis in patients with amyotrophic lateral sclerosis***

The cannabinoids found in cannabis have many pharmacologic mechanisms of action that can be immediately useful to help manage clinical symptoms in ALS. For example, cannabinoids been shown to produce an antiinflammatory effect by inhibiting the production and action of tumor necrosis factor and other acute-phase cytokines.[100] Additionally, cannabis may reduce pain sensation, through action at peripheral, spinal, and supraspinal levels. It likely also operates through a brain stem circuit that also contributes to the pain-suppressing effects of morphine.[122–124] Cannabinoids produce analgesia by modulating rostral ventromedial medulla neuronal activity in a manner similar to, but pharmacologically distinct from, that of morphine.[123,124] There are now multiple well-controlled clinical studies using cannabis to treat pain, showing ample evidence of analgesic efficacy.[125,126] A recent systematic review and meta-analysis of double-blind randomized controlled trials that compared any cannabis preparation with placebo among subjects with chronic pain showed a total of 18 completed trials. The studies indicate that cannabis is moderately efficacious for the treatment of chronic pain.[125,126] In the setting of ALS, cannabis use should be dose titrated to the point of comfort. If additional opiate medications are needed to get effective pain control, then the antiemetic effect of cannabis may help with the nausea sometimes associated with the use of opioids. The use of cannabis may lower the need for opiate medications and may be safely used concomitantly, as the opioid receptor system is distinct from the cannabinoid system. Additionally, the use of cannabis does not cause respiratory suppression or decreased gut motility, which are particularly helpful in this setting.

In addition to pain, spasticity is also a major problem for PALS. Cannabis has an inhibitory effect via augmentation of gamma-amino-butyric acid pathways in the CNS.[127–129] This effect produces motor neuron inhibition at spinal levels in mice. Several past studies have suggested that cannabinoid therapy provides at least a subjective reduction of spasticity, although virtually all of the studies have been done in patients with MS.[130–133] In addition to pain and spasticity, there are other pharmacologic effects of cannabis that may be useful for PALS. PALS and bulbar symptoms also usually have difficulty controlling and swallowing the saliva that is normally present in the oral cavity. Cannabis is a potent antisalivary compound that swiftly dries the oral cavity and upper airway, potentially reducing the risk for aspiration pneumonia and increasing patient comfort. Cannabis also increases appetite and may help prevent ALS cachexia, a phenomenon experienced by some patients whereby weight loss occurs in excess of that caused by muscle atrophy and reduced caloric intake. In addition to improving appetite, cannabis may also help with mood state and sleep. PALS previously have reported that cannabis is at least moderately effective at reducing symptoms of pain, spasticity, drooling, appetite loss, and depression.[102]

The AAN recently published excellent systematic literature reviews regarding the use of cannabis in neurologic disorders as well as specifically in another neurodegenerative disorder, MS.[132,133] The investigators concluded that, in patients with MS, oral cannabis extracts are effective to treat spasticity, painful spasms, as well as central pain. This pain included spasticity-related pain. The risk of serious adverse psychopathologic effects was estimated to be approximately 1%.

The route of administration is an important determinant of the pharmacokinetics of the various cannabinoids in cannabis, particularly absorption and metabolism.[134]

Cannabis does not need to be smoked to get a medical beneficial effect. Inhalation does have the advantage of rapid onset of effect and easy dose titration. However, because of their volatility, cannabinoids will vaporize at a much lower temperature than combustion, allowing them to be inhaled as a warm air mist, which is a much healthier option than smoking. Cannabinoids in the form of an aerosol in inhaled smoke or vapors are absorbed and delivered to the brain and circulation rapidly, as expected of a highly lipid-soluble drug. Cannabis may also be ingested orally, but this delivery route has markedly different pharmacokinetics compared with inhalation. The onset of action is delayed, and titration of dosing is more difficult. Maximum cannabinoid blood levels are only reached up to 6 hours after ingestion, with a much longer half-life, as long as 20 to 30 hours.[134] This delayed onset would also apply to any orally ingested cannabinoid, including dronabinol (Marinol). Dronabinol is available as a schedule III (CIII) controlled substance per the Drug Enforcement Agency's (DEA) guidelines.[134] The DEA still considers botanic cannabis as a schedule I (CI) controlled substance, dangerous, and without medical use,[135] though natural cannabis contains, at best, 20% THC. As noted previously, there are beneficial physiologic effects when the other cannabinoid forms are present, as is the case with natural cannabis plant material. Most PALS would likely find dronabinol too sedating and associated with too many psychoactive effects, and it is not an appropriate substitute for natural cannabis. Finally the cannabinoids may also be made into a liniment and absorbed through the skin, although this is the least efficient mode of delivery.

Although the medicinal use of cannabis is now allowed in a growing number of states in America, obtaining the medicine must be done through cooperatives, as it will not be available in a typical pharmacy. This circumstance may create varying degrees of psychological stress for PALS and their caregivers.[136] Moreover, third-party payers and insurance companies will not likely pay for cannabis use even for medical use as it is not FDA approved for any indication. As long as cannabis remains a schedule I compound, there will not likely be much interest from the pharmaceutical industry to finance the massive costs of clinical trials needed to get FDA approval for a given indication.

## *Acupuncture*

Acupuncture is a technique that involves the insertion of thin needles through the skin at specific points with the goal of achieving a therapeutic effect, most often pain reduction.[137] Acupuncture originated in ancient China and is a key component of traditional Chinese medicine (TCM). In the West, several different acupuncture schools and modalities are available. There are traditional Chinese and Japanese techniques and fusion contemporary Western approaches, and needle insertion is sometimes accompanied by the application of small electric currents (electroacupuncture) or injection of chemicals (acupuncture injection therapy).[137,138] Such diversity is a challenge when discussing the intended effects and results of acupuncture. It is also one of the reasons why few systematic studies exist on the topic as acupuncture treatments are highly individualized, dynamic, difficult to blind, and depend heavily on practitioner training and experience. Acupuncture has been proposed as both a symptomatic ALS treatment (pain control) and a way to slow, stop, or reverse progression.[139–141]

### *Mechanisms*

There are both traditional and modern theories on the mechanisms of acupuncture. TCM holds that an energy called *qi* flows along specific paths or meridians and regulates body functions.[137,138] Disease occurs when there are disruptions or blockages in the flow of this energy, and insertion of needles into specific locations (acupoints) restores energy flow and ameliorates disease.[137,138] Science has yet to find convincing evidence for qi, meridians, or acupoints.[138,142,143]

More theories start with needle insertions activating vasoactive substances and neuropeptides, such as histamine, calcitonin gene–related peptide, neuropeptide Y, enkephalin, beta-endorphin, and dynorphin.[138,144–147] In fact, the skin around the needles often becomes red, and a small weal can be seen under the skin. Needle manipulation by hand or addition of heat or electrical stimulation (electroacupuncture) may potentiate these effects. Some of these substances, in turn, are purported to have downstream effects on brain areas involved in pain perception.[146] These substances may also modulate the immune system[147–150]; in doing so, they could theoretically alter the progression of diseases whereby the immune system plays a pathogenic role, including ALS.[151,152] Indeed, elevated beta-endorphin levels,[146] altered functional MRI patterns,[152–157] and even altered inflammatory markers,[158–162] including in ALS animal models,[160,161] can occur following acupuncture. Opioid antagonists, such as naloxone or genetic downregulation of opioid receptors, can block the beneficial effects of acupuncture.[146]

However, even these modern theories have problems. They do not explain acupoints. Sham acupuncture using telescoping needles that do not break the skin can sometimes work as well as real acupuncture, raising the possibility that acupuncture works via a placebo effect.[138] The aforementioned mechanistic studies do not yield consistent results across investigators.[138]

#### *Potential uses in amyotrophic lateral sclerosis*

Although the underlying mechanisms of acupuncture have not been completely elucidated and may involve a significant placebo component, there is some evidence that it could help relieve 2 common ALS symptoms: pain[163–166] and spasticity.[167]

More controversial is the possibility that acupuncture could slow, stop, or reverse ALS progression. A small, flawed study in a mouse model of ALS showed that acupuncture was associated with improved motor neuron survival and delayed loss of motor performance compared with mice that did not receive any acupuncture.[160] This finding has yet to be independently replicated. There is only 1 published trial of acupuncture in patients with ALS.[168] In this trial, 18 patients were treated twice daily for 5 days, with before and after measurements of oxygen saturation, end-tidal carbon dioxide, respiratory rate, pulse rate, and ALSFRS-R. Acupuncture treatment was associated with statistically significant improvements in oxygen saturation and pulse rate. However, the size of these improvements (mean oxygen saturation increased from 95.42% to 95.58% and mean pulse rate increased from 82.49 to 80.08) is of dubious clinical significance.

More impressive than the animal study or the small trial are 2 published case series describing the effects of acupuncture on ALS.[169–172] Both these series describe improvements in motor function occurring with acupuncture. Unfortunately, these reports suffer from the use of other treatments (such as Chinese herbs or detoxification regimens) at the same time as the acupuncture, lack of detail regarding the ALS diagnoses, lack of a control group, lack of blinding, and failure to use validated ALS outcome measures.[173]

#### *Costs and risks*

Costs of acupuncture will vary greatly depending on the specific type and frequency. Within the online community PatientsLikeMe, members with ALS report a range of costs from less than $25 to more than $200 per month.[174]

Large series suggest that acupuncture is generally safe but not entirely without risk. Serious adverse events have been described, including cardiac tamponade,[138,175] pneumothorax,[138,176] and transmission of infections.[138,177] Mild adverse events, such as pain or bleeding, occur in 7% to 11% of patients.[138,178–180]

## Chelation

Chelation therapy is a medical procedure in which a chelating agent is administered to patients with the objective of removing a specific heavy metal from the body. The chelating agent binds to the heavy metal inactivating its toxic effect. This soluble compound is then excreted from the body. The chelating agent can be administered intravenously, orally, or intramuscularly.

### *Approved use*

Chelation therapy is the main treatment of heavy metal poisoning. The chelating agent used depends on the type of metal to which the patients have been exposed. For example, dimercaptosuccinic acid (DMSA) and EDTA are used in lead poisoning and dimercapto-propane sulfonate in arsenic and mercury poisoning.

### *Alternative use*

Chelation therapy has been and continues to be used as an alternative therapeutic approach in various conditions, including autism, cardiovascular disease, and cancer. This practice is not based on scientific studies and may lead to death.[181,182]

### *Use in patients with amyotrophic lateral sclerosis*

In spite of intense study over many years, there is no consistent evidence that any heavy metal toxicity can cause ALS.[183,184] It should not be surprising, then, that there is no evidence that chelation therapy is useful for the treatment of ALS. In fact, there is evidence to the contrary. One case report[185] described a PALS with an elevated blood level and massive urinary excretion of mercury, which did not respond to chelation treatment with DMSA. Another case report described a patient who developed bulbar-onset ALS in the setting of chronic lead intoxication from drinking water. Again, treatment with DSMA was administered for 6 months and had no effect on clinical course.[186] Finally, a study whereby 53 PALS or spinal muscular atrophy and a control group were given DMSA did not show a difference in the urinary excretion of lead and mercury between the 2 groups.[187] A search of the World Wide Web reveals many other individual reports of patients who did not benefit from chelation therapy.

### *Risks*

Chelation is generally thought to be a safe treatment when used properly. The use of sodium EDTA instead of calcium EDTA has resulted in severe hypocalcemia that lead to death in at least 3 reported patients.[188] Another reported side effect is elevated creatinine reflecting potential kidney damage.[182]

## Energy Healing

Energy healing, which also includes spiritual and faith healing, is a branch of alternative medicine whereby the healer channels healing energy onto a patient in order to cure them from a certain disease. This therapy is usually performed when the healer lays their hands on patients, although some healers do an off-hands method or even do remote healing with patients in different locations. There are many different types of energy healing. The most commonly used are spiritual healing and psychic healing, distant healing, intercessory prayer, therapeutic touch, healing touch, esoteric healing, Reiki, magnetic healing, qigong healing, Pranic healing, and crystal healing. Some forms of energy healing use an observable energy, such a magnet or light, although, in most cases, the energy is channeled via touch.

### *Energy healing in medicine*

Energy healing has been studied in randomized placebo-controlled trials in multiple diseases, such as asthma,[189] cardiac bypass surgery,[190] wound healing,[191] postoperative oral pain,[192] fatigue in patients with breast cancer undergoing radiation therapy,[193] and procedural pain in very preterm neonates.[194] These robust studies have all shown no effect on the disease progression or symptoms.

### *Energy healing in amyotrophic lateral sclerosis*

There are no trials on the effect of energy healing in PALS. However, there are individual testimonials of improvement in PALS with energy healing. One of these testimonials can be found on the Web page of Dean Kraft, one of the more famous energy healers in the United States. The following link depicts the story of Nelda Buss, a patient diagnosed with ALS in 1985: www.deankrafthealer.com/CaseHistory-NeldaBuss.html. Dean Kraft focused "a white stream of energy into her deteriorating respiratory system, her nerves..." She subsequently regained significant muscle strength, including regaining the ability to walk. The diagnosis and improvement in this patient were independently validated.[195] Many other healers have their own Web page with a story on curing ALS. In addition, there is a documentary film on healing ALS pending funding (http://healingals.com/). The movie's mission is to educate people diagnosed with ALS and their families about holistic protocols for ALS that can slow, stop, and even reverse the progression of ALS by showing multiple interviews with people who were diagnosed with ALS and had their disease cured through different holistic protocols. Unfortunately, along these claims of cure from ALS, there are many reports on ALS forums of a lack of benefit and high expenditure with different types of energy healing. The fact that ALS can sometimes reverse spontaneously has to be considered as an alternate explanation for the previously described improvements.[196–198]

### *Costs and risks*

The costs of energy healing vary depending on the practitioner, methods, and frequency. Dean Kraft charged Nelda Buss $75 per session and $25,000 overall.[195]

There seems to be no serious risks for energy healing on patients' health. However, some investigators argue that promoting energy healing could be detrimental to patients and health care systems.[199–201] According to the Ernst,[199–201] for example, healing can be expensive and might divert patients from effective treatments. He argues that spiritual healing might promote the belief in a supernatural healing energy, which undermines rationality in general and, hence, boosts pseudoscience. It could also potentially divert patients from adequate, scientifically studied treatments.

## OPTIONS FOR REVIEWING COMPLEMENTARY AND ALTERNATIVE MEDICINE WITH PEOPLE WITH AMYOTROPHIC LATERAL SCLEROSIS

There are at least 3 models by which decisions get made in the doctor-patient relationship. These models are all options for reviewing CAM with PALS in the clinic. Here the authors review these models and options.

### *Paternalism*

The oldest model, which has existed since the beginning of medicine, is paternalism. In this, the doctor acts as a parent or guardian and defines patients' goals and the methods for attaining them.[202] Here, a patient's question about an alternative therapy might be met with a response from the doctor: "That is not likely to help you and may even be harmful. I do not want you to pursue that." There are several problems with this approach. Although doctors do have many years of training and experience in evaluating care options, they may not always share the same goals, values, and an acceptable risk/benefit ratio with patients. This model ignores the fact that patients are different in terms of how they want their information presented.[203] Active seekers want to know everything right away about their condition and all its treatment options. Selective seekers just want a trickle of information, just enough to make the decisions they need to make today. Information avoiders want to have information and decisions filtered through someone else, often a family member or friend.[203] Finally, and worst of all, paternalism has been abused, both at the bedside and in clinical research, resulting in modern malpractice and informed consent laws.[204]

### *Autonomy*

A newer model, fueled by the Internet, is autonomy. Here the patients' goals and methods for achieving them are assumed to be central, correct, and absolute. The doctor becomes a vending machine, helping patients procure whatever it is they want. In this model, the doctor might answer a question about an alternative therapy as follows: "I understand what you want to do. How can I help?" Advantages of this model include respect for patient values and goals and allowance for different information-gathering preferences. Disadvantages include underutilization of physician education and experience and the fact that the information being used by the patients to make their decision may be flawed or inaccurate.[205]

### *Shared Decision Making*

In between paternalism and autonomy is shared decision making. Here the patients' values and goals are central but recognized to be fluid and potentially modifiable based on new information. Physicians help define the pros and cons of different treatment options being considered and may even make a suggestion based on their own synthesis of the data and their clinical experience. This model uses the talents and the skill set of the physician while still allowing patients to ultimately define their values, goals, and acceptable risks and benefits. There are data suggesting that shared decision making is preferred by both patients[206] and doctors[207] and associated with improved compliance and better health outcomes.[208] The biggest problem with shared decision making is that it takes significantly more physician time than paternalism or autonomy.

A group called ALSUntangled has developed a shared decision-making model that helps with this time issue.[205] There are 3 parts to this: inputs, reviews, and outputs. Inputs on alternative ALS therapies come from patients and families, either via face-to-face visits with clinicians that are part of the group or via e-mail or Twitter (@alsuntangled). Reviews follow a specific standard operating procedure, with a group of 100 investigators from across 10 countries grading each alternative therapy's mechanism, preclinical data, case reports, trials, and risk.[209] Outputs also follow a standard format and are published via free open access in the journal *Amyotrophic Lateral Sclerosis and Frontotemporal Degeneration* and on the Web site www.alsuntangled.org. Now when patients ask about an alternative therapy, a busy clinician that wants to engage in shared decision making can refer them to an ALSUntangled review rather than have to repeat the research themselves.

**Case Vignette**

*A 48-year-old university professor is newly diagnosed with ALS. She has no obvious cognitive or behavioral problems. She is presented with evidence-based, stage-appropriate options for treatment, including riluzole and multidisciplinary team care. She is also invited to participate in a research study. She accepts the first two but declines the research study because she has decided to pursue taking oral sodium chlorite, an alternative therapy she read about on the Internet.*

*Her clinician decides to engage in shared decision making and presents her with the ALSUntangled review of oral sodium chlorite.[210]*

*In reading this, she sees that oral sodium chlorite does not have a very plausible mechanism, any good preclinical data, or any good anecdotal data supporting its use in ALS; there are significant potential safety problems with it. She decides to forgo this initial decision and participate in the research study.*

## SUMMARY

PALS often consider CAM options, especially diets, nutritional supplements, cannabis, acupuncture, chelation, and energy healing. This article reviews these CAM options for patients and clinicians who opt to engage in shared decision making. ALSUntangled is an international program that uses shared decision making to objectively review CAM options, reducing some of the physician time burden while helping patients make more informed treatment decisions.

## REFERENCES


1. Available at: http://www.nlm.nih.gov/medlineplus/complementaryandalternativemedicine.html. Accessed February 21, 2015.
2. Wasner M, Klier H, Borasio G. The use of alternative medicine by patients with amyotrophic lateral sclerosis. J Neurol Sci 2001;191:151–4.
3. Vardeny O, Bromberg M. The use of herbal supplements and alternative therapies by patients with amyotrophic lateral sclerosis. J Herb Pharmacother 2005;5:23–31.
4. Miller RG, Jackson CE, Kasarskis J, et al. Practice parameter update: the care of the patient with amyotrophic lateral sclerosis: drug, nutritional, and respiratory therapies (an evidence-based review): report of the Quality Standards Subcommittee of the American Academy of Neurology. Neurology 2009;73:1218–26.
5. Miller RG, Jackson CE, Kasarskis J, et al. Practice parameter update: the care of the patient with amyotrophic lateral sclerosis: multidisciplinary care, symptom management, and cognitive/behavioral impairment (an evidence-based review). Neurology 2009;73:1227–33.
6. Karam C, Paganoni S, Joyce N, et al. Palliative care issues in amyotrophic lateral sclerosis: an evidence based review. Am J Hosp Palliat Care 2014. [Epub ahead of print].
7. Available at: https://www.google.com/#q=als+treatment. Accessed February 17, 2015.
8. Chew S, Khandji A, Montes J, et al. Olfactory ensheathing glia injections in Beijing: misleading patients with ALS. Amyotroph Lateral Scler 2007;8:314–6.
9. Piepers S, Van Den Berg L. No benefits from experimental treatment with olfactory ensheathing cells in patients with ALS. Amyotroph Lateral Scler 2010;11:328–30.

10. Bedlack RS, Pastula DM, Welsh E, et al. Scrutinizing enrollment in ALS trials: room for improvement? Amyotroph Lateral Scler 2008;9:257–65.
11. Kasarskis EJ, Berryman S, Vanderleest JG, et al. Nutritional status of patients with amyotrophic lateral sclerosis: relation to the proximity of death. Am J Clin Nutr 1996;63:130–7.
12. Desport JC, Preux PM, Truong CT, et al. Nutritional assessment and survival in ALS patients. Amyotroph Lateral Scler Other Motor Neuron Disord 2000;1: 91–6.
13. Heffernan C, Jenkinson C, Holmes T, et al. Nutritional management in MND/ALS patients: an evidence based review. Amyotroph Lateral Scler Other Motor Neuron Disord 2004;5:72–83.
14. Pedersen WA, Mattson MP. No benefit of dietary restriction on disease onset or progression in amyotrophic lateral sclerosis Cu/Zn-superoxide dismutase mutant mice. Brain Res 1999;833:117–20.
15. Hamadeh MJ, Rodriguez MC, Kaczor JJ, et al. Caloric restriction transiently improves motor performance but hastens clinical onset of disease in the Cu/Zn-superoxide dismutase mutant G93A mouse. Muscle Nerve 2005;31:214–20.
16. Zhao Z, Sui Y, Gao W, et al. Effects of diet on adenosine monophosphate-activated protein kinase activity and disease progression in an amyotrophic lateral sclerosis model. J Int Med Res 2015;43:67–79.
17. Mattson MP, Cutler RG, Camandola S. Energy intake and amyotrophic lateral sclerosis. Neuromolecular Med 2007;9:17–20.
18. Dupuis L, Oudart H, René F, et al. Evidence for defective energy homeostasis in amyotrophic lateral sclerosis: benefit of a high-energy diet in a transgenic mouse model. Proc Natl Acad Sci U S A 2004;27:11159–64.
19. Marin B, Desport JC, Kajeu P, et al. Alteration of nutritional status at diagnosis is a prognostic factor for survival of amyotrophic lateral sclerosis patients. J Neurol Neurosurg Psychiatry 2011;82:628–34.
20. Paganoni S, Deng J, Jaffa M, et al. Body mass index, not dyslipidemia, is an independent predictor of survival in amyotrophic lateral sclerosis. Muscle Nerve 2011;44:20–4.
21. Lindauer E, Dupuis L, Müller HP, et al. Adipose tissue distribution predicts survival in amyotrophic lateral sclerosis. PLoS One 2013;8:e67783.
22. Körner S, Hendricks M, Kollewe K, et al. Weight loss, dysphagia and supplement intake in patients with amyotrophic lateral sclerosis (ALS): impact on quality of life and therapeutic options. BMC Neurol 2013;13:84.
23. Symptom management and end of life care, in press.
24. Luu LCT, Kasarskis EJ, Tandan R. Nutritional treatment: theoretical and practical issues. In: Mitsumoto H, Przedborski S, Gordon PH, editors. Amyotrophic lateral sclerosis. New York: Taylor & Francis; 2006. p. 721–35.
25. Kasarskis EJ, Mendiondo MS, Wells S, et al, ALS Nutrition/NIPPV Study Group. The ALS Nutrition/NIPPV Study: design, feasibility, and initial results. Amyotroph Lateral Scler 2011;12:17–25.
26. Kasarskis EJ, Mendiondo MS, Matthews DE, et al, ALS Nutrition/NIPPV Study Group. Estimating daily energy expenditure in individuals with amyotrophic lateral sclerosis. Am J Clin Nutr 2014;99:792–803.
27. Available at: https://mednet.mc.uky.edu/alscalculator/. Accessed February 21, 2015.
28. Zhao Z, Lange DJ, Voustianiouk A, et al. A ketogenic diet as a potential novel therapeutic intervention in amyotrophic lateral sclerosis. BMC Neurosci 2006; 7:29.

29. Dorst J, Cypionka J, Ludolph AC. High-caloric food supplements in the treatment of amyotrophic lateral sclerosis: a prospective interventional study. Amyotroph Lateral Scler Frontotemporal Degener 2013;14:533–6.
30. Wills AM, Hubbard J, Macklin EA, et al, MDA Clinical Research Network. Hypercaloric enteral nutrition in patients with amyotrophic lateral sclerosis: a randomised, double-blind, placebo-controlled phase 2 trial. Lancet 2014;383:2065–72.
31. Yip PK, Pizzasegola C, Gladman S, et al. The omega-3 fatty acid eicosapentaenoic acid accelerates disease progression in a model of amyotrophic lateral sclerosis. PLoS One 2013;8(4):e61626.
32. Mathus-Vliegen LM, Louwerse LS, Merkus MP, et al. Percutaneous endoscopic gastrostomy in patients with amyotrophic lateral sclerosis and impaired pulmonary function. Gastrointest Endosc 1994;40:463–9.
33. Mazzini L, Corrà T, Zaccala M, et al. Percutaneous endoscopic gastrostomy and enteral nutrition in amyotrophic lateral sclerosis. J Neurol 1995;242:695–8.
34. Dorst J, Dupuis L, Petri S, et al. Percutaneous endoscopic gastrostomy in amyotrophic lateral sclerosis: a prospective observational study. J Neurol 2015;262:849–58.
35. Chio A, Galletti R, Finocchiaro C, et al. Percutaneous radiological gastrostomy: a safe and effective method of nutritional tube placement in advanced ALS. J Neurol Neurosurg Psychiatry 2004;75:645–7.
36. Available at: http://www.fda.gov/RegulatoryInformation/Legislation/FederalFoodDrugandCosmeticActFDCAct/SignificantAmendmentstotheFDCAct/ucm148003.htm. Accessed February 14, 2015.
37. Bradley WG, Anderson F, Gowda N, et al. Changes in the management of ALS since the publication of the AAN ALS practice parameter 1999. Amyotroph Lateral Scler Other Motor Neuron Disord 2004;5:240–4.
38. Rosenfeld J, Ellis A. Nutrition and dietary supplements in motor neuron disease. Phys Med Rehabil Clin N Am 2008;19:573.
39. ALSUntangled Group. ALS Untangled No. 20: the Deanna protocol. Amyotroph Lateral Scler Frontotemporal Degener 2013;14:319–23.
40. Available at: http://www.winningthefight.org/t/deanna-protocol. Accessed February 21, 2015.
41. Ari C, Poff AM, Held HE, et al. Metabolic therapy with Deanna Protocol supplementation delays disease, progression and extends survival in amyotrophic lateral sclerosis (ALS) mouse model. PLoS One 2014;9(7):e103526.
42. Ludolph A, Bendotti C, Blaugrund E, et al. Guidelines for preclinical animal research in ALS/MND: a consensus meeting. Amyotroph Lateral Scler 2010;11:38–45.
43. Xu Z, Chen S, Li X, et al. Neuroprotective effects of (-)-epigallocatechin-3-gallate in a transgenic mouse model of amyotrophic lateral sclerosis. Neurochem Res 2006;31:1263–9.
44. Matthews RT, Yang L, Browne S, et al. Coenzyme Q10 administration increases brain mitochondrial concentrations and exerts neuroprotective effects. Proc Natl Acad Sci U S A 1998;95:8892–7.
45. Ferrante KL, Shefner J, Zhang H, et al. Tolerance of high-dose (3,000 mg/day) coenzyme Q10 in ALS. Neurology 2005;65:1834–6.
46. Kaufmann P, Thompson JL, Levy G, et al. Phase II trial of CoQ10 for ALS finds insufficient evidence to justify phase III. Ann Neurol 2009;66:235–44.
47. Adhihetty PJ, Beal MF. Creatine and its potential therapeutic value for targeting cellular energy impairment in neurodegenerative diseases. Neuromolecular Med 2008;10:275–90.

48. Andreassen OA, Jenkins BG, Dedeoglu A, et al. Increases in cortical glutamate concentrations in transgenic amyotrophic lateral sclerosis mice are attenuated by creatine supplementation. J Neurochem 2001;77:383–90.
49. Derave W, Van Den Bosch L, Lemmens G, et al. Skeletal muscle properties in a transgenic mouse model for amyotrophic lateral sclerosis: effects of creatine treatment. Neurobiol Dis 2003;13:264–72.
50. Rosenfeld J, King RM, Jackson CE, et al. Creatine monohydrate in ALS: effects on strength, fatigue, respiratory status and ALSFRS. Amyotroph Lateral Scler 2008;9:266–72.
51. Groeneveld GJ, Veldink JH, van der Tweel I, et al. A randomized sequential trial of creatine in amyotrophic lateral sclerosis. Ann Neurol 2003;53:437–45.
52. Pastula DM, Moore DH, Bedlack RS. Creatine for amyotrophic lateral sclerosis/motor neuron disease. Cochrane Database Syst Rev 2012;(12):CD005225.
53. Atassi N, Ratai EM, Greenblatt DJ, et al. A phase I, pharmacokinetic, dosage escalation study of creatine monohydrate in subjects with amyotrophic lateral sclerosis. Amyotroph Lateral Scler 2010;11:508–13.
54. Erb M, Hoffmann-Enger B, Deppe H, et al. Features of idebenone and related short-chain quinones that rescue ATP levels under conditions of impaired mitochondrial complex I. PLoS One 2012;7:e36153.
55. Parkinson MH, Schulz JB, Giunti P. Co-enzyme Q10 and idebenone use in Friedreich's ataxia. J Neurochem 2013;126(Suppl 1):125–41.
56. Jaber S, Polster BM. Idebenone and neuroprotection: antioxidant, pro-oxidant, or electron carrier? J Bioenerg Biomembr 2015;47:111–8.
57. Gülçin I. Antioxidant and antiradical activities of L-carnitine. Life Sci 2006; 18(78):803–11.
58. Kira Y, Nishikawa M, Ochi A, et al. L-carnitine suppresses the onset of neuromuscular degeneration and increases the life span of mice with familial amyotrophic lateral sclerosis. Brain Res 2006;1070:206–14.
59. Beghi E, Pupillo E, Bonito V, et al, Italian ALS Study Group. Randomized double-blind placebo-controlled trial of acetyl-L-carnitine for ALS. Amyotroph Lateral Scler Frontotemporal Degener 2013;14:397–405.
60. Calder PC, Yaqoob P. Omega-3 polyunsaturated fatty acids and human health outcomes. Biofactors 2009;35:266–72.
61. Dyall SC, Michael-Titus AT. Neurological benefits of omega-3 fatty acids. Neuromolecular Med 2008;10:219–35.
62. Fitzgerald KC, O'Reilly ÉJ, Falcone GJ, et al. Dietary ω-3 polyunsaturated fatty acid intake and risk for amyotrophic lateral sclerosis. JAMA Neurol 2014;71: 1102–10.
63. Mancuso R, del Valle J, Modol L, et al. Resveratrol improves motoneuron function and extends survival in SOD1(G93A) ALS mice. Neurotherapeutics 2014;11:419–32.
64. Song L, Chen L, Zhang X, et al. Resveratrol ameliorates motor neuron degeneration and improves survival in SOD1(G93A) mouse model of amyotrophic lateral sclerosis. Biomed Res Int 2014;2014:483501.
65. Mancuso R, Del Valle J, Morell M, et al. Lack of synergistic effect of resveratrol and sigma-1 receptor agonist (PRE-084) in SOD1G$^{93}$A ALS mice: overlapping effects or limited therapeutic opportunity? Orphanet J Rare Dis 2014;9:78.
66. Park EJ, Pezzuto JM. The pharmacology of resveratrol in animals and humans. Biochim Biophys Acta 2015;31:S0925–4439.
67. Molina JA, de Bustos F, Jiménez-Jiménez FJ, et al. Serum levels of beta-carotene, alpha-carotene, and vitamin A in patients with amyotrophic lateral sclerosis. Acta Neurol Scand 1999;99:315–7.

68. Crochemore C, Virgili M, Bonamassa B, et al. Long-term dietary administration of valproic acid does not affect, while retinoic acid decreases, the lifespan of G93A mice, a model for amyotrophic lateral sclerosis. Muscle Nerve 2009;39:548–52.
69. Mattson MP, Shea TB. Folate and homocysteine metabolism in neural plasticity and neurodegenerative disorders. Trends Neurosci 2003;26:137–46.
70. Zoccolella S, Simone IL, Lamberti P, et al. Elevated plasma homocysteine levels in patients with amyotrophic lateral sclerosis. Neurology 2008;70(3):222–5.
71. Valentino F, Bivona G, Butera D, et al. Elevated cerebrospinal fluid and plasma homocysteine levels in ALS. Eur J Neurol 2010;17:84–9.
72. Zhang X, Chen S, Li L, et al. Folic acid protects motor neurons against the increased homocysteine, inflammation and apoptosis in SOD1 G93A transgenic mice. Neuropharmacology 2008;54(7):1112–9.
73. Hemendinger RA, Armstrong EJ 3rd, Brooks BR. Methyl vitamin B12 but not methylfolate rescues a motor neuron-like cell line from homocysteine-mediated cell death. Toxicol Appl Pharmacol 2011;251:217–25.
74. Song L, Gao Y, Zhang X, et al. Galactooligosaccharide improves the animal survival and alleviates motor neuron death in SOD1G93A mouse model of amyotrophic lateral sclerosis. Neuroscience 2013;246:281–90.
75. Poloni M, Patrini C, Rocchelli B, et al. Thiamin monophosphate in the CSF of patients with amyotrophic lateral sclerosis. Arch Neurol 1982;39:507–9.
76. Poloni M, Mazzarello P, Patrini C, et al. Inversion of T/TMP ratio in ALS: a specific finding? Ital J Neurol Sci 1986;7:333–5.
77. Moges H, Vasconcelos OM, Campbell WW, et al. Light therapy and supplementary riboflavin in the SOD1 transgenic mouse model of familial amyotrophic lateral sclerosis (FALS). Lasers Surg Med 2009;41:52–9.
78. Fitzgerald KC, O'Reilly EJ, Fondell E, et al. Intakes of vitamin C and carotenoids and risk of amyotrophic lateral sclerosis: pooled results from 5 cohort studies. Ann Neurol 2013;73:236–45.
79. Karam C, Scelsa SN. Can vitamin D delay the progression of ALS? Med Hypotheses 2011;76:643–5.
80. Camu W, Tremblier B, Plassot C, et al. Vitamin D confers protection to motoneurons and is a prognostic factor of amyotrophic lateral sclerosis. Neurobiol Aging 2014;35:1198–205.
81. Gianforcaro A, Hamadeh MJ. Dietary vitamin D3 supplementation at 10x the adequate intake improves functional capacity in the G93A transgenic mouse model of ALS, a pilot study. CNS Neurosci Ther 2012;18:547–57.
82. Gianforcaro A, Solomon JA, Hamadeh MJ. Vitamin D(3) at 50x AI attenuates the decline in paw grip endurance, but not disease outcomes, in the G93A mouse model of ALS, and is toxic in females. PLoS One 2013;8(2):e30243.
83. Solomon JA, Gianforcaro A, Hamadeh MJ. Vitamin D3 deficiency differentially affects functional and disease outcomes in the G93A mouse model of amyotrophic lateral sclerosis. PLoS One 2011;6:e29354.
84. Karam C, Barrett MJ, Imperato T, et al. Vitamin D deficiency and its supplementation in patients with amyotrophic lateral sclerosis. J Clin Neurosci 2013;20(11):1550–3.
85. ALSUntangled Group. ALSUntangled No. 24: vitamin D. Amyotroph Lateral Scler Frontotemporal Degener 2014;15:318–20.
86. Gurney ME, Cutting FB, Zhai P, et al. Benefit of vitamin E, riluzole, and gabapentin in a transgenic model of familial amyotrophic lateral sclerosis. Ann Neurol 1996;39:147–57.
87. Desnuelle C, Dib M, Garrel C, et al. A double-blind, placebo-controlled randomized clinical trial of alpha-tocopherol (vitamin E) in the treatment of amyotrophic

lateral sclerosis. ALS riluzole-tocopherol study group. Amyotroph Lateral Scler Other Motor Neuron Disord 2001;2:9–18.
88. Graf M, Ecker D, Horowski R, et al. High dose vitamin E therapy in amyotrophic lateral sclerosis as add-on therapy to riluzole: results of a placebo-controlled double-blind study. J Neural Transm 2005;112:649–60.
89. Wang H, O'Reilly EJ, Weisskopf MG, et al. Vitamin E intake and risk of amyotrophic lateral sclerosis: a pooled analysis of data from 5 prospective cohort studies. Am J Epidemiol 2011;173:595–602.
90. Carter GT, Bedlack R, Hardiman O, et al, ALSUntangled Group, Collaborators (79). ALSUntangled No. 16: cannabis. Amyotroph Lateral Scler 2012;13:400–4.
91. Kim K, Moore DH, Makriyannis A, et al. AM1241, a cannabinoid CB2 receptor selective compound, delays disease progression in a mouse model of amyotrophic lateral sclerosis. Eur J Pharmacol 2006;542(1–3):100–5.
92. Shoemaker JL, Seely KA, Reed RL, et al. The CB2 cannabinoid agonist AM-1241 prolongs survival in a transgenic mouse model of amyotrophic lateral sclerosis when initiated at symptom onset. J Neurochem 2007;101(1):87–98.
93. Raman C, McAllister SD, Rizvi G, et al. Amyotrophic lateral sclerosis: delayed disease progression in mice by treatment with a cannabinoid. Amyotroph Lateral Scler Other Motor Neuron Disord 2004;5(1):33–9.
94. Weydt P, Hong S, Witting A, et al. Cannabinol delays symptom onset in SOD1 (G93A) transgenic mice without affecting survival. Amyotroph Lateral Scler Other Motor Neuron Disord 2005;6(3):182–4.
95. Rossi S, De Chiara V, Musella A, et al. Abnormal sensitivity of cannabinoid CB1 receptors in the striatum of mice with experimental amyotrophic lateral sclerosis. Amyotroph Lateral Scler 2009;19(1):1–8.
96. Bilsland LG, Dick JR, Pryce G, et al. Increasing cannabinoid levels by pharmacological and genetic manipulation delay disease progression in SOD1 mice. FASEB J 2006;20(7):1003–5.
97. Bilsland LG, Greensmith L. The endocannabinoid system in amyotrophic lateral sclerosis. Curr Pharm Des 2008;14(23):2306–16.
98. Zhao P, Ignacio S, Beattie EC, et al. Altered presymptomatic AMPA and cannabinoid receptor trafficking in motor neurons of ALS model mice: implications for excitotoxicity. Eur J Neurosci 2008;27(3):572–9.
99. Witting A, Weydt P, Hong S, et al. Endocannabinoids accumulate in spinal cord of SOD1 transgenic mice. J Neurochem 2004;89(6):1555–7.
100. Carter GT, Rosen BS. Marijuana in the management of amyotrophic lateral sclerosis. Am J Hosp Palliat Care 2001;18(4):264–70.
101. Gelinas D, Miller RG, Abood ME. A pilot study of safety and tolerability of Delta 9-THC (Marinol) treatment for ALS. Amyotroph Lateral Scler Other Motor Neuron Disord 2002;3(suppl 1):23.
102. Amtmann D, Weydt P, Johnson KL, et al. Survey of cannabis use in patients with amyotrophic lateral sclerosis. Am J Hosp Palliat Care 2004;21:95–104.
103. Carter GT, Abood ME, Aggarwal SK, et al. Cannabis and amyotrophic lateral sclerosis: practical and hypothetical applications, and a call for clinical trials. Am J Hosp Palliat Care 2010;27(5):347–56.
104. Di Iorio G, Lupi M, Sarchione F, et al. The endocannabinoid system: a putative role in neurodegenerative diseases. Int J High Risk Behav Addict 2013;2(3):100–6.
105. Abood ME. Molecular biology of cannabinoid receptors. Handb Exp Pharmacol 2005;168:81–115.
106. McAllister SD, Hurst DP, Barnett-Norris J, et al. Structural mimicry in class A G protein-coupled receptor rotamer toggle switches: the importance of the

F3.36(201)/W6.48(357) interaction in cannabinoid CB1 receptor activation. J Biol Chem 2004;279(46):48024–37.
107. Kapur A, Samaniego P, Thakur GA, et al. Mapping the structural requirements in the CB1 cannabinoid receptor transmembrane helix II for signal transduction. J Pharmacol Exp Ther 2008;325(1):341–8.
108. Anavi-Goffer S, Fleischer D, Hurst DP, et al. Helix 8 Leu in the CB1 cannabinoid receptor contributes to selective signal transduction mechanisms. J Biol Chem 2007;282(34):25100–13.
109. Abood ME, Rizvi G, Sallapudi N, et al. Activation of the CB1 cannabinoid receptor protects cultured mouse spinal neurons against excitotoxicity. Neurosci Lett 2001;309(3):197–201.
110. Klein TW, Lane B, Newton CA, et al. The cannabinoid system and cytokine network. Proc Soc Exp Biol Med 2000;225(1):1–8.
111. Pertwee RG. Cannabinoid receptor ligands: clinical and neuropharmacological considerations, relevant to future drug discovery and development. Expert Opin Investig Drugs 2000;9(7):1553–71.
112. Aizpurua-Olaizola O, Omar J, Navarro P, et al. Identification and quantification of cannabinoids in Cannabis sativa L. plants by high performance liquid chromatography-mass spectrometry. Anal Bioanal Chem 2014;406(29):7549–60.
113. Mechoulam R, Hanuš LO, Pertwee R, et al. Early phytocannabinoid chemistry to endocannabinoids and beyond. Nat Rev Neurosci 2014;15(11):757–64.
114. De Petrocellis L, Di Marzo V. Non-CB1, non-CB2 receptors for endocannabinoids, plant cannabinoids, and synthetic cannabimimetics: focus on G-protein-coupled receptors and transient receptor potential channels. J Neuroimmune Pharmacol 2010;5(1):103–21.
115. Russo EB. Taming THC: potential cannabis synergy and phytocannabinoid-terpenoid entourage effects. Br J Pharmacol 2011;163(7):1344–64.
116. Pertwee RG. Pharmacological actions of cannabinoids. Handb Exp Pharmacol 2005;168:1–51.
117. Gonçalves TC, Londe AK, Albano RI, et al. Cannabidiol and endogenous opioid peptide-mediated mechanisms modulate antinociception induced by transcutaneous electrostimulation of the peripheral nervous system. J Neurol Sci 2014;347(1–2):82–9.
118. Stout SM, Cimino NM. Exogenous cannabinoids as substrates, inhibitors, and inducers of human drug metabolizing enzymes: a systematic review. Drug Metab Rev 2014;46(1):86–95.
119. Castaneto MS, Gorelick DA, Desrosiers NA, et al. Synthetic cannabinoids: epidemiology, pharmacodynamics, and clinical implications. Drug Alcohol Depend 2014;1(144):12–41.
120. Adams IB, Martin BR. Cannabis: pharmacology and toxicology in animals and humans. Addiction 1996;91(11):1585–614.
121. Romero J, Orgado JM. Cannabinoids and neurodegenerative diseases. CNS Neurol Disord Drug Targets 2009;8(6):440–50.
122. Meng ID, Manning BH, Martin WJ, et al. An analgesia circuit activated by cannabinoids. Nature 1998;395(6700):381–3.
123. Zeltser R, Seltzer Z, Eisen A, et al. Suppression of neuropathic pain behavior in rats by a non-psychotropic synthetic cannabinoid with NMDA receptor-blocking properties. Pain 1991;47(1):95–103.
124. Elikottil J, Gupta P, Gupta K. The analgesic potential of cannabinoids. J Opioid Manag 2009;5(6):341–57.

125. Martín-Sánchez E, Furukawa TA, Taylor J, et al. Systematic review and meta-analysis of cannabis treatment for chronic pain. Pain Med 2009;10(8): 1353–68.
126. Lynch ME, Campbell F. Cannabinoids for treatment of chronic non-cancer pain; a systematic review of randomized trials. Br J Clin Pharmacol 2011;72(5): 735–44.
127. Fine PG, Rosenfeld MJ. The endocannabinoid system, cannabinoids, and pain. Rambam Maimonides Med J 2013;4(4):e0022.
128. Fitzgerald PB, Williams S, Daskalakis ZJ. A transcranial magnetic stimulation study of the effects of cannabis use on motor cortical inhibition and excitability. Neuropsychopharmacology 2009;34(11):2368–75.
129. Lichtman AH, Martin BR. Spinal and supraspinal components of cannabinoid-induced antinociception. J Pharmacol Exp Ther 1991;258: 517–23.
130. Collin C, Davies P, Mutiboko IK, et al, Sativex Spasticity in MS Study Group. Randomized controlled trial of cannabis-based medicine in spasticity caused by multiple sclerosis. Eur J Neurol 2007;14(3):290–6.
131. Corey-Bloom J, Wolfson T, Gamst A, et al. (2012) Smoked cannabis for spasticity in multiple sclerosis: a randomized, placebo-controlled trial. CMAJ 2012; 184(10):1143–50.
132. Koppel BS, Brust JC, Fife T, et al. Systematic review: efficacy and safety of medical marijuana in selected neurologic disorders: report of the Guideline Development Subcommittee of the American Academy of Neurology. Neurology 2014; 82(17):1556–63.
133. Yadav V, Bever C Jr, Bowen J, et al. Summary of evidence-based guideline: complementary and alternative medicine in multiple sclerosis: report of the Guideline Development Subcommittee of the American Academy of Neurology. Neurology 2014;82(12):1083–92.
134. Carter GT, Weydt P, Kyashna-Tocha M, et al. Medical marijuana: rational guidelines for dosing. IDrugs 2004;7(5):464–70.
135. Schedules of controlled substances: rescheduling of the Food and Drug Administration approved product containing synthetic dronabinol[(-) - [DELTA] less than 9 greater than - (trans)-tetrahydrocannabinol] in sesame oil and encapsulated in soft gelatin capsules from schedule II to schedule III. Department of Justice (DOJ), Drug Enforcement Administration (DEA). Final rule. Fed Regist 1999;64(127):35928–30.
136. Aggarwal SK, Carter GT, Sullivan MD, et al. Enforcement in a series of medical cannabis patients. J Nerv Ment Dis 2013;201(4):292–303.
137. Available at: http://en.wikipedia.org/wiki/Acupuncture. Accessed March 3, 2015.
138. Ernst E. Acupuncture-a critical analysis. J Intern Med 2006;259:125–37.
139. Available at: http://www.drmihaly-acupuncture.com/chinese-scalp-acupuncture-als.html. Accessed March 7, 2015.
140. Available at: http://www.hughsacupuncture.com/als-treatment-by-acupuncture-and-traditional-chinese-medicine/. Accessed March 7, 2015.
141. Available at: http://www.taoiststudy.com/content/use-qigong-herbal-medicine-achieve-cure-als. Accessed March 7, 2015.
142. Ramey D. Acupuncture points and meridians do not exist. Sci Rev Alternative Med 2001;5:143–8.
143. Gorski D. Integrative oncology: really the best of both worlds? Nat Rev Cancer 2014;2014:692–700.

144. Dawidson I, Angmar-Mansson B, Blom M, et al. The influence of sensory stimulation (acupuncture) on the release of neuropeptides in the saliva of healthy subjects. Life Sci 1998;63:659–74.
145. Yu JS, Zeng BY, Hsieh CL. Acupuncture stimulation and neuroendocrine regulation. Int Rev Neurobiol 2013;111:125–40.
146. Han J-S. Acupuncture and endorphins. Neurosci Lett 2004;361:236–40.
147. Lee HJ, Lee JH, Lee EO, et al. Substance P and beta-endorphin mediate electro-acupuncture induced analgesia in mouse cancer pain model. J Exp Clin Cancer Res 2009;28:102.
148. Eisenstein T. Opioids and the immune system: what is their role? Br J Pharmacol 2011;16:1826–8.
149. Panerai AE, Radulovic J, Monastra G, et al. Beta-endorphin concentrations in brain areas and peritoneal macrophages in rats susceptible and resistant to experimental allergic encephalomyelitis: a possible relationship between tumor necrosis factor alpha and opioids in the disease. J Neuroimmunol 1994;51:169–76.
150. McCarthy L, Wetzel M, Sliker JK, et al. Opioids, opioid receptors and the immune response. Drug Alcohol Depend 2001;62:111–23.
151. Murdock BJ, Bender DE, Segal BM, et al. The dual roles of immunity and ALS: injury overrides protection. Neurobiol Dis 2015;77:1–12.
152. Hooten KG, Beers DR, Zhao W, et al. Protective and toxic neuroinflammation in amyotrophic lateral sclerosis. Neurotherapeutics 2015;12(2):364–75.
153. Napadow V, Makris N, Liu J, et al. Effects of electroacupuncture versus manual acupuncture on the human brain as measured by fMRI. Hum Brain Mapp 2005;24:193–205.
154. Wu MT, Sheen JM, Chuang KH, et al. Neuronal specificity of acupuncture response: an fMRI study with electroacupuncture. Neuroimage 2002;16:1028–37.
155. Fang JL, Krings T, Weidemann J, et al. Functional MRI in healthy subjects during acupuncture; different effects of needle rotation in real and false acupoints. Neuroradiology 2004;46:359–62.
156. Cho ZH, Chung SC, Jones JP, et al. New findings of the correlation between acupoints and corresponding brain cortices using functional MRI. Proc Natl Acad Sci U S A 1998;95:2670–3.
157. Yan B, Li K, Xu J, et al. Acupoint-specific fMRI patterns in human brain. Neurosci Lett 2005;383:236–40.
158. Zillstra F, van den Berg-de-Lange I, Huygen F, et al. Anti-inflammatory actions of acupuncture. Mediators Inflamm 2003;12:59–69.
159. Kim ST, Doo AR, Kim SRN, et al. Acupuncture suppresses kainic acid-induced neuronal death and inflammatory events in mouse hippocampus. J Physiol Sci 2012;62:377–83.
160. Yang E, Jiang J, Lee S, et al. Electroacupuncture reduces neuroinflammatory responses in symptomatic amyotrophic lateral sclerosis model. J Neuroimmunol 2010;223:84–91.
161. Jiang J, Yang E, Baek M, et al. Anti-inflammatory effects of electroacupuncture in the respiratory system of a symptomatic amyotrophic lateral sclerosis model. Neurodegener Dis 2011;8:504–14.
162. Chapman C, Benedetti C, Colpitts Y, et al. Naloxone fails to reverse pain thresholds elevated by acupuncture. Pain 1983;16:13–31.
163. Lam M, Galvin R, Curry P. Effectiveness of acupuncture for nonspecific chronic low back pain: a systematic review and meta-analysis. Spine (Phila Pa 1976) 2013;38:2124–38.

164. Wilke J, Vogt L, Niederer D, et al. Short-term effects of acupuncture and stretching on myofascial trigger point pain of the neck: a blinded, placebo-controlled RCT. Complement Ther Med 2014;22:835–41.
165. Crespin DJ, Griffin KH, Johnson JR, et al. Acupuncture provides short-term pain relief for patients in a total joint replacement program. Pain Med 2015;16(6): 1195–203.
166. Iacobone M, Citton M, Zanella S, et al. The effects of acupuncture after thyroid surgery: a randomized, controlled trial. Surgery 2014;156:1605–12 [discussion: 1612–3].
167. Lim SM, Yoo J, Lee E, et al. Acupuncture for spasticity after stroke: a systematic review and meta-analysis of randomized controlled trials. Evid Based Complement Alternat Med 2015;2015:870398.
168. Lee S, Kim S. The effects of sa-am acupuncture treatment on respiratory parameters in amyotrophic lateral sclerosis. Evid Based Complement Alternat Med 2013;2013:506317.
169. Yongde C. Formulating a therapeutic program with the governing vessel in treating 46 cases of ALS. Shanghai Journal of Moxibustion 1998;17:43.
170. Yongde C. Clinical observation on 46 cases of ALS in consideration of the treatment principal breaking through the Dumai. Zhejiang Journal of Integrating Traditional Chinese and Western Medicine 1999;9:16–7.
171. Available at: http://www.itmonline.org/arts/als.htm. Accessed March 19, 2015.
172. Liang S, Christner D, DuLaux S, et al. Significant neurological improvement in two patients with amyotrophic lateral sclerosis after 4 weeks of treatment with acupuncture injection point therapy using enercel. J Acupunct Meridian Stud 2011;4:257–61.
173. ALSUntangled Group. ALSUntangled 28: acupuncture. Amyotroph Lateral Scler Frontotemporal Degener 2015;16(3–4):286–9.
174. Available at: http://www.patientslikeme.com/treatment_evaluations/browse?brand=f&condition_id=9&id=213-acupuncture-side-effects-and-efficacy. Accessed March 21, 2015.
175. Ernst E, Zhang J. Cardiac tamponade caused by acupuncture: a review of the literature. Int J Cardiol 2011;149:287–9.
176. Demir M, Oruc M, Dalli A, et al. A rare complication of acupuncture: pneumothorax. Tuberk Toraks 2014;62:316–8.
177. Ernst E, Sherman KJ. Is acupuncture a risk factor for hepatitis? Systematic review of epidemiological studies. J Gastroenterol Hepatol 2003;18:1231–6.
178. White A, Hayhoe S, Hart A, et al. Adverse events following acupuncture: a prospective survey of 32000 consultations with doctors and physiotherapists. BMJ 2001;323:485–6.
179. Melchart D, Weidenhammer W, Streng A, et al. Prospective investigation of adverse events in 97,733 patients. Arch Intern Med 2004;164:104–5.
180. MacPherson H, Scullion A, Thomas KJ, et al. Patient reports of adverse events associated with acupuncture treatment: a prospective national survey. Qual Saf Health Care 2004;13:349–55.
181. Villarruz MV, Dans A, Tan F. Chelation therapy for atherosclerotic cardiovascular disease. Cochrane Database Syst Rev 2002;(4):CD002785.
182. Seely DM, Wu P, Mills EJ. EDTA chelation therapy for cardiovascular disease: a systematic review. BMC Cardiovasc Disord 2005;5:32.
183. Sutedja NA, Veldink JH, Fischer K, et al. Exposure to chemicals and metals and risk of amyotrophic lateral sclerosis: a systematic review. Amyotroph Lateral Scler 2009;10(5–6):302–9.

184. Callaghan B, Feldman D, Gruis K, et al. The association of exposure to lead, mercury, and selenium in the development of amyotrophic lateral sclerosis and the epigenetic implications. Neurodegener Dis 2011;8:1–8.
185. Praline J, Guennoc AM, Limousin N, et al. ALS and mercury intoxication: a relationship? Clin Neurol Neurosurg 2007;109(10):880–3.
186. Couratier P, Bernet-Bernady P, Truong T, et al. Lead intoxication and amyotrophic lateral sclerosis. Rev Neurol (Paris) 1998;154(4):345–7 [in French].
187. Louwerse ES, Buchet JP, Van Dijk MA, et al. Urinary excretion of lead and mercury after oral administration of meso-2,3-dimercaptosuccinic acid in patients with motor neurone disease. Int Arch Occup Environ Health 1995;67(2):135–8.
188. Available at: http://www.cdc.gov/mmwr/preview/mmwrhtml/mm5508a3.htm. Accessed March 25, 2015.
189. Cleland JA, Price DB, Lee AJ, et al. A pragmatic, three-arm randomised controlled trial of spiritual healing for asthma in primary care. Br J Gen Pract 2006;56(527):444–9.
190. Benson H, Dusek JA, Sherwood JB, et al. Study of the Therapeutic Effects of Intercessory Prayer (STEP) in cardiac bypass patients: a multicenter randomized trial of uncertainty and certainty of receiving intercessory prayer. Am Heart J 2006;151(4):934–42.
191. O'Mathúna DP, Ashford RL. Therapeutic touch for healing acute wounds. Cochrane Database Syst Rev 2014;(7):CD002766.
192. Kundu A, Lin Y, Oron AP, et al. Reiki therapy for postoperative oral pain in pediatric patients: pilot data from a double-blind, randomized clinical trial. Complement Ther Clin Pract 2014;20(1):21–5.
193. FitzHenry F, Wells N, Slater V, et al. A randomized placebo-controlled pilot study of the impact of healing touch on fatigue in breast cancer patients undergoing radiation therapy. Integr Cancer Ther 2014;13(2):105–13.
194. Johnston C, Campbell-Yeo M, Rich B, et al. Therapeutic touch is not therapeutic for procedural pain in very preterm neonates: a randomized trial. Clin J Pain 2013;29(9):824–9.
195. ALSUntangled Group. ALSUntangled 12: Dean Kraft, energy healer. Amyotroph Lateral Scler 2011;12:389–91.
196. Miyoshi K, Ohyagi Y, Amano T, et al. A patient with motor neuron syndrome clinically similar to amyotrophic lateral sclerosis presenting a spontaneous recovery. Rinsho Shinkeigaku 2000;40:1090–5.
197. Tsai CP, Ho HH, Yen DJ, et al. Reversible motor neuron disease. Eur Neurol 1993;33:387–9.
198. Tucker T, Layzer R, Miller R, et al. Subacute, reversible motor neuron disease. Neurology 1991;41:1541–4.
199. Ernst E. Distant healing–an "update" of a systematic review. Wien Klin Wochenschr 2003;115(7–8):241–5.
200. Ernst E. Complementary treatment: who cares how it works, as long as it does? Lancet Oncol 2005;6(3):131–2.
201. Ernst E. Spiritual healing: more than meets the eye. J Pain Symptom Manage 2006;32(5):393–5.
202. Emanuel E, Emanuel L. Four models of the physician-patient relationship. JAMA 1992;267:2221–6.
203. O'Brien MR. Information-seeking behavior among people with motor neuron disease. Br J Nurs 2004;13:964–8.
204. Osman H. History and development of the doctrine of informed consent. Int Electron J Health Educ 2001;4:41–7.

205. Bedlack R, Hardiman O. ALSUntangled: a scientific approach to off-label treatment options for patients with ALS using tweets and twitters. Amyotroph Lateral Scler 2009;3:129–30.
206. Deber R, Kraetschmer N, Urowitz S, et al. Do people want to be autonomous patients? Preferred roles in treatment decision-making in several patient populations. Health Expect 2007;3:248–58.
207. Murray E, Pollck L, White M, et al. Clinical decision-making: physicians' preferences and experiences. BMC Fam Pract 2007;8:10.
208. Joosten E, DeFuentes-Merillas L, de Weert G, et al. Systematic review of the effects of shared decision-making on patient satisfaction, treatment adherence and health status. Psychother Psychosom 2008;77:219–26.
209. The ALSUntangled Group. ALSUntangled: introducing the table of evidence. Amyotroph Lateral Scler Frontotemporal Degener 2015;16:142–5.
210. ALSUntangled Group. ALSUntangled No. 19: sodium chlorite. Amyotroph Lateral Scler Frontotemporal Degener 2013;14(3):236–8.

# The Dilemma of the Clinical Trialist in Amyotrophic Lateral Sclerosis

## The Hurdles to Finding a Cure

Jonathan S. Katz, MD[a,*], Richard J. Barohn, MD[b], Mazen M. Dimachkie, MD[b], Hiroshi Mitsumoto, MD, DSc[c]

**KEYWORDS**

- Amyotrophic lateral sclerosis • Clinical trialists • Drug development • Treatment

**KEY POINTS**

- ALS is a condition that lacks any markedly effective treatment.
- Because of the poor understanding of the disease, it is not unreasonable to predict that there are currently no effective agents within the research pipeline, yet clinical trials are frequent. In this scenario, false-positive outcomes are not uncommon, and create a dilemma for ALS trialists.
- Research trials are still done because they provide hope and because there is a strong desire for patients to try treatments even when there is a low chance of success.
- It is important to create infrastructure that allows for robust screening trials. These should be cost effective and large enough to identify effective agents, while quickly eliminating drugs that are destined for failure.

## REPORT

Amyotrophic lateral sclerosis (ALS) is a disease that currently has no treatment that dramatically alters its course. Given the uncertain physiology, even the best scientist is hard pressed to state how neurons begin to degenerate, how the disease spreads, or whether these processes are the same in every patient. The excitement that accompanied the codiscoveries of the SOD1 gene mutation and the drug riluzole in the mid-1990s has been followed by a steady increase in the number of ALS clinical trials, with

[a] Department of Neurology, Forbes Norris MDA/ALS Center, California Pacific Medical Center, 2324 Sacramento Street, Suite 111, San Francisco, CA 94115, USA; [b] Department of Neurology, The University of Kansas Medical Center, 3901 Rainbow Boulevard, Mail Stop 2012, Kansas City, KS 66160, USA; [c] Department of Neurology, Eleanor and Lou Gehrig MDA/ALS Research Center, Columbia University Medical Center, 710 West 168th Street, New York, NY 10032, USA
* Corresponding author.
*E-mail address:* Katzjs@sutterhealth.org

Neurol Clin 33 (2015) 937–947
http://dx.doi.org/10.1016/j.ncl.2015.07.014 neurologic.theclinics.com

an expansion in the breadth of targets, delivery methods, and types of designs. Yet two decades have passed, and riluzole remains the only treatment, with its slight effect on survival[1] and nearly imperceptible effect on day-to-day life (**Fig. 1**). During the summer of 2014, the ice bucket challenge greatly increased the level of funding for ALS research, and brought a new surge in hope. In the aftermath, investigators and the Amyotrophic Lateral Sclerosis Association, the primary benefactor of that serendipitous campaign, are faced with the pragmatic question of exactly how to go about directing resources to increase the chances of finding a cure, or whether these funds should be invested to improve current care of ALS patients. The focus here is on research opportunities in ALS.

There have been nearly 50 randomized controlled trials for disease-modifying treatments over the past half-century (**Box 1**). The first modern clinical trial in ALS was designed to determine whether treatment of poliovirus infection could alter the course of the disease.[2] At the time, latent polio was suspected as a key underlying cause. Subsequent trials have tested readily available agents, such as minocycline,[3] vitamin E,[4] celebrex,[5] lithium,[6] and creatine,[7] to name a few, which are already on the market. As science has moved on, these look increasingly like treatments that would not or should not (in the case if minocycline) be attempted based on current understanding. ALS trialists have tested drugs targeting varied underlying hypothesized mechanisms including excitotoxicity, growth factors, neuroinflammation, neurotrophic factors, apoptosis, growth factors, protein aggregation, viruses, astrocyte dysfunction, autophagocytic vesicles, and underlying genetic defects.[2] A better understanding of ALS genetics over recent years has led to newer targets including RNA processing, protein toxicity, and repeat expansion pathology.[8] But the many past failures still reflect that there is an imprecise grasp of the disorder. As a result, it still remains impossible to know exactly when it will be possible to predict that there is a reasonable likelihood of success for any new candidate treatment when it is first proposed for study.

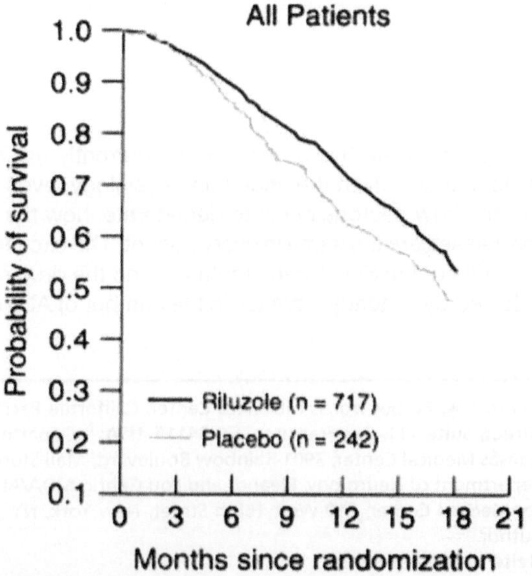


**Fig. 1.** The effect of riluzole in ALS. (*From* Lacomblez L, Bensimon G, Leigh PN, et al. A confirmatory dose-ranging study of riluzole in ALS. ALS/Riluzole Study Group-II. Neurology 1996;47(6 Suppl 4):S247; with permission.)

**Box 1**
**List of potential targets in ALS trials**

*Potential Targets and Treatment Trials*

- Antiglutamate
  - Riluzole
  - Gabapentin
  - Topiramate
  - Dextromethorphan
  - Talampanel
  - Ceftriaxone
  - Memantine[a]
- Growth factors
  - Brain-derived neurotrophic factor
  - Ciliary neurotrophic factor
  - Insulinlike growth factor-1
  - Xaliproden
  - Vascular endothelial growth factor
  - Skin cells[a]
- Protein aggregation
  - Arimoclomol
- Antioxidant/bioenergetics
  - Creatine (5 and 10 g)
  - Vitamin E
  - Selegiline
  - Acetylcysteine
  - Coenzyme Q
  - R-pramipexole
  - Cytokinetics[a]
  - Rasagiline[a]
  - Mexiletine[a]
  - Ozanezumab[a]
- Anti-inflammatory
  - Celebrex
  - Minocycline
  - Neuraltus
  - Toclizumab
  - Acthar[a]
- Antiapoptotic
  - TCH386
  - Pentoxyfilline
  - Glatiramer acetate
  - Lithium
  - Stem cell[a]
  - Antisense oligos[a]
  - Mexiletine[a]

[a] Active.

The more cynical trialist might suggest that it is reasonable to entertain the hypothesis that there is no effective agent in the pipeline, or anywhere under the sun. In this scenario, the only feasible "positive result" of a clinical trial is a false-positive. In fact, type I errors are expected intermittently, and are relatively common if many smaller trials are designed. This is because small trials are susceptible to chance results, particularly in a disease with a variable clinical course. In this environment, the false-positive results intermittently raise hope, and lead to larger, more definitive trials, which are destined to fail.

A slightly more positive trialist might postulate the existence of at least a few effective agents, but with relatively small effect sizes. In this scenario, the task of finding the few effective agents is extremely difficult. Even if an investigator was able to design and select the right agent, pass it through preclinical testing, and then secure start up funding for a small trial, the hill to climb is still steep. Because the drug has only a small effect, screening trials are susceptible to false-negative results and even if the small study correctly demonstrates the outcome (or better), it is still hard to distinguish this positive trial from an erroneous positive result from one of many ineffective drugs that might be tested. It follows that investors and funding agencies might be hesitant to provide further support, which makes it difficult to perform a large definitive study. A second small trial might be required to "de-risk" the investment in preparation for the larger study, but that would again risk a false-negative result. There is a general understanding that the risk of a false-negative result is reduced by enrolling larger numbers of patients, but this requires resources that might not be available.

Looking back at outcomes of ALS trials over the last few decades, it is safe to assume that we live in a universe a lot like the ones described previously. Dream drugs, of the type that are game changing, have not been discovered. Drugs that halt progression or actually lead to recovery would be easy to identify using any trial methodology. But the reality is that ALS investigators are looking for small clues. In fact, many investigators believe that small treatment effects mean that clinicians will ultimately have to rely on combination drug treatments.[2,9,10] Yet, many trialists recognize that this adds another level of complexity and makes the task even more difficult.[11]

Negative trials not only reflect a poor understanding of the disease, but demonstrate the willingness of the ALS community to test new agents, despite the general understanding that this is a low-probability universe. The ALS community values treatments because of intangible benefits that may be rationale, despite the steep scientific challenge of finding a cure. Trials allow clinicians to take part in a fight for a cure and, without trials, patients would seek out obscure treatments anyway. Because the disease is fatal, patients are willing to take risks or entertain new ideas and hypotheses. It is valuable for trialists to work with patients rather than leave them to wrestle with a constant bombardment of media and chatter about untested therapies. These factors have all led to repeated cycles of hope and hype, where scientific arguments are able to gain momentum when bolstered by the general feeling that potential treatments should be tested expeditiously. Sadly, these cycles have nearly uniformly ended in disappointment, followed by retrenchment, and further cycles.

It is hard to enumerate the exact factors that bring one candidate treatment to the forefront and into the active trial pipeline.[12] Looking back, no potential treatment has ever been close to a sure thing, so other factors must play a role in the selection process. Common to all studies is a reasonable hypothesis that the agent will have an effect on a disease mechanism, but beyond this, positive results in the SOD1 mouse model, an effective response in an in vitro assay, a positive response in a different neurodegenerative disease, or success in a small human trial are required. On the near horizon, treatments like antisense oligonucleotides that block the production of toxic proteins are a good example of a rational approach but these early phase 1 trials are just beginning.

Finding small treatment effects requires better tools of detection. The SOD1 mouse model has been used as the "gate keeper" for drug development. Drugs that have been considered for human trials have typically showed benefits in the mouse model first. Some investigators believe this model is the best way to screen new agents at this time, but most negative human studies were initially misled by positive studies in the SOD1 mice. Conversely, there is no way ensure that the model is not screening out potentially effective agents. The argument against relying on the mouse model has three premises: (1) it is a different species; (2) many mouse studies are done in the preclinical phase, before the onset of disease; and (3) many mouse studies have not been replicated by other preclinical investigators.[2,13] Contrarians also point out that testing has used sample sizes that are too small to be statistically significant and that familial ALS associated with SOD1 mutations tends to be an outlier disease that differs pathologically from sporadic ALS and other forms of familial ALS with respect to the content of the pathologic inclusions. SOD1-related disease also has divergent clinical presentations that raise questions about heterogenous pathophysiology (eg, certain mutations lead to very rapid progression).

ALS is a heterogeneous disease, where patients have different rates of disease progression, patterns of spread, and various sites of onset. The disease is also associated with a variety of different genetic mutations.[8] It is reasonable to postulate that a treatment might not fit all patients. If this is true, trialists must figure out how to identify small responder groups within larger populations. Moreover, most modern trials have been designed to enroll patients with "moderate" rates of disease progression. This is accomplished by excluding individuals with long disease durations (typically more than 2 or 3 years from onset at the time of enrollment). Such cases are, by definition, slow progressors whose flat progression slopes representing their functional decline make it hard to detect differences between treatment groups. Patients who have developed advanced respiratory or bulbar disease are also excluded because of the risk that they would not be able to complete the study. This leaves an already limited population eligible for trials. As trialists begin to focus on specific markers of disease, the available population who can enroll in trials will become even smaller, and novel recruitment strategies may be needed.[14]

Target engagement, cerebrospinal fluid penetration, and delivery methods are areas that are actively undergoing transformation. Trials that ignore the question of whether a treatment interacted with its presumed target cannot resolve whether a poor response stemmed from underlying disease pathways or from pharmacologic factors. These "failed" studies leave the door open to retesting drugs, and waste future resources. Finding more relevant biomarkers would enhance the power to test disease pathways directly.[15,16] They could be used to detect disease changes, aid in rapid diagnosis, provide information about prognosis, enable selection of specific patients, and improve on stratification strategies. However, the discovery of biomarkers remains complicated by the same poor understanding of the disease, and at this time an ideal set of biomarkers remains elusive. One current strategy is to invest in small trials that aim to look for effects on blood or electrophysiologic markers. Several trials are also testing novel routes for treatment administration. These include the intrathecal injections of antisense oligonucleotides[17] and direct spinal injections of stem cells.[18] Stem cells are being engineered to produce specific neurotrophic factors, potentially allowing delivery of treatments directly to the spinal cord.[19]

These innovative discoveries are setting the field in a direction where future studies will target subsets of patients, with specific clinical, laboratory, or genetic features. The concern is that subgroup analysis can easily create even more false-positive outcomes when subgroups are sliced and diced into ever increasing numbers of smaller populations, again bringing up the risks of false-positive outcomes. Subgroup analyses introduce analytical challenges that can lead to overstated and misleading results.[20] This exact dilemma has already been seen in the aftermath of the very large, phase III Biogen trial.[21] Here, a report of subgroup analyses pointed to benefits for short duration, El Escorial Criteria–definite, riluzole-treated patients. Top ALS statisticians debated the meaning of this report, with some stating that this was the expected finding when analyzing too many subgroups. Others believed it could be a clue that the drug may be valuable and deserved further testing. The answer may lie in the observation that the drug was not studied further. The likelihood is that this was a case of overanalyzing. Again, false-positive results are a statistical likelihood when studying many smaller cohorts. In contrast, an actual effective treatment of ALS would be unusual.

Currently used outcome measures in clinical trials include survival; functional scales (ALS Functional Rating Scale-revised [ALSFRS-R]); various strength measures; and pulmonary testing, such as forced vital capacity. These measures are adequate in large-scale clinical trials, conducted over long periods of time, but they are too variable for early phase trials, where small numbers of patients and shorter treatment periods risk random errors.[15] Survival end points require long periods of observation and may be affected by supportive therapies, so they have been mostly abandoned for smaller trials. The most commonly used primary end point has been the rate of functional decline, as measured by the ALSFRS-R. Trials have also used other end points, including one that combined survival and functional decline into a single end point,[21] time to reach a specified drop in function,[22] or the percentage of patients showing no functional decline over a specified time (the responder rate).[23] If a treatment slowed progression, all of these measures would tend to move in the same direction. In traditional analyses, the primary outcome measure and the size of the study are selected a priori such that the subsequent result would determine futility or success. For larger, definitive trials, this is a rational approach that is essentially mandated by the Food and Drug Administration (FDA). In smaller trials, a priori end points help in determining the number of patients needed to reach a solid statistical conclusion, but they do not help in deciding whether a drug should be tested further. In fact, investigators often work backward to justify small trial budgets. They can enroll relatively small numbers of patients if they power trials to detect relatively large treatment effects. But large effect sizes do not fit the history and the understanding of pathophysiology, which suggests that such treatments do not exist. Moreover, where there is no guarantee of further funding or drug access, one can be certain that several outcome measures will ultimately be scrutinized to determine if larger studies are warranted. This is particularly true when individuals or companies have invested in a treatment or when a trialist who already has secured funding considers an interim analysis that could potentially stop a trial. It would be only natural to point to the most favorable outcome, rather than the a priori primary end point. For these insiders, it is only rational to scavenge the entire set of data and to make the best case to secure further funding. Thus, for smaller trials, it is really the data as a whole that serve as the discussion point for funding next steps.

Over the last decade, the field has been successful at performing large-scale, industry or National Institutes of Health funded trials.[21,24,25] Recruitment has been rapid and many of these trials have enrolled quickly. However, costs for these trials are tens of million dollars, and when there are failures, such trials are potentially perceived as poor financial ventures. It follows that earlier-stage trials must shed enough information to lower this risk. To ensure this, those "smaller trials" must still be powered so they are large enough to avoid the risk of reaching incorrect conclusions. The other concern is that by incorporating biomarker testing or "precision medicine" tools into current studies, the cost of a trial adds up even further. Most trials are performed at a relatively fixed cost. In essence, this is a zero-sum game, where resources used on safety, training, biomarkers, dose ranging, or longer durations of therapy make it more difficult to enroll sufficient numbers of patients (**Fig. 2**).

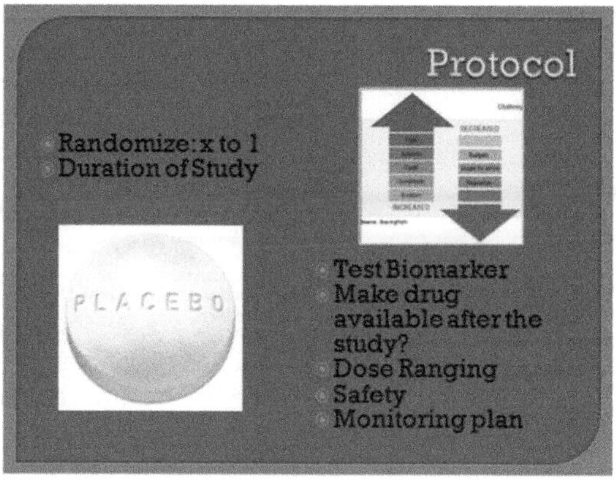


**Fig. 2.** Choices in an ALS protocol that may influence costs.

The case can be made that when an agent is available, known to be safe, and when the primary outcome measure is functional decline, the costs of a trial do not have to be high. Because of social media, patients are calling for access to many types of therapies. In many cases this occurs even when there is essentially no clinical testing. The budding right-to-try movement argues that patients with terminal diseases, such as ALS, should be allowed access to safe drugs. In a field such as ALS, this may require new infrastructure, where trialists are better able to test agents, while at the same time quickly eliminate most therapies that are destined to failure. Improved infrastructure would be defined as tools that lower costs of screening treatments in humans.

One current direction is to find algorithms that predict outcomes based on baseline clinical features, laboratory testing, or perhaps some yet to be discovered biomarker. Taken to an extreme, knowing the expected outcome for a given patient with certainty would make it simple to determine if a treatment altered that course. It follows that investing in predictive algorithms would eventually reduce the number of patients needed in a trial. Thus far, such tools, using advanced mathematics, have been derived from historical databases of patients who have enrolled in trials.[26] Along the same lines, historical placebo databases from prior clinical trials have been used as placebo control for later studies.[27] The next step is to develop additional databases that can collect data from ALS patients across the full spectrum of the disease. This adds the ability to study lead-in progression by providing access to standard pretrial data. This offers a deeper, less homogenous population for developing biomarkers. Efforts are already underway to collect data, at the bedside, for all patients who attend ALS clinics (**Fig. 3**). Other efforts are underway to reduce administrative and data costs by forming cohesive working groups. These efforts must overcome current barriers that drive up costs and waste time related to fragmented funding mechanisms, indirect costs required by universities, and working with the multiple inefficient institutions where many ALS clinics are centered.

## CASE EXAMPLES OF TRIAL CHALLENGES

In 2008, Fornai and colleagues[6] reported that lithium was effective in slowing the progression of ALS. The report was based on the treatment of a small cohort over 15 months. However, investigators found improvements over placebo in strength, survival, function, and respiratory function. The report went on to describe a positive response in the mouse model and a scientific rationale for lithium as a therapy.

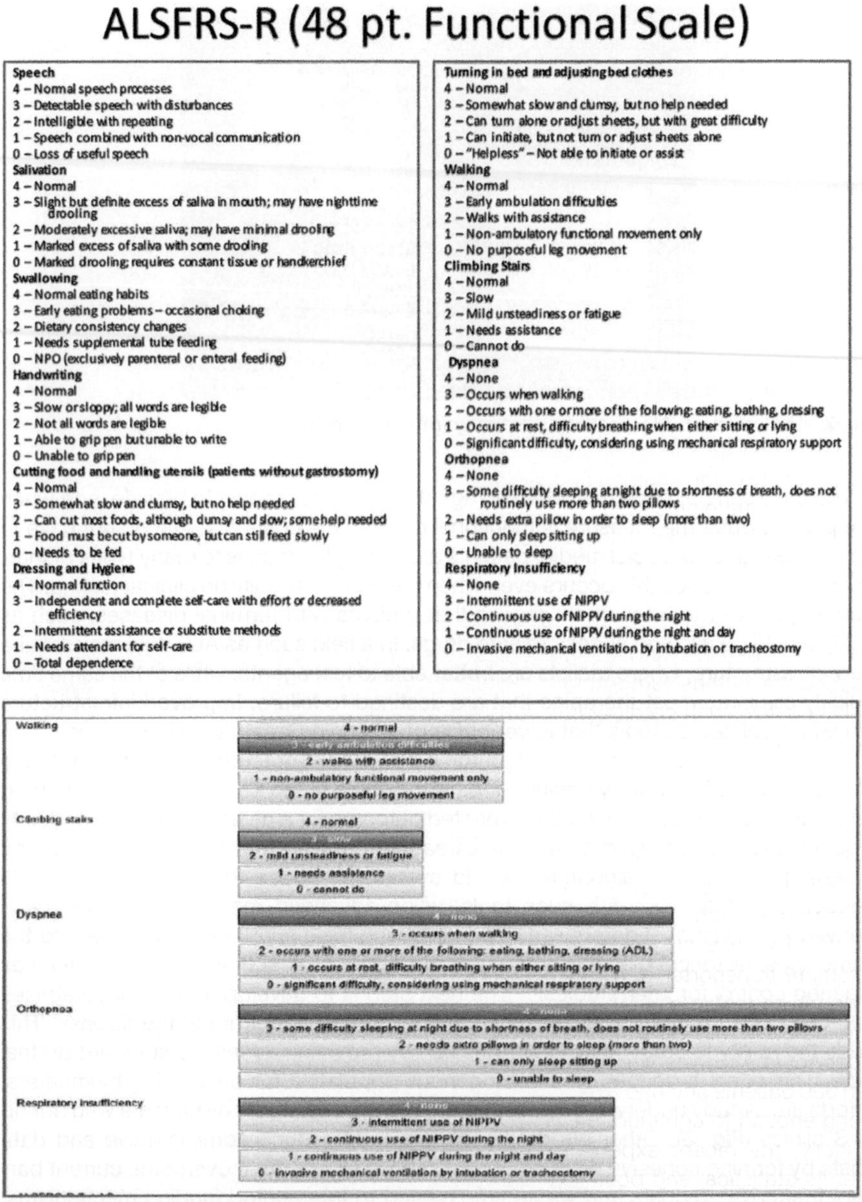
ALSFRS-R (48 pt. Functional Scale)
Speech
4 – Normal speech processes
3 – Detectable speech with disturbances
2 – Intelligible with repeating
1 – Speech combined with non-vocal communication
0 – Loss of useful speech
Salivation
4 – Normal
3 – Slight but definite excess of saliva in mouth; may have nighttime drooling
2 – Moderately excessive saliva; may have minimal drooling
1 – Marked excess of saliva with some drooling
0 – Marked drooling; requires constant tissue or handkerchief
Swallowing
4 – Normal eating habits
3 – Early eating problems – occasional choking
2 – Dietary consistency changes
1 – Needs supplemental tube feeding
0 – NPO (exclusively parenteral or enteral feeding)
Handwriting
4 – Normal
3 – Slow or sloppy; all words are legible
2 – Not all words are legible
1 – Able to grip pen but unable to write
0 – Unable to grip pen
Cutting food and handling utensils (patients without gastrostomy)
4 – Normal
3 – Somewhat slow and clumsy, but no help needed
2 – Can cut most foods, although clumsy and slow; some help needed
1 – Food must be cut by someone, but can still feed slowly
0 – Needs to be fed
Dressing and Hygiene
4 – Normal function
3 – Independent and complete self-care with effort or decreased efficiency
2 – Intermittent assistance or substitute methods
1 – Needs attendant for self-care
0 – Total dependence
Turning in bed and adjusting bed clothes
4 – Normal
3 – Somewhat slow and clumsy, but no help needed
2 – Can turn alone or adjust sheets, but with great difficulty
1 – Can initiate, but not turn or adjust sheets alone
0 – "Helpless" – Not able to initiate or assist
Walking
4 – Normal
3 – Early ambulation difficulties
2 – Walks with assistance
1 – Non-ambulatory functional movement only
0 – No purposeful leg movement
Climbing Stairs
4 – Normal
3 – Slow
2 – Mild unsteadiness or fatigue
1 – Needs assistance
0 – Cannot do
Dyspnea
4 – None
3 – Occurs when walking
2 – Occurs with one or more of the following: eating, bathing, dressing
1 – Occurs at rest, difficulty breathing when either sitting or lying
0 – Significant difficulty, considering using mechanical respiratory support
Orthopnea
4 – None
3 – Some difficulty sleeping at night due to shortness of breath, does not routinely use more than two pillows
2 – Needs extra pillow in order to sleep (more than two)
1 – Can only sleep sitting up
0 – Unable to sleep
Respiratory Insufficiency
4 – None
3 – Intermittent use of NIPPV
2 – Continuous use of NIPPV during the night
1 – Continuous use of NIPPV during the night and day
0 – Invasive mechanical ventilation by intubation or tracheostomy
Walking
4 - normal
2 - walks with assistance
1 - non-ambulatory functional movement only
0 - no purposeful leg movement
Climbing stairs
4 - normal
2 - mild unsteadiness or fatigue
1 - needs assistance
0 - cannot do
Dyspnea
3 - occurs when walking
2 - occurs with one or more of the following: eating, bathing, dressing (ADL)
1 - occurs at rest, difficulty breathing when either sitting or lying
0 - significant difficulty, considering using mechanical respiratory support
Orthopnea
3 - some difficulty sleeping at night due to shortness of breath, does not routinely use more than two pillows
2 - needs extra pillows in order to sleep (more than two)
1 - can only sleep sitting up
0 - unable to sleep
Respiratory insufficiency
3 - intermittent use of NIPPV
2 - continuous use of NIPPV during the night
1 - continuous use of NIPPV during the night and day
0 - invasive mechanical ventilation by intubation or tracheostomy

**Fig. 3.** A standard functional score as a tool for collecting standard data. (*Top*) The ALS Functional Rating Scale Revised. (*Bottom*) Data are captured at the bedside using smart forms linked to a standard database. Different centers using this interface have identical data that can be sent to a central repository. (*From* Cedarbaum JM, Stambler N, Malta E, et al. The ALSFRS-R: a revised ALS functional rating scale that incorporates assessments of respiratory function. BDNF ALS Study Group (Phase III). J Neurol Sci 1999;169(1–2):14–5; with permission.)

Immediately after the report, patients started asking for the drug, which was available by prescription. Despite the report, there was a large amount of skepticism about the methodology and results of the initial study. The response by the field was rapid with eight studies completed over the next 2 years. These trials were uniformly negative.[22,27–29] The effort was completed using relatively small cohorts (27–220 patients) where the basic goal was to disprove the original study. The studies were completed with moderately low budgets and creative designs where investigators were willing to discontinue trials for futility at very early stages, use historical controls, or novel end points. One trial simply powered their study to disprove the Italian study, which allowed for a faster exit. The period of multiple trials demonstrates how the approach changes if trials are not accompanied by optimism about a drug. There was little fear of a false-negative result, which allowed the investigators to take shortcuts.

In contrast to the trials of lithium, studies of dexpramiprexole,[30–32] just a year later, show how the opposite approach may occur under different circumstances. Dexpramiprexole is an enantomer of the Parkinson disease drug pramiprexole, and is thought to have beneficial effects on mitochondria. It was owned by Knopp pharmaceuticals. There were two early human studies, both relatively small.[30,31] The first of these was a short study where placebo and three doses were compared. The findings were strong and this was followed by a larger trial comparing a high (300 mg) and low dose (50 mg). The latter study again pointed to improvements in vital capacity, function, and survival up to 2 years. With these results, the company was able to secure large amounts of funding for a phase III trial that enrolled 943 patients at 81 sites in 11 countries. The trial was expensive and carried out to completion. Just before the results were released, the enthusiasm within the field was palpable, but the outcome was spectacularly negative, with no difference between the treatment and placebo group.[32] Subsequent to the release of data, the owners of dexpramiprexole argued that patients with definite ALS had better outcomes than less severe forms of the disease, but subset analysis never led to further studies. It may have also been instructive to notice that in the earlier human trial the decline ALSFRS-R score of the low-dose group seemed to be rapid compared with what one would have expected from historical placebo controls. This could potentially have raised flags that would have decreased the enthusiasm for the treatment before the phase III study.

Ceftriaxone was also studied in ALS after it turned out to be the best upregulator of a glutamate transporter of all FDA-approved medications. The competitive preclinical work, which tested all FDA-approved drugs, had to pick the most promising candidate, so eventually ceftriaxione was selected.[33] The idea that glutamate toxicity was important in ALS was vogue at the time of the clinical trial. The study enrolled more than 500 patients and had a negative result, although interim analyses were apparently strong enough to continue the trial to its conclusion.[24]

Finally, the recent experience with the anti-inflammatory drug NP-001 did not meet its statistical end point, but did find a slight slowing of disease progression in a moderately sized study.[25,34] However, the study found, in a post hoc analysis, that a large percentage of patients were nonprogressors. Nearly 30% of patients on the high dose showed no progression of disease compared with about 10% in a usual trial. This led to the reasonable hypothesis that the drug had helped some patients, but this had been diluted by patients who progressed at normal rates. The hypothesis was further supported by finding that a large percentage of the responders had high levels of inflammatory biomarkers in serum. Despite these findings, Neuraltus Pharmaceuticals was not able to gain additional private sector funding for a follow-up trial for more than 2 years after trial completion. However, a trial sponsored by the Amyotrophic Lateral Sclerosis Association is under way.

## REFERENCES

1. Bensimon G, Lacomblez L, Meininger V, et al. A controlled trial of riluzole in amyotrophic lateral sclerosis. N Engl J Med 1994;330:585–91.
2. Mitsumoto H, Brooks BR, Silani V. Clinical trials in amyotrophic lateral sclerosis: why so many negative trials and how can trials be improved? Lancet Neurol 2014;13:1127–38.
3. Gordon PH, Moore DH, Miller RG, et al. Efficacy of minocycline in patients with amyotrophic lateral sclerosis: a phase III randomised trial. Lancet Neurol 2007; 6:1045–53.
4. Graf M, Ecker D, Horowski R, et al. High dose vitamin E therapy in amyotrophic lateral sclerosis as add-on therapy to riluzole: results of a placebo-controlled double-blind study. J Neural Transm 2005;112:649–60.
5. Cudkowicz ME, Shefner JM, Schoenfeld DA, et al. Trial of celecoxib in amyotrophic lateral sclerosis. Ann Neurol 2006;60:22–31.
6. Fornai F, Longone P, Cafaro L, et al. Lithium delays progression of amyotrophic lateral sclerosis. Proc Natl Acad Sci U S A 2008;105(6):2052–7.
7. Rosenfeld J, King RM, Jackson CE, et al. Creatine monohydrate in ALS: effects on strength, fatigue, respiratory status and ALSFRS. Amyotroph Lateral Scler 2008;9:266–72.
8. Sreedharan J, Brown RH Jr. Amyotrophic lateral sclerosis: problems and prospects. Ann Neurol 2013;74:309–16.
9. Gordon PH, Cheung YK, Levin B, et al. A novel, efficient, randomized selection trial comparing combinations of drug therapy for ALS. Amyotroph Lateral Scler 2008;9:212–22.
10. Weiss MD, Weydt P, Carter GT. Current pharmacological management of amyotrophic lateral sclerosis and a role for rational polypharmacy. Expert Opin Pharmacother 2004;5:735–46.
11. Shefner JM, Leigh N. Commentary on 'a novel, efficient, randomized selection trial comparing combinations of drug therapy for ALS'. Amyotroph Lateral Scler 2008;9:254–6.
12. Turner MR, Hardiman O, Benatar M, et al. Controversies and priorities in amyotrophic lateral sclerosis. Lancet Neurol 2013;12:310–22.
13. Rothstein JD. Of mice and men: reconciling preclinical ALS mouse studies and human clinical trials. Ann Neurol 2003;53:423–6.
14. Benatar M, Polak M, Kaplan S, et al. Preventing familial amyotrophic lateral sclerosis: is a clinical trial feasible? J Neurol Sci 2006;251:3–9.
15. Nicholson KA, Cudkowicz ME, Berry JD. Clinical trial designs in amyotrophic lateral sclerosis: does one design fit all? Neurotherapeutics 2015;12:376–83.
16. Bakkar N, Boehringer A, Bowser R. Use of biomarkers in ALS drug development and clinical trials. Brain Res 2015;1607:94–107.
17. Miller TM, Pestronk A, David W, et al. An antisense oligonucleotide against SOD1 delivered intrathecally for patients with SOD1 familial amyotrophic lateral sclerosis: a phase 1, randomised, first-in-man study. Lancet Neurol 2013;12: 435–42.
18. Brainstorm-Cell Therapeutics. Phase 2, randomized, double blind, placebo controlled multicenter study of autologous MSC-NTF cells in patients with ALS (NurOwn). Available at: https://www.clinicaltrials.gov/ct2/show/NCT02017912. Accessed July 15, 2015.
19. Thomsen GM, Gowing G, Svendsen S, et al. The past, present and future of stem cell clinical trials for ALS. Exp Neurol 2014;262:127–37.

20. Wang R, Lagakos SW, Ware JH, et al. Statistics in medicine—reporting of subgroup analyses in clinical trials. N Engl J Med 2007;357:2189–94.
21. Cudkowicz ME, van den Berg LH, Shefner JM, et al. Dexpramipexole versus placebo for patients with amyotrophic lateral sclerosis (EMPOWER): a randomised, double-blind, phase 3 trial. Lancet Neurol 2013;12:1059–67.
22. Aggarwal SP, Zinman L, Simpson E, et al. Safety and efficacy of lithium in combination with riluzole for treatment of amyotrophic lateral sclerosis: a randomised, double-blind, placebo-controlled trial. Lancet Neurol 2010;9(5):481–8.
23. Pascuzzi RM, Shefner J, Chappell AS, et al. A phase II trial of talampanel in subjects with amyotrophic lateral sclerosis. Amyotroph Lateral Scler 2010;11:266–71.
24. Berry JD, Shefner JM, Conwit R, et al. Design and initial results of a multi-phase randomized trial of ceftriaxone in amyotrophic lateral sclerosis. PLoS One 2013;8(4):e61177.
25. Miller RG, Block G, Katz JS, et al, Phase 2 Trial NP001 Investigators. Randomized phase 2 trial of NP001-a novel immune regulator: safety and early efficacy in ALS. Neurol Neuroimmunol Neuroinflamm 2015;2(3):e100.
26. Zach N, Ennist DL, Taylor AA, et al. Being PRO-ACTive: what can a clinical trial database reveal about ALS? Neurotherapeutics 2015;12(2):417–23.
27. Miller RG, Moore DH, Forshew DA, et al. Phase II screening trial of lithium carbonate in amyotrophic lateral sclerosis: examining a more efficient trial design. Neurology 2011;77(10):973–9.
28. Verstraete E, Veldink JH, Huisman MH, et al. Lithium lacks effect on survival in amyotrophic lateral sclerosis: a phase IIb randomised sequential trial. J Neurol Neurosurg Psychiatry 2012;83(5):557–64.
29. UKMND-LiCALS Study Group, Morrison KE, Dhariwal S, et al. Lithium in patients with amyotrophic lateral sclerosis (LiCALS): a phase 3 multicentre, randomised, double-blind, placebo-controlled trial. Lancet Neurol 2013;12(4):339–45.
30. Wang H, Larriviere KS, Keller KE, et al. R+ pramipexole as a mitochondrially focused neuroprotectant: initial early phase studies in ALS. Amyotroph Lateral Scler 2008;9(1):50–8.
31. Cudkowicz M, Bozik ME, Ingersoll EW, et al. The effects of dexpramipexole (KNS-760704) in individuals with amyotrophic lateral sclerosis. Nat Med 2011;17(12):1652–6.
32. Bozik ME, Mitsumoto H, Brooks BR, et al. A post hoc analysis of subgroup outcomes and creatinine in the phase III clinical trial (EMPOWER) of dexpramipexole in ALS. Amyotroph Lateral Scler Frontotemporal Degener 2014;15(5–6):406–13.
33. Rothstein JD, Patel S, Regan MR, et al. Beta-lactam antibiotics offer neuroprotection by increasing glutamate transporter expression. Nature 2005;433(7021):73–7.
34. Miller RG, Zhang R, Block G, et al. NP001 regulation of macrophage activation markers in ALS: a phase I clinical and biomarker study. Amyotroph Lateral Scler Frontotemporal Degener 2014;15(7–8):601–9.

# Index

*Note:* Page numbers of article titles are in **boldface** type.




Neurol Clin 33 (2015) 949–958
http://dx.doi.org/10.1016/S0733-8619(15)00095-X

**D**



**E**

## F



## G

## P



## R

## S

**United States Postal Service**

# Statement of Ownership, Management, and Circulation
## (All Periodicals Publications Except Requestor Publications)

| | | |
|---|---|---|
| 1. Publication Title<br>Neurologic Clinics | 2. Publication Number<br>0 0 0 - 7 1 2 | 3. Filing Date<br>9/18/15 |
| 4. Issue Frequency<br>Feb, May, Aug, Nov | 5. Number of Issues Published Annually<br>4 | 6. Annual Subscription Price<br>$300.00 |
| 7. Complete Mailing Address of Known Office of Publication (*Not printer*) (*Street, city, county, state, and ZIP+4®*)<br>Elsevier Inc.<br>360 Park Avenue South<br>New York, NY 10010-1710 | | Contact Person<br>Stephen R. Bushing<br>Telephone (Include area code)<br>215-239-3688 |

8. Complete Mailing Address of Headquarters or General Business Office of Publisher (*Not printer*)

Elsevier Inc., 360 Park Avenue South, New York, NY 10010-1710

9. Full Names and Complete Mailing Addresses of Publisher, Editor, and Managing Editor (*Do not leave blank*)

Publisher (*Name and complete mailing address*)

Linda Belfus, Elsevier Inc., 1600 John F. Kennedy Blvd., Suite 1800, Philadelphia, PA 19103

Editor (*Name and complete mailing address*)

Lauren Boyle, Elsevier Inc., 1600 John F. Kennedy Blvd., Suite 1800, Philadelphia, PA 19103-2899

Managing Editor (*Name and complete mailing address*)

Adrianne Brigido, Elsevier Inc., 1600 John F. Kennedy Blvd., Suite 1800, Philadelphia, PA 19103-2899

10. Owner (*Do not leave blank. If the publication is owned by a corporation, give the name and address of the corporation immediately followed by the names and addresses of all stockholders owning or holding 1 percent or more of the total amount of stock. If not owned by a corporation, give the names and addresses of the individual owners. If owned by a partnership or other unincorporated firm, give its name and address as well as those of each individual owner. If the publication is published by a nonprofit organization, give its name and address.*)

| Full Name | Complete Mailing Address |
|---|---|
| Wholly owned subsidiary of | 1600 John F. Kennedy Blvd, Ste. 1800 |
| Reed/Elsevier, US holdings | Philadelphia, PA 19103-2899 |
| | |
| | |

11. Known Bondholders, Mortgagees, and Other Security Holders Owning or Holding 1 Percent or More of Total Amount of Bonds, Mortgages, or Other Securities. If none, check box → ☐ None

| Full Name | Complete Mailing Address |
|---|---|
| N/A | |
| | |
| | |
| | |

12. Tax Status (*For completion by nonprofit organizations authorized to mail at nonprofit rates*) (*Check one*)
The purpose, function, and nonprofit status of this organization and the exempt status for federal income tax purposes:
☐ Has Not Changed During Preceding 12 Months
☐ Has Changed During Preceding 12 Months (*Publisher must submit explanation of change with this statement*)

| | |
|---|---|
| 13. Publication Title<br>Neurologic Clinics | 14. Issue Date for Circulation Data Below<br>August 2015 |

PS Form **3526**, July 2014 (Page 1 of 3 (Instructions Page 3)) PSN 7530-01-000-9931 **PRIVACY NOTICE**: See our Privacy policy in www.usps.com

| 15. Extent and Nature of Circulation | | | Average No. Copies Each Issue During Preceding 12 Months | No. Copies of Single Issue Published Nearest to Filing Date |
|---|---|---|---|---|
| a. Total Number of Copies (*Net press run*) | | | 748 | 654 |
| b. Legitimate Paid and Or Requested Distribution (By Mail and Outside the Mail) | (1) | Mailed Outside County Paid/Requested Mail Subscriptions stated on PS Form 3541. (*Include paid distribution above nominal rate, advertiser's proof copies and exchange copies*) | 319 | 238 |
| | (2) | Mailed In-County Paid/Requested Mail Subscriptions stated on PS Form 3541. (*Include paid distribution above nominal rate, advertiser's proof copies and exchange copies*) | | |
| | (3) | Paid Distribution Outside the Mails Including Sales Through Dealers And Carriers, Street Vendors, Counter Sales, and Other Paid Distribution Outside USPS® | 152 | 186 |
| | (4) | Paid Distribution by Other Classes of Mail Through the USPS (e.g. First-Class Mail®) | | |
| c. Total Paid and or Requested Circulation (*Sum of 15b (1), (2), (3), and (4)*) ► | | | 471 | 424 |
| d. Free or Nominal Rate Distribution (By Mail and Outside the Mail) | (1) | Free or Nominal Rate Outside-County Copies included on PS Form 3541 | 86 | 85 |
| | (2) | Free or Nominal Rate in-County Copies included on PS Form 3541 | | |
| | (3) | Free or Nominal Rate Copies mailed at Other classes Through the USPS (e.g. First-Class Mail®) | | |
| | (4) | Free or Nominal Rate Distribution Outside the Mail (*Carriers or Other means*) | | |
| e. Total Nonrequested Distribution (Sum of 15d (1), (2), (3) and (4) | | | 86 | 85 |
| f. Total Distribution (Sum of 15c and 15e) ► | | | 557 | 509 |
| g. Copies not Distributed (See instructions to publishers #4 (page #3)) ► | | | 191 | 145 |
| h. Total (Sum of 15f and g) | | | 748 | 654 |
| i. Percent Paid and/or Requested Circulation (15c divided by 15f times 100) ► | | | 84.56% | 83.30% |
| * If you are claiming electronic copies go to line 16 on page 3. If you are not claiming Electronic copies, skip to line 17 on page 3 | | | | |

| *16. Electronic Copy Circulation* | *Average No. Copies Each Issue During Preceding 12 Months* | *No. Copies of Single Issue Published Nearest to Filing Date* |
|---|---|---|
| *a. Paid Electronic Copies* | | |
| *b. Total paid Print Copies (Line 15c) + Paid Electronic copies (Line 16a)* | | |
| *c. Total Print Distribution (Line 15f) + Paid Electronic Copies (Line 16a)* | | |
| *d. Percent Paid (Both Print & Electronic copies) (16b divided by 16c X 100)* | | |
| ***I certify that 50% of all my distributed copies (electronic and print) are paid above a nominal price*** | | |

*17. Publication of Statement of Ownership*
*If the publication is a general publication, publication of this statement is required. Will be printed in the* ***November 2015*** *issue of this publication.*

| 18. Signature and Title of Editor, Publisher, Business Manager, or Owner | Date |
|---|---|
| Stephen R. Bushing<br>Stephen R. Bushing – Inventory Distribution Coordinator | September 18, 2015 |

**I certify that all information furnished on this form is true and complete. I understand that anyone who furnishes false or misleading information on this form or who omits material or information requested on the form may be subject to criminal sanctions (including fines and imprisonment) and/or civil sanctions (including civil penalties).**

**PS Form 3526, July 2014 (Page 3 of 3)**

Printed and bound by CPI Group (UK) Ltd, Croydon, CR0 4YY
03/10/2024
01040490-0007